ARIF A. CHOWDHURY, M.D., P.C.
1660 W. ANTELOPE DR. STE 230
LAYTON, UT 84041

CLINICAL EXAMINATION OF THE NERVOUS SYSTEM

CLINICAL EXAMINATION OF THE NERVOUS SYSTEM

EDITOR

SID GILMAN, MD

Chairman, Department of Neurology
University of Michigan
Ann Arbor, Michigan

McGraw-Hill
HEALTH PROFESSIONS DIVISION

New York St. Louis San Francisco Auckland Bogotá Caracas Lisbon London Madrid
Mexico City Milan Montreal New Delhi San Juan Singapore Sydney Tokyo Toronto

McGraw-Hill

A Division of The **McGraw·Hill** *Companies*

CLINICAL EXAMINATION OF THE NERVOUS SYSTEM
Copyright © 2000 by *The* **McGraw-Hill** *Companies,* Inc. All rights reserved.
Printed in the United States of America. Except as permitted under the United
States Copyright Act of 1976, no part of this publication may be reproduced or
distributed in any form or by any means, or stored in a data base or retrieval
system, without prior written permission of the publisher.

1234567890 DOCDOC 9987

ISBN 0-07-024252-6

This book was set in Times Roman by Progressive Information Technologies, Inc.
The editors were Joseph Hefta and Steven Melvin.
The production supervisor was Helene G. Landers.
The cover and text were designed by Marsha Cohen/Paralellogram.
R.R. Donnelley & Sons, Inc. was the printer and binder.

This book is printed on acid-free paper.

Library of Congress Cataloging-in-Publication Data
Clinical examination of the nervous system / editor, Sid Gilman.
     p.   cm.
   Includes bibliographical references and index.
   ISBN 0-07-024252-6
   1. Neurologic examination.   I. Gilman, Sid.
   [DNLM: 1. Neurologic Examination.   2. Nervous System Diseases-
-diagnosis.   WL   141 C6409 1999]
RC348.C635   2000
616.8'0475--dc21
DNLM/DLC
for Library of Congress   99-19468
                                       CIP

CONTENTS

CONTRIBUTORS

James W. Albers, MD, PhD
Professor, Departments of Neurology, Physical Medicine
  and Rehabilitation, and Environmental and Industrial
  Health
University of Michigan Medical Center
Ann Arbor, MI

Roger L. Albin, MD
Associate Professor of Neurology
University of Michigan
Chief, Neuroscience Research
Geriatrics Research, Education and Clinical Center
Department of Veterans Affairs Medical Center
Ann Arbor, MI

Kenneth L. Casey, MD
Professor of Neurology
Professor of Physiology
Chief, Neurology Service
Veterans Administration Medical Center
Ann Arbor, MI

David M. Dawson, MD
Professor of Neurology
Harvard Medical School
Boston, MA

Ivo Drury, MB BCh
Professor and Chairman, Department of Neurology
The Henry Ford Health System
Detroit, MI

Sid Gilman, MD
Chairman, Department of Neurology
University of Michigan
Ann Arbor, MI

Gary W. Goldstein, MD
Professor, Departments of Neurology and Pediatrics
Johns Hopkins University School of Medicine and
  The Kennedy Krieger Institute
Professor, Environmental Health Sciences, Johns Hopkins
  University School of Hygiene and Public Health
Baltimore, MD

Michael V. Johnston, MD
Professor, Departments of Neurology and Pediatrics

Johns Hopkins University School of Medicine and The
  Kennedy Krieger Institute
Baltimore, MD

Larry Junck, MD
Associate Professor of Neurology
University of Michigan Medical Cetner
Ann Arbor, MI

David Knopman, MD
Associate Professor of Neurology
University of Minnesota
Minneapolis, MN

Adriana A. Kori, MD
Department of Neurology
University Hospitals
Cleveland, OH

R. John Leigh, MD
Professor of Neurology
Case Western Reserve University
Staff Physician, Cleveland Veterans Affairs Medical
  Center
Cleveland, OH

Joel C. Morgenlander, MD
Assistant Professor of Medicine (Neurology)
Director, Neurology Residency Training Program
Duke University Medical Center
Durham, NC

Frisso A. Potts, MD
Brockton-West Roxbury VA Medical Center
Neurology Service
West Roxbury, MA

Bruce K. Shapiro, MD
The Kennedy Krieger Institute
Department of Pediatrics
Baltimore, MD

John J. Wald, MD
Clinical Assistant Professor of Neurology
University of Michigan Medical Center
Ann Arbor, MI

PREFACE

Evaluation of a patient with symptoms referable to the nervous system is an exciting and interesting aspect of medicine. The process required consists of the sequential steps of obtaining a full and complete history of the patient's neurological complaint, followed by other relevant current and past medical history, the system review, family history, and social history. A general physical examination followed by a neurological examination provides the additional data needed.

The next step of the process consists of deductive reasoning based upon the clinician's knowledge of neuroanatomy. Based upon the results of the neurological examination, the clinician first localizes the disease process to a particular part of the nervous system. Then, based upon the history, the clinician determines the type of neuropathological process that would explain the mode of onset and progression of the disorder. After these initial steps have been completed, in most cases a differential diagnosis can be constructed and the appropriate laboratory studies can be planned. Clinicians who attempt to bypass these initial steps in the evaluation and move immediately to laboratory studies often become frustrated when multiple costly laboratory studies do not clarify the nature of the patient's symptoms.

This book was developed to describe the methods of examining the nervous system clinically in a succinct volume. It is intended for the instruction of trainees and practitioners of clinical neurology, pediatric neurology, and neurosurgery, as well as for trainees and practitioners in related fields, such as physiatry, psychiatry, and internal medicine. The book provides a guide to obtaining a neurological history and to performing a neurological examination and an appropriate general medical examination. It includes discussion of the principles of localization of disease processes in the nervous system and presents the clinically relevant neuroanatomy.

The book is organized in approximately the order that many neurologists follow in evaluating their patients. Hence, the initial chapters deal with the neurological and medical history and the general physical examination. Next come chapters concerning the neurological examination, beginning with the mental status, and moving on to the cranial nerves, motor system, reflexes, and then sensation. Additional chapters concern methods of clinically testing the autonomic nervous system and examination of the child's nervous system. The final chapter provides up-to-date information concerning laboratory studies that are helpful in neurological diagnosis.

I have selected the contributors to this book based not only upon their expertise as clinical neurologists, but also upon their abilities as teachers and writers. I am greatly indebted to them for the excellent quality of their work, to Wendy Jackelow for her wonderful new illustrations, and to Joseph Hefta of McGraw-Hill for his patience and skill.

Sid Gilman, M.D.
Ann Arbor, Michigan

CLINICAL EXAMINATION OF THE NERVOUS SYSTEM

CHAPTER 1

THE NEUROLOGIC HISTORY

For patients with symptoms referable to the nervous system, evaluation involves an exercise in deductive logic. The process begins when you establish essential facts about your patient as clearly as possible, beginning with the chief complaint and continuing through a full chronologic sequence of the patient's history of the present illness. You supplement this with the history of past medical disorders, a review of systems, family history, and social history, focusing principally on the current problem but also assessing the risk factors for neurologic diseases. You follow this with a general physical examination and then a neurologic examination. Having completed this aspect of data collection, you review the findings and determine the location of a lesion that could be responsible for the neurologic disorder and the type of pathology in this location. Assessment of the location of the lesion depends on the findings of the neurologic examination, although the history usually focuses your attention on the relevant part of the nervous system. Next, you use the history to deduce the type of pathologic process involved. For example, the sudden onset of a disorder involving the central nervous system such as paralysis of the arm and leg on one side of the body often indicates a vascular process such as ischemic infarction or hemorrhage. The gradual evolution of neurologic impairment suggests a neurodegenerative or neoplastic disease. A disorder with exacerbations and remissions commonly results from demyelinative diseases such as multiple sclerosis.

After deducing the location of the lesion and the type of pathologic process involved, you can develop a short list of possible diagnoses and then determine the additional testing needed to move the evaluation along. You should follow the sequence outlined above in evaluating patients and not yield to the temptation to leap immediately into a request for an imaging study; this type of shortcut frequently yields negative results, leading to frustration on your part and waste of both time and resources. Without first determining the most likely location and type of pathology, you cannot plan the appropriate laboratory evaluation.

In planning the laboratory evaluation, begin with the simplest, most minimally invasive, and least costly tests required. If they would be helpful in establishing the diagnosis, consider a blood count, test panel, urinalysis, chest x-ray, electrocardiogram, electroencephalogram, or other inexpensive studies before you turn to computed tomography scanning, magnetic resonance imaging, magnetic resonance angiography, catheter arteriography, or spinal puncture. In evaluating patients with acute neurologic illnesses, particularly those with acute infections of the nervous system, you will waste valuable time by sending the patient for a radiologic evaluation before completing your evaluation and determining the safest and most helpful procedure for establishing the diagnosis and initiating treatment.

INTERACTIONS WITH THE PATIENT

When you initially encounter a patient, do your utmost to develop good rapport, to demonstrate your interest in the patient, and to create an atmosphere of trust. To this end, it is essential that you devote your entire attention to the patient and avoid distractions. If possible, turn off your pager to prevent interruptions during the encounter. Particularly with new patients, but also with those you have seen previously, begin your interview with a few friendly open-ended questions such as, "How are you today?"; "Did you have any difficulty finding this office?"; "Was parking difficult?" It is important that you make eye contact with the patient and pay full attention to the patient's initial words. Commonly, new patients bring records and films from previous evaluations and present them to you immediately. You should look through this material after your initial greeting and friendly interactions with the patient, and it is best to say, "Excuse me for a few minutes while I review this material." Do not ignore that material and begin taking the history; this could make the patient angry when you ask questions that have answers contained in the material presented to you. Once you have looked through the material, ask whether you can keep the material to study it further, and again turn your full attention to the patient and begin taking the history.

Do your best not to look at your wristwatch or a clock on the wall while interacting with the patient, particularly when taking the history. This may give the impression that you are hurrying through the encounter, perhaps leading the patient to believe that you want to complete the interview quickly. During your initial interactions with the patient, avoid questions related to sexual orientation, sexual function, or marital status. These questions can come later in context during the history-taking process after you have developed some rapport. Any initial focus on these issues could be misinterpreted to suggest that you have a bias about the patient's sexual orientation or marital status.

In providing a history, patients often begin by telling you how frustrated they are with their previous physician and their difficulty obtaining information about their problems, and they may attempt to tell you about myriad other problems that are irrelevant to the task that you face. To maintain rapport, you need to listen to these complaints, express understanding, but make no judgmental statements, and in particular avoid making comments about physicians the patient has seen previously. Comments such as "I can understand why you are so frustrated," or "This must be a very difficult situation for you" indicate empathy and demonstrate that you are listening attentively but will not add to difficulties between the patient and the referring physician. There are several reasons to avoid making judgmental comments about other physicians the patient has seen. The judgments may be incorrect; the patient may have misinterpreted comments from the physicians and may be relaying incorrect information to you. For example, the physicians may have attempted to tell the patient the facts about the patient's medical problems, but the comments may have been threatening to the patient or presented in overly complex language. Moreover, you may find later that the patient has difficulty understanding your comments and may pass on complaints about you, irrespective of your attempts to inform the patient fully and to manage the patient effectively. In addition, many patients carry back to the referring physicians comments that you make about them, placing them in a difficult position and fostering anger at you. Finally, the patient might consider initiating a lawsuit against the previous physicians based on your comments, and you may be named in the suit.

Managing an angry patient requires patience and skill. The most important aspect of the interaction is for you to listen to all the patient has to say while maintaining eye contact. Comments such as "I see" as the patient speaks indicate that you are listening and understand the patient's concerns. It is important not to interrupt unless the patient's monologue goes on so long that you will have insufficient time to evaluate the medical problem. Simply listening to the problems and demonstrating that you understand them can be helpful. If the patient's anger is directed to you, you need to respond directly, honestly, and appropriately. Often, a simple explanation will be all that is necessary. If you have made a mistake, you should acknowledge the mistake and apologize. If personnel in your institution are responsible for the patient's anger, you should assure the patient that you will look into the matter and contact the patient later with an explanation or a description of the action you took. It is important for you to follow through when patients have complaints. Do your best not to be defensive and do not be overly swift to accept responsibility or "blame." At times patients and their families have unrealistic expectations of their physicians.

Often, patients with neurologic problems wish to have a spouse, family member, or friend in the examination room with them for the entire evaluation. Some patients appear with several family members. Some gay or lesbian patients want to have their partners accompany them. You should encourage patients to have their family members and partners stay with them through the evaluation. Usually, this provides support and reassurance, allowing patients to feel more at ease and often to be more accurate in describing the history. In evaluations of patients with limited capacity to provide a history such as those with mental retardation or cognitive disorders, a history from family members can be essential. The presence of other people in the room can be distracting, however, particularly when family members speak frequently, contradict the patient's history, and want to present their own recollections of the history. At times family members will want to tell you about their own health problems, even as you attempt to focus on the patient's problem. Although this can be frustrating and slow the evaluation, family members can often provide valuable additions and corrections to the history. If the interactions with family members become overly distracting and do nothing more than waste time, you can ask politely that they withhold their comments until you have completed the history. Then they can comment on the history as you recite it back.

As you take the history, do your best to continue making eye contact with the patient and family members in the room. If you take notes during the history, which is usually essential, look directly at the patient periodically to indicate that you are fully in touch with the narrative. Moreover, frequent acknowledgments that you understand the history help assuage the patient's concerns about the level of attention you are devoting to the problem. Once you have completed the history, if time permits, repeat the history for the patient and family for verification and to assure them that you have the facts straight.

TABLE 1-1.   Outline of the Neurologic History

Identifying information: name, age, sex, marital status, occupation.
Referral information: name and address of referring physician(s).
Chief complaint
History of the present illness
Past medical history
Review of systems
Family history
Social history

PURPOSES OF THE HISTORY

A clear and accurate history serves many purposes. First and foremost, it provides you with data to formulate the patient's complaints and proceed with the diagnostic evaluation. Second, if taken and recorded properly, the history provides valuable documentation that other physicians can use in managing the patient's medical problems in the future. In providing continuing care, physicians frequently refer back to the initial history and examination, which usually contain the most complete review of the patient's medical problems. Third, a written history is required by third-party carriers, many of whom must have documentation supporting the level of billing. Fourth, the history provides the means for you to develop an independent view of the patient's disorder. It is essential that you avoid focusing excessively on impressions by other physicians, previous diagnoses, or previous laboratory data. Your opinion based on the facts of the patient's history and examination is the most valuable contribution you can make to the patient's care. Table 1-1 provides an outline of the neurologic history.

THE CHIEF COMPLAINT

Begin taking the history by obtaining the patient's full name (if it is not already on the registration material), age, and occupation. If the patient's complaints involve cognitive dysfunction or a language disorder, ask about the patient's handedness to help assess hemisphere dominance for language. Obtain the full name, relevant degree (M.D., D.O., R.N., or Ph.D.), address, and telephone number of the physicians or other health care professionals who should receive a copy of your evaluation. You may also wish to ask your patients if they want to receive a copy of the evaluation as well. If they do, obviously you will need their full address.

Record the principal complaint in the patient's own words using quotation marks, if possible. If the patient has multiple complaints, list them in order of importance to the patient, once again using the patient's own words with quotations. If the patient has been referred by another physician for a problem but the patient presents a different chief complaint, list both complaints. If the patient has no complaint because of a cognitive disorder or for other reasons, obtain from the family or referring physician the patient's principal symptoms or the reason for the referral.

Note the duration of each principal complaint. Patients often have difficulty identifying the precise onset of a symptom, but you should urge them to come as close to the time of onset as possible. A good leading question is, "When were you last entirely well?" For patients with multiple complaints, list the duration of each. State the source of the history as part of the Chief Complaint.

THE PRESENT ILLNESS

Obtain and record the history of the present illness chronologically, beginning with the initial presentation of the symptoms and proceeding through to the present. If the patient has a single complaint, ascertain when the symptoms began and how they evolved over time. If the patient has multiple complaints, explore the evolution of each complaint chronologically before moving on to others. If the patient's complaints all appear to be interrelated, obtain the history chronologically from the outset with a full description of each complaint as it occurred, information about the subsequent development of that complaint, then the time of onset and the evolution of each additional complaint. Bring all components of the history up to the present. Do your best to allow the patient to explain the history without interruption. If necessary, you should interrupt for focused questions or to keep the patient on track. Table 1-2 contains a guide to specific areas of inquiry

TABLE 1-2. Specific Areas of Inquiry in the Neurologic History Organized by Functional Systems

1. Higher cerebral functions
   a. Disorders of memory, judgment, insight, concentration
   b. Disorientation in time and space (loss of awareness of day, date, year; getting lost when driving)
   c. Disturbances of consciousness, including blackouts or seizures and head injury
   d. Speech disorders (trouble finding correct words or stammering with preserved comprehension; rambling, irrelevant or meaningless speech; or difficulty understanding spoken or written language)
   e. Sleep disturbances (difficulty falling asleep or remaining asleep, early morning awakening with inability to return to sleep, nightmares or night terrors, excessive limb movements during sleep, snoring and apnea during sleep)
   f. Psychologic disturbances, including anxiety, depression, elation, loss of body weight or gain of weight
2. Cranial nerve and brainstem functions
   a. Visual disorders, including loss of vision and double vision
   b. Headache
   c. Dizziness (attempt to differentiate vertigo from light-headedness)
   d. Deafness
   e. Tinnitus
   f. Difficulty with articulation

(continued)

TABLE 1-2. Specific Areas of Inquiry in the Neurologic History Organized by Functional Systems *(Continued)*

3. Motor functions
   a. Weakness or paralysis
   b. Slowness or stiffness of movement, including difficulty getting out of a chair or turning over in bed
   c. Involuntary movements, including tremors or twitches
   d. Unsteadiness in standing and walking
   e. Falling
4. Sensory functions
   a. Loss of sensation
   b. Numbness, including decreased sensation or tingling ("pins and needles")
   c. Pain
5. Autonomic functions
   a. Disturbances in the control of urination and defecation
   b. Light-headedness upon standing
   c. Nausea and vomiting

in the neurologic history to help you explore the history fully. The table is organized by neurologic functional systems corresponding to the major components of the neurologic examination.

As you inquire about each complaint, obtain as full a description as possible. Some complaints require extensive questioning to comprehend the patient's experience, notably dizziness, numbness, and weakness. The complaint of "dizziness" requires a thorough evaluation of the patient's experience. This term can be used to describe vertigo (a sensation of spinning of the environment around the patient or spinning of the patient in an immobile environment), light-headedness (a feeling of faintness), momentary loss of vision, generalized weakness, or even imbalance with walking. A history of "numbness"

TABLE 1-3. Questions Relevant to Complaints of Pain

1. Location (and sites of radiation)
2. Quality (sharp, dull, shooting, burning, aching)
3. Severity (on a scale of 1–10 in which 10 is the worst pain the patient ever experienced)
4. Duration (of each episode of pain)
5. Frequency (average number of episodes of pain per day, week, or month)
6. Timing (times of day or night when pain usually occurs)
7. Context (situations that appear to be associated with development or worsening of pain)
8. Associated features (erythema, swelling, nausea, vomiting)
9. Modifying factors (maneuvers that provoke or worsen pain such as changes of posture; deep breathing; performing the Valsalva maneuver as by straining at stool, coughing, or sneezing; decreases in sensory input, as when lying awake in bed at night; methods of obtaining relief, including rubbing, cooling, or warming the affected site; medications used and their effectiveness)

TABLE 1-4. Questions Relevant to Headache

1. Location (hemicranial, frontal, temporal, parietal, occipital) and radiation sites
2. Quality (sharp, dull, pounding, constricting)
3. Severity (on a scale of 1 to 10)
4. Duration (of the average attack, with a range)
5. Frequency (average number of attacks per day, week, month)
6. Timing with respect to time of day, day of the week, or day of the month (and for women, in relation to the menstrual cycle)
7. Context (developing with stressful events during the day or on awakening in the morning after a stressful day)
8. Associated features
   a. Autonomic disorders (pallor, sweating, drowsiness, nausea, vomiting, weakness)
   b. Visual disturbances (fortification spectra, visual blurring, loss of central vision)
9. Modifying factors
   a. Stimuli that provoke headache: foods (citrus fruits and fruit juices, spiced meats, pickles, spiced mushrooms, cheeses, caffeine, alcoholic beverages, particularly red wine); changes in the weather (exposure to wind and changes in barometric pressure); effects of sleep (both excessive amounts and inadequate amounts); a visual environment containing stripes
   b. Methods of treating headache: sleep, caffeine intake, medications (types and effectiveness)

can indicate diminished sensation, absence of sensation, tingling, or even pain. The term "weakness" can be used to describe loss of muscle strength, but also imbalance, incoordination, generalized fatigue, or a sensory disturbance. For each complaint in which these descriptors are relevant, ask about the location, quality, severity, duration, frequency, timing, context, associated features, and modifying factors. As examples, Table 1-3 provides guidance in obtaining a history about pain, and Tables 1-4, 1-5, and 1-6 about headache, dizziness, and loss of consciousness.

TABLE 1-5. Questions Relevant to Complaints of Dizziness

1. Location (i.e., visual, motor, or sensory symptoms)
2. Quality
   a. Vertigo (a sense of spinning of the patient or the environment)
   b. Faintness (light-headedness)
   c. Blurred vision
   d. Incoordination
   e. Fear of falling
3. Severity (on a scale of 1 to 10)
4. Duration of each episode
5. Frequency of episodes
6. Timing (during specific parts of the day or night)
7. Context (associated with rising from a recumbent or seated position or with rapid head turning)

(continued)

TABLE 1-5.   Questions Relevant to Complaints of Dizziness *(Continued)*

8. Associated features
   a. Visual disturbances (diplopia, blurred vision, total loss of vision)
   b. Autonomic symptoms (nausea, vomiting)
   c. Auditory symptoms (tinnitus, hearing loss)
   d. Headache
9. Modifying factors (provocation of symptoms by rapid changes of body or head position and by medications that might cause orthostatic hypotension or light-headedness; improvement of symptoms by sitting or lying down at the onset of symptoms or by avoiding rapid head movements)

Complete the Present Illness by obtaining a list of all medications the patient currently receives. If the patient has brought along the bottles of medications, obtain from the labels the name, dosage, and frequency of administration of each. If the medication containers are not available, obtain as complete information as possible from the patient. It is astonishing to find, particularly with older patients, that physicians prescribe medications without knowing the other medications the patient takes. Commonly, elderly people take

TABLE 1-6.   Questions Relevant to Complaints of Loss of Consciousness

I. Quality
   A. Onset (events at the beginning of the episode such as hyperventilation; numbness; tingling; visual disorders; feelings of floating or spinning; a strong feeling that the surroundings seem strangely familiar or unfamiliar)
   B. Progression (examples)
      1. Loss of consciousness with falling without movements of body or limbs
      2. Loss of consciousness with falling followed by stiffening of the body and shaking of all limbs, with or without urinary incontinence
      3. Initial turning of head and eyes followed by involuntary movements such as twitching of the face and shaking of the limbs, with progression of shaking movements from face to upper limb and then lower limb or in some other sequence, then shaking movements of the limbs on the opposite side of the body, with or without incontinence
      4. Unresponsiveness with staring and smacking movements of the lips, with or without subsequent falling, generalized stiffening, and generalized shaking of the limbs, with or without incontinence
   C. Offset (mode of termination of the episode)
II. Severity (mild or abortive forms of the episode)
III. Duration (of each component and from onset to full termination of the episode)
IV. Frequency (episodes per week, month, or year)
V. Timing (with respect to the time of day, day of the week, and week of the month)
VI. Context (when the patient is alone or only with others present)
VII. Associated features (apnea, tongue biting, injuries)
VIII. Modifying factors (sleep deprivation, stress levels, medications)

TABLE 1-7. Past Medical History

Operations
Trauma
Allergies
Major illnesses

10 or more medications, at times including duplicating types, and often excessive medications lead to symptoms such as cognitive dysfunction that can be managed effectively by simply eliminating one or more of the medications.

THE PAST MEDICAL HISTORY

The degree to which you will need to obtain the past medical history depends on the extent of the previous medical evaluation. If another physician already has obtained a thorough medical history and you have written documentation of it, you can review the written account and verify its accuracy with the patient, asking for further details if needed. If no previous historical information is available, proceed by asking for the dates and inquiring about any complications from previous operations; injuries, particularly craniocerebral and spinal trauma, including the duration of unconsciousness if applicable; allergies, past and present, including untoward reactions to medications; and major illnesses, especially those involving the nervous system (Table 1-7).

REVIEW OF SYSTEMS

Begin by inquiring about constitutional symptoms such as changes in personality or mood, fatigue, lassitude, weight loss or gain, and sleep disorders (Table 1-8). Proceed to ask about the head, eyes, ears, nose, mouth, and throat. Inquire about cardiovascular, respiratory, gastrointestinal, genitourinary, musculoskeletal, skin, endocrinologic, and hematologic/lymphatic systems. Finally, ask about allergic or immunologic disorders, psychiatric symptoms, and if indicated, sexual disturbances and menstrual functions.

To evaluate the head, eyes, ears, nose, mouth, and throat, ask about visual disturbances, including dimness or loss of vision, double vision, and use of glasses; difficulty with hearing, tinnitus, and vertigo; and difficulty with speaking, chewing, or swallowing. For the cardiovascular and respiratory systems inquire about exercise tolerance, shortness of breath, wheezing, frequent respiratory infections, difficulty lying flat in bed, ankle swelling, irregular heartbeat, previously detected heart murmurs, chest pain, and myocardial infarction ("heart attack"). Concerning the gastrointestinal system, ask about abdominal pain, indigestion ("heartburn"), acid eructations, nausea, vomiting, constipation, diarrhea, bloody or black stools, and use of medications such as antacids. In taking the genitourinary history, ask about urinary frequency, dysuria (burning or pain), infections,

TABLE 1-8.   Review of Systems

Constitutional
Head
Eyes
Ears, nose, mouth, throat
Cardiovascular
Respiratory
Gastrointestinal
Genitourinary
Musculoskeletal
Dermatologic
Endocrinologic
Hematologic/lymphatic
Allergic/immunologic
Psychiatric
Sexual
Menstrual

incontinence, dribbling, difficulty starting or stopping the stream, and nocturia. To evaluate the musculoskeletal system, inquire about muscle weakness, stiffness, difficulty walking, and joint pain, and the factors that exacerbate and relieve pain. Ask about skin lesions, changes in the size of moles and the results of biopsies of such lesions, itching or flaking of skin, and previous treatment for skin problems. Evaluate endocrinologic problems with inquiries about generalized weakness; changes in skin texture, skin pigmentation, or body weight; hair loss; and discomfort in cold or warm environments. For the hematologic/lymphatic system, ask about pallor, fatigue, easy bruising, excessive bleeding, and any history of anemia. Ask for any history of hay fever, asthma, and food and drug allergies, and medications used for these problems. For the psychiatric history, ask about anxiety, depression, difficulty with concentration, sleep disorders, periods of elation cycling with depression, lassitude, obsessive thoughts, and compulsive behavior.

It may be important to take a sexual history, particularly if the history leads you to suspect an autonomic disorder or a spinal cord lesion. Reserve the sexual history for the last part of the history, when hopefully you will have established good rapport with the patient. Frequently, physicians are reluctant to embarrass patients and themselves by taking this history, but it can be extremely important in formulating a diagnosis. You may wish to ask family members to leave the room if the questions will be embarrassing to the patient or family members. Often, however, it is helpful to have the spouse present. For men, ask whether the patient has erections adequate for sexual intercourse, morning erections, and difficulty with intercourse, such as premature ejaculation or inability to achieve ejaculation. For women, ask about appropriate levels of vaginal lubrication with sexual stimulation, pain with intercourse, and whether the patient achieves orgasm. To obtain a history of menstrual functioning, ask women the age of menarche, frequency of menses, and if appropriate, the age of menopause. Inquire about pain, excessive bleeding, and irregularity of the cycle.

TABLE 1-9. Family History

Neurologic diseases in family
Ages of parents at death, if not living
Siblings: number and ages
Inherited disorders

FAMILY HISTORY

Many neurologic disorders are inherited, and in others a positive family history constitutes a risk factor. Examples of inherited disorders are those with autosomal dominant inheritance such as Huntington disease and those with autosomal recessive inheritance such as Friedreich's ataxia. An example of a neurologic disorder that includes a positive family history as a risk factor is Alzheimer disease of the late-onset "sporadic" type. Accordingly, a full family history (Table 1-9) can be the key to a correct diagnosis. Begin taking the family history by asking whether any family members have or have had neurologic disorders similar to those the patient is experiencing. Next ask whether the parents are living and ask for their state of health. If they have died, ask about the age and cause of death of both the mother and father. Determine the number of siblings and ask about their health. Ask about children, including their ages and state of health. If you find evidence of a disorder in a parent suggesting a dominantly inherited disease, draw a diagram of a full family tree, including both parents, grandparents on the side of the affected parent, including siblings of grandparents and parents along with the patient's siblings and children. Take the family tree back through as many previous generations as possible.

SOCIAL HISTORY

Begin the social history (Table 1-10) by determining the highest level of education the patient attained and, if important in the assessment, asking about performance in school and any degrees granted. Obtain a history of current employment and previous occupations. Inquire about marital status. Ask about personal habits, including use of alcohol and tobacco, and exposure to "street drugs." The inquiry about alcohol should include the number of alcoholic drinks consumed per day in the past and at present and, if the patient consumes more than about four drinks daily, ask about the preferred drink, the time of day for the first drink, weekend binge drinking, loss of time from work because of

TABLE 1-10. Social History

Education
Occupation
Marital
Habits: alcohol, tobacco, "street drugs"

drinking, frequency of early morning drinking, and any consequences of excessive alcohol intake such as arrests for intoxication or drunk driving, limb tremors, and episodes of delirium tremens. If you obtain a history of alcohol abuse (six or more alcoholic drinks daily), obtain a detailed history about nutrition. Ask whether the patient goes without food for one or more days at a time owing to the constant consumption of alcohol. If the patient has at least one meal per day, ascertain the average types and amounts of food consumed. For the history of tobacco use, record the age the patient began smoking, the approximate number of packages of cigarettes or other forms of tobacco used per day, and the total number of years of smoking. In reviewing exposure to drugs, ask about the use of marijuana, heroin, cocaine, "uppers" and "downers," and other commonly used substances, obtaining a history of the age at first exposure, frequency of exposure, and current use.

INTERPRETATION OF THE HISTORY

A clear, concise history will assist you in determining the type of pathology that may be responsible for the patient's complaints. The chapters that follow provide detailed information concerning the interpretation of the history and physical findings. Accordingly, this account will be limited to a succinct presentation of points that may be helpful in understanding the significance of the patient's symptoms.

Complaints of difficulty with memory raise the possibility of a dementing disease such as Alzheimer disease, multi-infarct dementia, or dementia with Lewy bodies. Disorders of language can result from structural lesions of the left cerebral hemisphere if the disorder involves difficulty finding the correct words to express thoughts (which raises the possibility of an anterior left cerebral hemisphere lesion), trouble comprehending spoken or written speech (which usually results from a posterior left cerebral hemisphere lesion), or inability to articulate clearly (which can occur with bilateral internal capsule, basal ganglia, brainstem, or cerebellar lesions). Disturbances in the comprehension or execution of speech and language can also result from widespread cerebral lesions as part of a dementia such as Alzheimer disease. Difficulty in managing spatial information (as in getting lost when driving an automobile) can occur with right cerebral hemisphere lesions, principally those involving the parietal lobe, but also as part of a dementing disease with widespread cerebral pathology. Defective judgment raises the possibility of a dementing illness, but also can reflect focal lesions bilaterally in the prefrontal cerebral cortex.

A history of visual disorders can help focus on examination of the visual system, and the results often permit precise localization of the site of pathology. Tinnitus usually results from disease of the inner ear and not the central nervous system. The complaint of dizziness requires multiple questions to determine the precise symptom experienced. Vertigo usually reflects peripheral vestibular apparatus disease, though at times brainstem disorders can present with a rocking type of sensation of movement. Light-headedness may result from postural hypotension, particularly with onset on standing, and is a common side effect of medications, notably beta blockers. When inquiring about blackouts, attempt to determine whether the patient loses consciousness but remains upright or loses postural tone and falls. Loss of consciousness without falling can result from many causes, but distracted thoughts, medication effects, and conversion reactions may produce this symptom. Loss of consciousness with falling can result from orthostatic hypotension, cardiac arrhythmia, or seizures. A history of stiffening of the body before or after falling, with or without subsequent clonic movements of the limbs, raises the likely possibility of a seizure disorder. If you suspect this, ask about subjective experiences preceding the loss of consciousness, including déjà vu (a feeling that the surroundings are strangely familiar), *jamais vu* (a feeling that the surrounds are strangely unfamiliar), feelings of depersonalization, floating, macropsia (viewing objects as abnormally large), and micropsia (viewing objects as abnormally small), all of which raise the possibility of a seizure disorder, particularly complex partial seizures.

In evaluating complaints of headache, the history provides strong clues to the diagnosis. A headache upon awakening in the morning with relief after standing and walking about can result from increased intracranial pressure as with a brain tumor. A bilateral pressure sensation feeling as if a tight band had been placed around the head often results from muscle tension headache. Migraine headaches can be hemicranial or bilateral and often are accompanied by visual disorders (usually fortification spectra), nausea, vomiting, pallor, light-headedness, or mild vertigo. Common provocative factors for migraine headache are exposure to spiced meats or vegetables, ripe cheeses, citrus fruits or juices, wind, dropping barometric pressure, excessive or inadequate amounts of sleep, and rows of lines or stripes in the visual environment.

Complaints of weakness need to be evaluated to determine whether the patient suffers from loss of muscular strength or from generalized fatigue, loss of coordination, muscle stiffness, or imbalance and a tendency to fall. Loss of muscular strength usually indicates a lesion of the motor pathways, affecting upper motor neuron connections if accompanied by spasticity, hyperactive muscle stretch reflexes and extensor plantar responses, and involving the lower motor neuron pathway if accompanied by decreased resistance to passive movement, decreased muscle stretch reflexes, and fasciculations (indicating motor neuron disease, as in amyotrophic lateral sclerosis) or sensory loss (indicating peripheral nerve or spinal root disease). Imbalance and a tendency to fall commonly result from disease of the brainstem, cerebellum, or basal ganglia.

REFERENCES

Gelb DJ: *Introduction to Clinical Neurology.* Boston, Butterworth-Heinemann, 1995.

Gilman S, Newman SW: *Manter and Gatz's Essentials of Clinical Neuroanatomy and Neurophysiology,* 9th ed. Philadelphia, FA Davis, 1996.

Haerer AF: *DeJong's The Neurologic Examination,* 5th ed. Philadelphia, JB Lippincott, 1992.

Isselbacher KJ, Braunwald E, Wilson JD, et al: *Harrison's Principles of Internal Medicine,* 14th ed. New York, McGraw-Hill, 1998.

Joynt R, Griggs R: *Clinical Neurology.* Philadelphia, Lippincott-Raven, 1996.

Rosenberg RN, Pleasure DE: *Comprehensive Neurology,* 2d ed. New York, Wiley-Liss, 1998.

Watts RL, Koller WC: *Movement Disorders. Neurologic Principles and Practice.* New York, McGraw-Hill, 1997.

SID GILMAN

THE PHYSICAL AND NEUROLOGIC EXAMINATION

Clinical diagnosis in neurologic disease begins with the history and continues with the neurologic examination. As described in Chap. 1, the history gives evidence about the kind of pathology responsible for the symptoms, and the neurologic examination about the location of the pathology. After completing these steps, the clinician can use the information obtained to formulate the case, developing a differential diagnosis and a plan for further evaluation, management, and treatment. Long experience indicates the wisdom of a parsimonious approach to neurologic diagnosis, which requires from the outset the assumption that the patient's symptoms can be explained by a single type of pathology in a single location in the nervous system. While not infallible, this approach is consistently useful.

The neurologic examination must be supplemented by a general physical examination (Table 2-1) to look for medical disorders responsible for or contributing to the neurologic problem, and the extent of this examination depends on the information available at the time of the evaluation. Patients recently examined by physicians who provided records of thorough physical examinations may need little additional examination, whereas patients without such records may require a full examination. This chapter concerns the general physical examination that should be conducted in evaluation of patients without records of previous examinations, and it also provides an overall guide to the neurologic

TABLE 2-1. Outline of the General Physical Examination

General appearance
Vital signs
Skin
Head, neck, extremities, and spine
Eyes
Ear, nose, mouth, and throat
Lungs
Heart
Abdomen
Genitalia and anus

examination, which is thoroughly explored in the remaining chapters of this book. The chapter concludes with comments about interpretation of the neurologic examination in determining the site of the pathology.

GENERAL APPEARANCE

The physical and neurologic examinations begin when you first encounter the patient, whether in an outpatient waiting room or in a hospital bed. Observe the patient's facial expression and look for signs of distress, anger, depression, or apathy. Determine whether the patient appears younger or older than the stated age. Premature balding in men or graying in men and women is usually hereditary, but frontal balding occurs with myotonic dystrophy and early graying can be seen in pernicious anemia. Observe the patient's body habitus and nutrition, skin color, amount and distribution of hair, grooming of hair and nails, and posture of the trunk and limbs. Many chronic illnesses are associated with pallor and weight loss, leading to emaciation. Diffuse hyperpigmentation occurs with Addison disease, hemochromatosis, pernicious anemia, pellagra, folic acid deficiency, and Whipple disease. Drugs can cause many pigmentary changes in the skin; phenothiazines can be deposited in the skin and cause a slate-gray color; antimalarials induce a gray or yellow pigmentation; and phenytoin can produce light brown pigmented spots in women. Look for dysmorphic features such as an excessively large head, short neck, or short legs and for any obvious deformity of the head, limbs, and trunk. Dysmorphic features can be associated with a number of disorders, including endocrinopathies, premature closure of the skull sutures, and malformations such as the Chiari types.

Observe the responsiveness of the patient's facial expression and look for asymmetry of the patient's face, particularly with smiling. Parkinson disease results in a poverty of facial expression termed "masking," and facial asymmetry can be a subtle indication of facial weakness. Look for ptosis and proptosis and note the size of the pupils. When you initially listen to the patient speak, determine whether the speech is clear and fluent or dysarthric or hesitant, and whether the patient has difficulty finding correct words to express thoughts. As you walk the patient to the examination room, note the patient's posture, steadiness, and gait and look for tremor and lack of arm swing, either unilaterally or bilaterally. In Parkinson disease the posture is stooped, the arms and legs are flexed, and the gait is unsteady, consisting of small, shuffling steps with little arm swing. Cerebellar disorders cause an ataxic gait; the patient takes irregularly sized steps and frequently bumps into walls, particularly when rounding corners. With an early or mild spastic hemiparesis the affected arm is adducted at the shoulder and flexed at the elbow, wrist, and fingers and does not swing with walking. The affected leg is extended at the hip, knee, and ankle and circumducts with walking.

VITAL SIGNS

Measure height and weight and obtain an oral temperature. Measure the blood pressure, pulse rate, and respiratory rate with the patient seated or standing. If the history includes light-headedness or blackouts on standing or in other ways suggests an autonomic disorder, measure the blood pressure and pulse rate after the patient has been supine for 2 to 3 min. Then have the patient stand up, wait 2 to 3 min, and again measure the blood pressure and pulse rate. A decline of 20 mmHg systolic or 10 mmHg diastolic with movement from the supine to the standing position constitutes postural hypotension. In evaluating the significance of the decrease of blood pressure with standing, factors to consider include medications that induce postural hypotension (e.g., beta blockers), dehydration, and some acute systemic illnesses.

THE SKIN

Examine the skin of the face, extremities, trunk, and legs and note the color, temperature, moisture, and dryness. In Parkinson disease the face is often oily. Look for sebaceous adenomas of the face, which usually follow a butterfly area distribution over the bridge of the nose and suggest tuberous sclerosis. Observe the face for a port-wine nevus, usually on the forehead in the first division of the trigeminal nerve, which may indicate ipsilateral cortical cerebral angiomas (encephalotrigeminal angiomatosis or Sturge-Weber syndrome). Look for cutaneous nevi in a segmental (nerve-root) distribution, which may be associated with a hemangioma of the spinal cord. Examine for cafe´ au lait spots, subcutaneous neurofibromas, and pedunculated polyps, which occur with neurofibromatosis. Inspect the lumbosacral region for shagreen patches, which are yellowish-brown elevated plaques with the texture of pig skin and are found in tuberous sclerosis.

HEAD, NECK, EXTREMITIES, AND SPINE

Examine the head, looking for an abnormally large (macrocephalic) or small (microcephalic) skull. Note the shape and symmetry of the head to detect skull deformities such as scaphocephaly (an oblong-shaped skull), brachycephaly (a skull with a broad biparietal diameter), or oxycephaly (a tower-shaped skull). Inspect the scalp to look for old incisions and palpate the skull to detect deformities such as burr holes and bony abnormalities suggesting previous surgery or fractures. Palpate the temporal arteries and listen for bruits over them and over the globes. To listen over the globes, have the patient close both eyes, place the stethoscope on one, then ask the patient to open the other eye and fix on an object across the room. This will reduce noise from movements of the lids and eyes. Inspect and palpate the neck to seek an enlarged thyroid gland and cervical adenopathy. Note whether the head is tilted to the right or left and whether the chin is rotated to the right or left (torticollis). Passively flex the neck to detect pain or limitation of movement suggesting meningeal irritation. Palpate the carotid arteries and listen for bruits over both. Inspect the wrists, hands, and fingers to detect joint swelling or deformity from arthritis and observe the fingernails to look for pallor, cyanosis, bitten nails, ungual fibromas, and bifid nails. Multiple ungual fibromas are a primary feature of tuberous sclerosis, and bifid nails can occur. Look for Meese lines, which consist of narrow white bands laterally crossing the nails resulting from arsenic intoxication. Palpate the radial arteries bilaterally.

Examine the legs to detect genu valgus or varus, abnormally high arches, and hammer toe deformity. Friedreich's ataxia and some of the hereditary sensorimotor neuropathies are associated with high arches and hammer toes. Palpate the dorsalis pedis and posterior tibial arteries. Observe the hair distribution over the lower portions of the legs. Loss of hair from these regions occurs with autonomic neuropathies, frequently diabetic neuropathy. Inspect the spine to look for kyphosis and scoliosis. Note whether the patient carries one shoulder higher than the other and determine whether one hip is higher than the other by placing your hands on the dorsolateral margins of the pelvis on each side. Many dystonias are associated with asymmetric positions of the shoulders and hips and with scoliosis. Inspect and palpate the spine and adjacent muscles to detect tenderness or muscle spasm. Look at the base of the spine for a dimple in the skin or tuft of hair suggesting spina bifida or meningocele, which can be a component of a Chiari malformation.

EYES

Measure the width of the palpebral fissures to detect differences on the two sides and note any ptosis or proptosis. Inspect the corneas for Kayser-Fleischer rings, which often can be seen without a slit lamp and are diagnostic of Wilson disease. These rings usually consist of golden-brown pigment at the periphery of the cornea, characteristically broader superiorly and inferiorly than medially and laterally. Look for an arcus senilis and for scleral icterus and chemosis. Measure the size of the pupils and their responses to light both directly and consensually. The remaining parts of the eye examination are described with the cranial nerves below.

EARS, NOSE, MOUTH, AND THROAT

Note any malformations of the auricles and look for tophi, then use an otoscope to observe the canals and tympanic membranes. Examine the nose for deformities, obstruction, discharge, and septal deviation. Inspect the lips for cyanosis or pallor, then look at the gingivae and teeth to detect gingival hyperplasia, pyorrhea, redness or erosion, malocclusion, or abnormally shaped teeth. Examine the gums for hyperplasia, which occurs with phenytoin ingestion and ascorbic acid deficiency, and for discoloration, which can result from heavy metals, notably copper and arsenic, antimalarial drugs, and adrenocorticotrophic hormone. Note the color of the tongue and determine whether it is abnormally red, smooth, or fissured. Several vitamin deficiencies, notably niacin, riboflavin, and cyanocobalamin, are associated with a red, smooth tongue. Examine the throat to detect redness and tonsillar hypertrophy.

LUNGS

Look for dyspnea, orthopnea, or shortness of breath with minor exertion. Inspect the thorax for increased anterior-posterior diameter and note whether the chest expands equally on both sides with breathing. Look for guarding and for pain with breathing. If indicated, percuss over the back to detect dullness and to determine whether the diaphragm descends equally on each side. As the patient takes deep breaths listen over the lung fields for rales, rhonchi, or wheezes. Palpate the axillae to detect lymphadenopathy. If a breast examination of a woman is indicated, it is prudent to do this with a nurse in the room. Inspect the contour of the breasts and look for dimpling, or orange skin appearance; retraction of the nipples; and discharge from the nipples. Palpate the breasts in each of the four quadrants.

HEART

Inspect and palpate the chest to detect the cardiac point of maximum impulse. If indicated, percuss the left anterior thorax to determine the size of the heart, then use a stethoscope to listen at the apex, along the left sternal border, and at the base of the heart on each side of the sternum. Note the rate, rhythm, and tone of the heart sounds and listen for murmurs. If you hear a murmur, track it into the neck and listen for a bruit over the carotid arteries. A carotid bruit transmitted from the chest is less likely to indicate significant atherosclerotic carotid artery disease than a bruit not transmitted from the heart. Examine the jugular veins with the patient recumbent to detect venous distention and examine the extremities for edema.

ABDOMEN

Inspect and palpate the abdomen to detect tenderness, muscle spasm, masses, and abnormal pulsations. Determine the size of the liver by percussing and palpating the liver edge with a deep breath. Examine the spleen by palpation and percussion. Palpate to detect costovertebral angle tenderness and examine for a fluid wave when indicated. Listen for bowel sounds.

GENITALIA AND ANUS

Examination of the genitalia in men and pelvic examination in women should be performed when indicated, though a nurse must be present for examination of women. The anus should be examined when indicated. For this, inspect the anal orifice to determine whether it is closed or patulous. Using a disposable pin, scratch the lateral margin of the skin successively on each side of the anus to detect the superficial anal (anal wink) reflex, which consists of contraction of the external anal sphincter in response to each stimulus. Insert a gloved finger moistened with lubricant to determine the integrity of the anal sphincter, to probe for masses, and, in men, to palpate the prostate gland.

NEUROLOGIC EXAMINATION

The neurologic examination can be divided into five parts, mental status, cranial nerves, motor system, reflexes, and sensation. We discuss each of these parts in detail in the

TABLE 2-2. Examination of Mental Status

Orientation
Attention and state of consciousness
Memory
Retention and immediate recall
Calculations
Grasp of general information
Proverb interpretation
Similarities
Insight

remaining chapters of this book. Hence this account will provide only a brief summary in outline form of the principal elements to examine.

Mental Status

In taking the history from your patient, you have already developed an impression of the mental status. If the patient is alert, provides a clear history, and has no complaints relevant to higher cognitive function, the mental status can be evaluated with a few simple tests such as memory, calculations, and proverb interpretation. If you suspect cognitive dysfunction, use all the tests (Table 2-2) outlined below and, if indicated, supplement the examination with the appropriate neuropsychologic test batteries.

ORIENTATION   Determine whether the patient is oriented to time, place, and person.

ATTENTION AND STATE OF CONSCIOUSNESS   Describe the level of alertness and capacity to attend to the examination.

MEMORY   Test remote memory by asking for the patient's date of birth, dates of completing various schools, and date of marriage. Test intermediate memory by asking for events of the previous three to five years, either with personal history or with national events. Test recent memory with descriptions of the events of the past couple of days pertaining to the present illness, events since hospitalization, and travel to the office to see you. You will need to have a family member or friend present to verify at least some of the answers.

RETENTION AND IMMEDIATE RECALL   Verbally present three digits at a rate of about one per second and ask the patient to repeat the digits forward and then backward. Increase the number of digits sequentially until the patient fails to repeat the digits correctly backward and then forward. Record the number of digits repeated successfully forward and backward. Most normal adults can repeat seven digits forward and five backward. Present three unrelated objects verbally such as "desk, airplane, carrot" and ask the patient to repeat the objects immediately and again after 5 min. Record the number of objects recalled at 5 min. Tell a brief story and ask the patient to repeat the story as accurately as possible. Record the story you told and the version repeated.

CALCULATIONS Present the following problems: subtract 7 from 100, give the answer, then sequentially subtract 7 from the remainder; count from 1 to 20 and backwards to 1; multiply 3 times 16; compute the interest on $200 at 10% annually for 18 months.

GRASP OF GENERAL INFORMATION Ask for the names of the U.S. President, Vice-President, and Secretary of State, and the local mayor and governor; the names of the five largest cities in the United States; the dates of Christmas and Washington's birthday; the dates of the beginning and end of the world wars, the Korean war, or the Vietnam conflict.

PROVERB INTERPRETATION Verbally present a proverb such as, "people who live in glass houses shouldn't throw stones" and ask for an interpretation of the proverb. The interpretation should be abstract as, for example, "nobody is perfect, so people should not criticize others." Partially or fully concrete interpretations (such as, "they will break the windows") indicate cognitive impairment. Other useful proverbs are: "a new broom sweeps clean"; "every cloud has a silver lining"; and "a rolling stone gathers no moss."

SIMILARITIES Verbally present two objects such as apple and lemon and ask in what way they are similar. The response should be abstract such as, "both are fruit" and not concrete such as, "they are round." Other pairs of objects that can be used are bicycle and truck and bird and airplane.

INSIGHT Describe finding a stamped, addressed, sealed envelope on the street and ask what should be done with it. The response should be to drop it in a mailbox or give it to a postal carrier. Responses such as "open it to find out what is inside" or "throw it away" indicate cognitive impairment. Ask what the patient would do upon detecting a fire when seated in a theater. The response should be to walk to the nearest exit and notify responsible attendants or the fire department. Responses such as "Shout fire" or "Run out fast" may indicate cognitive impairment. If the patient presents such a response, ask additional questions to determine whether the patient can grasp the hazards of this type of behavior. Seek the patient's level of understanding of the illness, plans to assist the recovery process, and planned activities after recovery.

Cranial Nerves

For screening purposes, usually you do not need to test the olfactory nerves or corneal reflexes or use the Rinne or Weber test. The remaining parts of the cranial nerve examination (Table 2-3) can be completed rapidly. Test the olfactory nerves if the patient has a history of a serious head injury, complaints of loss of the sense of taste or smell, or frontal headaches. Test the corneal reflexes if the patient has decreased sensation on the face. Use the Rinne and Weber tests if the patient has complaints of hearing loss.

I. OLFACTORY NERVES Test the sense of smell in each nostril using oil of lemon, cloves, or coffee. Do not use noxious fumes such as ammonia vapor as they stimulate cranial nerve V.

TABLE 2-3.   Examination of the Cranial Nerves

I. Olfactory nerves
II. Optic nerves: visual acuity, visual fields, optic fundi
III, IV, VI. Extraocular muscle function: pupils, lids, eye movements
V. Trigeminal nerves: motor division, sensory division
VII. Facial nerves: motor division, sensory division
VIII. Auditory nerves
IX, X. Glossopharyngeal nerves
XI. Spinal accessory nerves
XII. Hypoglossal nerves

II. OPTIC NERVES

Visual Acuity   Measure visual acuity with a Snellen chart or a handheld test card such as the Rosenbaum Pocket Vision Screener or the Jaeger card. Have the patient hold the card 14 in. from the eye being tested while keeping the other eye closed. Record visual acuity for each eye separately with and without glasses. Record the results in distance equivalent numbers: VOD (vision in the right eye) = 20/size read, VOS (vision in the left eye) = 20/size read.

Visual Fields   For office or bedside screening, have the patient cover one eye at a time and test each of the four quadrants in the uncovered eye by moving your finger and asking the patient to determine when movement occurs. If the patient complains of a visual disorder or if you detect a field disorder by testing with movement of your fingers, repeat the test by plotting the fields using a 4-mm, round, white object or the head of a red match by confrontation. This can be done at the bedside or in the office. Confirm the findings with perimetry or tangent screen examination. If you suspect a disorder of the parietal or occipital regions of the cerebral cortex, test for extinction with double simultaneous stimulation with both eyes open. To do this, hold your right hand in the temporal half of the patient's left visual field and your left hand in the temporal half of the patient's right visual field. Then quickly move your right index finger and then your left index finger to determine whether the patient can detect movement on each side when presented separately. Next quickly move your right and left index fingers simultaneously to determine whether the patient detects movement on both sides or only on one side. Extinction is defined by detection of movement on each side separately, but on one side alone with dual simultaneous stimulation.

Optic Fundi   Examine the fundus of each eye with an ophthalmoscope and describe the optic disc, retina, veins, and arteries.

III, IV, VI. EXTRAOCULAR MUSCLE FUNCTION

Pupils   Measure the size of each pupil in dim, ambient light and the change in size with bright illumination applied directly to the eye (the direct reaction to light). Next shine the light in the right eye and determine the change in size of the left pupil, then repeat the test with illumination of the left eye (the consensual reaction to light). Measure the size of each pupil as the patient gazes in the distance, then at a focal point about 14 in. from the nose (reaction to accommodation). Inspect the pupils for regularity to determine whether they are round, oval, or irregular, and whether the margins are smooth or scalloped.

Lids   Look for unilateral or bilateral lid retraction or drooping, noting the positions of the lids on the sclerae or irises on each side.

Eye Movements   Inspect the axis of the eyes with straight-ahead gaze to determine whether they are parallel. Then ask the patient to fixate on an object such as a light or your finger as you move the object to the right, to the left, upward, and downward. Note any limitation of movement and any change in the axis of each eye in any direction. Look for nystagmus, which consists of repetitive beating movements of the eyes with gaze in any of the four cardinal directions.

V. TRIGEMINAL NERVES

Motor Division   Inspect and palpate the masseter muscles bilaterally with clenching of the jaw to detect differences in bulk or contraction on the two sides. Attempt to open the jaw with clenching to assess the strength of the masseter muscles and then, with the mouth open, attempt to close the jaw to assess the strength of the pterygoid muscles.

Sensory Division   Test sensation in all three divisions on the face with a cold object, light touch with cotton wool, and pinprick. Test the corneal reflex by touching each cornea with a wisp of cotton as the patient gazes upward and determine whether the eyelid quickly closes.

VII. FACIAL NERVES

Motor Division   Inspect the face to detect any asymmetry and determine whether the face is expressive or impassive (a "masked" face is common in Parkinson disease). Ask the patient to move the facial muscle by frowning, closing the eyes forcefully, baring the teeth, and smiling. Upper motor neuron disorders cause weakness of the lower facial muscles whereas lower motor neuron or peripheral nerve disorders cause weakness of upper and lower facial muscles.

Sensory Division   Test taste on the anterior two-thirds of the tongue with a solution of sugar or salt in water. Apply the solution to the lateral margin of the tongue with a moistened cotton swab.

VIII. AUDITORY NERVES   Test hearing with a whispered voice or a ticking watch near each ear independently. Using a 128-Hz tuning fork, determine whether air conduction exceeds bone conduction by tapping one of the prongs, then holding the base of the tuning fork on the mastoid process. Ask when the sound no longer can be heard, then hold the prongs, which will still be vibrating, next to the ear to determine whether the patient can detect the sound. This is the Rinne test, and normally air conduction can be heard after bone conduction can be heard no longer. Using the same tuning fork, set the prongs in motion with a tap and hold the base of the tuning fork on the center of the forehead, asking the patient whether the sound volume is louder in one ear than the other. This is the Weber test, and normally sound should be detected as equal on the two sides. Tests of vestibular function are seldom needed in a clinical examination, but can be performed with cold-water calorics in awake, cooperative patients and with the doll's-eye maneuver in comatose patients.

IX, X. GLOSSOPHARYNGEAL NERVES   Inspect the soft palate with the mouth open and the patient at rest and then with vocalization of "ahh." Determine whether the uvula is in the midline at rest and whether the palate elevates symmetrically with articulation.

XI. SPINAL ACCESSORY NERVES   Test the strength of the sternomastoid muscles by asking the patient to turn the head to the right and the left against resistance. Test the strength of the trapezius by asking the patient to shrug the shoulders against resistance.

XII. HYPOGLOSSAL NERVES   Ask the patient to protrude the tongue in the midline and then to move it from side to side rapidly. Look for deviation of the tongue to the right or left on protrusion and for atrophy of the tongue on one side or both. You will have heard enough speech by listening as you take history. You can supplement this examination with specific tasks such as vocalizing "pa-pa-pa" for labial sounds, "ta-ta-ta" for lingual, and "ka-ka-ka" for palatal. Speech disorders can be divided into ataxic, hypokinetic, spastic, and flaccid. Ataxic speech is associated with cerebellar disorders, hypokinetic speech with basal ganglia diseases, spastic speech with corticobulbar disorders, and flaccid speech with diseases of the lower motor neurons or peripheral branches of the IXth, Xth, and XIIth cranial nerves.

Motor System

You begin the motor system examination when you enter a patient's hospital room or encounter the patient in an outpatient waiting room. Observe the entire person, looking for asymmetries of posture and movement, involuntary movements, facial twitching, imbalance in walking, and shuffling steps. Then focus on individual components of the motor system (Table 2-4) as described below.

POSTURE   Observe the patient's posture to detect asymmetries in the position of the head, height of the shoulders, attitudes of the arms and hands, and positions of the legs and feet. If the patient is lying in a hospital bed, note whether the chin is deviated to the right or left and the eyes to the right or left and observe the postures of the arms and legs. Hemiparesis from a cerebral hemisphere lesion results in flattening of the lower face, flexion of the arm, and extension with external rotation of the leg on the side contralateral to the lesion. Subtle asymmetries may give a clue to such a lesion when the hemiparesis is early or mild. Look for tremor or spasm of the face or limbs at rest. Ask the patient to extend both

TABLE 2-4. Examination of the Motor System

Posture
Muscle atrophy
Resistance to passive manipulation of the limbs
Muscle strength
Coordination
Gait
Involuntary movements

arms with the hands open and fingers spread, first in the pronated and then in the supinated position, to look for asymmetry of upper limb posture. Ask the patient to maintain this position with the eyes closed to determine whether one arm drifts downward, indicating subtle limb weakness. In patients with upper motor neuron diseases affecting the upper limb, the weak arm descends and pronates. In patients with conversion reactions manifested as limb weakness, the arm presumed to be weak descends but does not pronate.

ATROPHY Inspect the musculature for atrophy and fasciculations before testing muscle strength, as in some people without neurologic disease muscle contraction can evoke fasciculations. Inspect the bulk of the muscles in each limb and the trunk and abdominal musculature to detect focal or generalized muscle atrophy. Inspect the arms, legs, and back for fasciculations, which are involuntary contractions of the muscles of single motor units manifested as fine flickering movements of the skin, usually insufficient to cause movements about joints.

RESISTANCE TO PASSIVE MANIPULATION ("TONE") Evaluate resistance to passive manipulation before testing strength to promote patient relaxation. Ask the patient not to oppose your movements. Grasp the patient's hand with one of your hands and the patient's forearm with your other hand. Move the patient's hand up and then down rapidly at the wrist to detect abnormal resistance. Test the forearm by taking the patient's hand as if to shake hands, then rapidly move the hand from full pronation to full supination. Passively flex and extend the arm at the elbow and at the shoulder. Similarly dorsiflex and plantarflex each foot at the ankle, flex and extend the lower leg at the knee, and flex and extend the entire leg at the hip. A sensitive means of detecting spasticity in the legs is to flex one leg at the knee rapidly with the patient lying supine and relaxed. A catch followed by a release of resistance with passive manipulation indicates spasticity and is usually accompanied by hyperactive muscle stretch (deep tendon) reflexes. A sequential series of resistances to manipulation during a single excursion of passive flexion or extension, each followed by release of resistance, indicates cogwheel rigidity, which is common in parkinsonism. This is best detected at the wrist. A smooth, even resistance throughout movement is termed plastic rigidity. A progressively increasing resistance through the range of passive manipulation is termed dystonic rigidity. Spasticity usually results from disorders of the corticospinal pathways and rigidity from disease of the basal ganglia and their connections. Decreased resistance to passive manipulation (hypotonia) is difficult to detect when bilateral, but can be demonstrated by observing the motions of the joints as you passively shake a limb. The joints will appear to be abnormally loose. Hypotonia results from diseases of the cerebellum and its connections and disorders of peripheral nerve or root innervation of muscle. Hypotonia also occurs acutely after a sudden lesion of the corticospinal projections.

STRENGTH   Test the power of muscle contraction at each joint, proceeding from the shoulders to the elbows, wrists, and fingers, then from the hips to the knees, ankles, and toes. Test flexion and extension and, where possible, adduction and abduction. Evaluate the strength of the intercostal muscles by observing chest movement with deep breaths. Determine the power of the abdominal muscles by asking the patient to raise the head from the examining table while in the supine position. Test the strength of the back muscles by asking the patient to bend forward, then straighten up against resistance. Use a 5-point scale for power as follows: 0 = no contraction; 1 = detectable contraction; 2 = weak contraction insufficient to overcome gravity; 3 = weak contraction that overcomes gravity, but that the examiner can overcome easily; 4 = moderately strong contraction still demonstrating some weakness; and 5 = full strength.

COORDINATION   Ask the patient alternately to use the index finger of one hand to touch the patient's nose and then your index finger, maintaining your finger a full arm's length away from the patient (the finger-nose-finger test). Have the patient place the heel of one leg on the knee of the other, then slide the heel smoothly down the front of the lower leg in a straight line, terminating the movement at the ankle (the heel-knee-shin test). Ask the patient to tap the palm of the left hand with the palm and then the dorsum of the right hand repetitively and rapidly. Repeat the test, tapping the right hand with the left. Have the patient maintain the heel of a foot immobile on the floor, then rapidly rotate the foot to the right and left, successively tapping the ball of the foot on the floor after full rotation to the right, and then upon full rotation to the left. In disorders of cerebellar function these movements show abnormalities of rate and trajectory with poor or incomplete sequences of movement. The finger-nose-finger test and heel-knee-shin test show that the limbs take a veering course and develop a tremor that is generated at the proximal joints of the limb. In basal ganglia diseases such as parkinsonism, these movements are accurate but slow and at times halting.

GAIT   Ask the patient to walk slowly down the hall while you observe the posture of the head, positions of the shoulders, swing of the arms, size and directions of the steps, and direction of the movement. Observe whether the head is straight, the shoulders are equal in height, the arms swing equally, stride length is equal with each leg, and the direction of the movement is straight. Next have the patient walk on the balls of the feet and then on the heels, then walk in a straight line heel-to-toe, that is, alternately touching the heel of one foot against the toes of the other. In hemiplegia, the arm flexes at the elbow and does not swing with walking, and the leg extends stiffly at the knee and plantarflexes at the ankle so that the ball of the foot scrapes on the floor, and the entire leg circumducts with each step. In cerebellar diseases, the stance is on a wide base and the steps are irregular in size and direction so that the patient deviates or reels, and then staggers on attempting to turn. In Parkinson disease the posture is stooped, the steps are short, and stepping accelerates as walking continues. In conversion reactions many abnormalities can be seen, but the disturbances of gait are inconsistent with the ability to move the limbs in other tests of coordination, and exaggerated balancing occurs commonly.

INVOLUNTARY MOVEMENTS Observe the patient sitting quietly to detect a parkinsonian tremor, which consists of a distal 4- to 5-Hz rhythmic alternating flexion-extension of the fingers with adduction-abduction of the thumb and of the lips and eyelids when lightly closed. The tremor occurs with the limbs at rest and disappears briefly with active movement. Heredofamilial or senile tremor consists of a fine distal trembling movement of the fingers when extended. A shaking tremor of the head is also common in this disorder, and classically the tremor abates markedly with ingestion of even a single alcoholic drink. Cerebellar tremor consists of rhythmic lateral movements of the proximal joints of the limbs with posture holding and active movement. Severe cerebellar tremor can affect the trunk and head, causing a titubation (back-and-forth or side-to-side rhythmic movements). Rubral tremor consists of a combined proximal tremor characteristic of cerebellar disease and a distal tremor similar to heredofamilial tremor, usually with both flexion-extension and adduction-abduction components to the movements of the fingers. Myoclonus consists of a sudden brief (lightning-like) jerk of muscle groups causing limb or trunk movement. Athetosis consists of a slow series of movements involving the limbs, face, and trunk, usually appearing in combination with dystonic (relatively fixed abnormal) postures. Athetosis is frequently seen in cerebral palsy. Athetotic movements consist of repeated cycles of limb extension with supination and then flexion with pronation. At times rapid jerking movements accompany the slower athetotic movements, a combination labeled choreoathetosis. Chorea is best seen in Huntington disease and in patients with Parkinson disease overdosed with levodopa-containing medication. The movements are moderately rapid, flowing constantly between face, limbs, and trunk, involving facial grimacing, sweeping movements of the chin across the chest, piano-playing movements of the fingers, and elevation and depression of the shoulders and hips. Often, these movements make it appear that the patient is performing a complex dance. Hemiballismus consists of a flinging movement of the whole arm at the shoulder and the leg at the hip. Tics are stereotyped, regularly repeated movements occurring at irregular intervals. The movements include blinking of the eyes, twitching of the facial muscles, elevation of one shoulder, coughing loudly, and twitching of the body. In Tourette's syndrome, verbalization (usually coprolalia) or gutteral sounds accompany the stereotyped tics.

Reflexes

The reflexes (Table 2-5) provide objective measures that are highly useful in neurologic diagnosis, as they do not depend on subjective responses from the patient. Patients with conversion reactions experience weakness and put out poor effort with testing, often showing "give-way" weakness. This consists of an initially strong muscle contraction against resistance during strength testing, but quickly the muscle contraction weakens, letting the limb give way. These patients may complain of sensory loss, and sensory testing may show abnormalities (though usually the areas affected are inconsistent and do not follow anatomic boundaries). In such patients, reflex testing usually shows no abnormalities, and thereby can assist in diagnosis.

TABLE 2-5.   Examination of the Reflexes

Muscle stretch reflexes
    Jaw reflex
    Biceps reflex
    Brachioradialis reflex
    Triceps reflex
    Finger reflexes
    Hoffmann's sign
    Patellar reflex
    Achilles reflex
Superficial reflexes
    Abdominal reflexes
    Cremaster reflexes
    Superficial anal reflex
Plantar reflex

MUSCLE STRETCH (DEEP TENDON) REFLEXES   These reflexes are sensitive indicators of the level of excitability of the afferent pathway from stretch receptors in the striated skeletal muscle excited by the stimulus, the motor neurons in the spinal cord activated by these receptors, and the efferent pathway to muscle. Muscle stretch reflexes become hyperactive after injury to upper motor neuron pathways, and hypoactive with disease of the relevant lower motor neurons, spinal roots, or peripheral nerves. Reflex testing provides useful information that can be used in conjunction with other parts of the examination. Normal reflex responses show wide variability, from absent to +++; only reflexes with clonus can be considered definitely abnormal. Clonus consists of repetitive contraction of the muscles activated by muscle stretch and can be tested conveniently at the ankle. For this, place the patient in a comfortable position, flex the knee to about a right angle, then rapidly dorsiflex the foot and maintain the foot in dorsiflexion. The response is repetitive contraction of the calf muscles as long as you maintain the foot in dorsiflexion. Clonus can be demonstrated at the knee by pushing sharply down on the rostral part of the patella and maintaining the patella in the same position. The response is repetitive contraction of the quadriceps muscle as long as you keep pressure on the patella. In some patients, clonus can be demonstrated in the upper limbs with equivalent maneuvers. In the absence of demonstrable clonus, asymmetries of the reflexes on the two sides of the body provide the most useful information concerning pathologic changes in the nervous system; however, asymmetric reflexes can result from pathologically decreased responses on one side or pathologically increased responses on the other. Test the reflexes with the patient relaxed, and if you find an absent response, test the reflex again, asking the patient to clench the teeth strongly or to pull the curled fingers of one hand against the curled fingers of the other hand as you tap the tendon. This is the Jendrassik maneuver, which provides an excitatory barrage to the motor neuron pools, enhancing reflex responses. Grade the reflexes on a five-point scale: 0 = absent even with reinforcement; + = barely detectable; ++ = normal amplitude and speed; +++ = larger than normal amplitude and speed or spread of muscle contraction beyond the zone of muscles usually activated; ++++ = larger than normal amplitude and speed with clonus.

Jaw Reflex   With the patient's mouth slightly open, place your index finger on the patient's chin, then tap your finger with a reflex hammer. The response is closure of the jaw from contraction of the masseter muscles.

Biceps Reflex   Place your thumb on the biceps tendon with the arm loosely flexed and tap your thumb with a reflex hammer. The response is contraction of the biceps muscle.

Brachioradialis Reflex   With the arm loosely flexed and supported, tap the brachioradialis tendon with a reflex hammer. The response is contraction of the brachioradialis muscle and at times the biceps muscle as well.

Triceps Reflex   With the arm flexed to a right angle at the elbow, tap the triceps tendon with a reflex hammer. The response is contraction of the triceps muscle.

Finger Reflexes   With the patient's hand relaxed and the fingers slightly curled, place the palmar surface of your fingers against the palmar surface of the patient's fingers and tap your fingers lightly with a reflex hammer. The response is contraction of the patient's fingers.

Hoffmann's Sign   Stretch the patient's middle finger slightly in extension and flick the fingernail upward quickly. A flexion response of all the patient's fingers constitutes Hoffmann's sign. This sign can be found in normal subjects, but then it is symmetric on the two sides. The sign is most helpful when found unilaterally, in which case it indicates corticospinal pathway injury.

Patellar Reflex (Knee Jerk)   With the leg flexed to a right angle at the knee, tap the patellar tendon with a reflex hammer. The response is contraction of the quadriceps muscles.

Achilles Reflex (Ankle Jerk)   With the foot supported to form a right angle with the leg, tap the Achilles tendon with a reflex hammer. The response is contraction of the calf muscles.

SUPERFICIAL REFLEXES   The abdominal and cremaster reflexes are decreased or absent on the side affected by a corticospinal tract lesion and, thus, serve as adjuncts to the muscle stretch and plantar reflexes. The abdominal reflex is less reliable than the muscle stretch or plantar reflexes, however, and consequently less useful. The superficial anal reflex is important and useful for detecting lesions affecting the sacral spinal segments or their afferent or efferent limbs.

Abdominal Reflexes   With the patient lying supine and the abdomen exposed, lightly scratch the skin of each of the four quadrants of the abdomen from the ribs to the epigastrium. The response is contraction of the musculature underlying the skin following each stroke.

Cremaster Reflexes   These reflexes can be tested only in men. With the scrotum and upper legs exposed, lightly scratch the skin of the medial portion of the upper leg lightly on each side of the body. The response is contraction of the scrotal sac on the side of the stimulus.

Superficial Anal ("Anal Wink") Reflex   Spread the buttocks to expose the anus, then move the tip of a disposable pin lightly along the skin on the left and then the right side of the anus. The response to the stimulus on each side is contraction of the levator ani and related perineal muscles, seen as narrowing of the anal orifice.

PLANTAR REFLEX   This is one of the most useful clinical signs in the neurologic examination. The reflex becomes abnormal when the corticospinal pathway has been injured. To examine for this reflex, place the patient in a comfortable position with the legs relaxed and the feet warm. Ask the patient to avoid making any movement in response to the stimulus. Slowly move an object with a blunt-pointed end such as a key slowly along the outer border of the sole of the foot beginning from the heel and terminating at the ball of the great toe. If the patient withdraws the limb, lighten the intensity of the stimulus. A normal response is slow flexion (plantarflexion) of the great toe. An abnormal response is extension (dorsiflexion) of the great toe, also termed the Babinski response. Do not refer to the response as a "positive" or "negative" Babinski, as this is confusing. State that plantar stimulation evoked flexion or extension of the great toe to communicate the findings most clearly. Many ancillary tests have been described (the Oppenheim and Chaddock, for example) but all have higher thresholds than plantar stimulation, and none is as useful.

Sensation

Sensory testing (Table 2-6) is difficult, even in the most cooperative patient, and anxiety can make testing even more difficult. Testing is also difficult in patients with conversion reactions, as the responses often are inconsistent from moment to moment. If you suspect a conversion reaction in a patient who reports a decrease of all forms of sensation on one side of the body, test vibration sense by placing the base of a vibrating 128-Hz tuning fork on the temple of the affected side. If the patient reports decreased or absent sensation, move the vibrating tuning fork on the forehead of the affected side about 1 cm from the midline and ask whether the sensory disturbance persists. If so, move the vibrating tuning fork to the unaffected side about 1 cm from midline and ask about the intensity of sensation. If the patient claims that it is normal, the patient probably has a nonorganic disorder. Conduction of vibration through periosteum is so rapid that vibration should be detected equally on both sides of the skull close to the midline. Similar testing can be applied to the sternum.

If the patient has no sensory symptoms, use screening tests of cold, position, and vibration sense in all four limbs. This may pick up asymptomatic sensory abnormalities. If the patient has sensory symptoms, focus the testing on the region affected and use screening tests for the remaining areas. Test sensation carefully also if you find localized atrophy, weakness, ataxia, or trophic changes such as ulcers and blisters. Test sensation thoroughly

TABLE 2-6. Sensation

Cold
Pinprick
Position sense
Vibration sense
Light touch
Discriminative sensation
Joint position sense
Two-point discrimination
Complex pattern recognition
Tactile localization
Stereognosis

also if you find evidence of a cerebral cortical lesion, then focus on the discriminative modalities and tests for extinction on the two sides of the body. If you suspect a spinal cord lesion, test sensation on the trunk, looking for a level demarcating normal from diminished sensation. Testing with a cold object or a pin is a useful means of beginning this examination.

COLD   For screening, one prong of a 128-Hz tuning fork is usually sufficiently cool as to evoke a sense of coolness. Apply the object over each of the four limbs, comparing the intensity of coolness on the distal as compared to the proximal parts of the limb. There should be no difference in the intensity of cold in these locations. For testing areas showing sensory abnormalities, use the external surface of a small tube of ice water.

PINPRICK   Use a disposable pin and lightly touch the skin with the tip, moving from the distal to the proximal parts of the limbs. Move slowly from one stimulus site to the next to avoid spatial summation, and do not apply pinprick rapidly or you will evoke temporal summation. Compare sensation on the two sides of the body.

POSITION SENSE   Grasp the great toe on the medial and lateral sides and, with the patient's eyes closed, bend the toe firmly upward and hold it steady. Ask whether you displaced the toe up or down. Next move the toe firmly down and ask for the position again. Repeat the test until you are convinced that the patient's responses are reliable. The Romberg sign is a test of position sense in the lower extremities, particularly in the proximal joints. Have the patient stand with both legs together, feet touching, eyes open, and note whether the patient is steady. If so, ask the patient to close the eyes and wait to see whether the position can be maintained. Be prepared for the possibility of a fall. A positive Romberg sign is when the patient becomes unsteady and is about to fall provided the stance is steady with the eyes open. Markedly ataxic patients usually cannot be tested because they are unsteady standing with their legs together with the eyes open. In most cases, if you evoke a positive Romberg sign in a patient with intact position sense, you have conducted the test incorrectly or the patient has a nonorganic disorder.

VIBRATION SENSE   Strike one prong of a 128-Hz tuning fork and apply the base of the fork firmly to the great toe. Ask the patient to describe the sensation, which should be perceived as "vibration" or "buzzing." If vibration sense is absent in the great toe, place the vibrating tuning fork successively on the calcaneus, dorsal tibia, patella, and lateral trochanter. Vibration sense can be detected on skin but is best appreciated when applied to bony prominences.

LIGHT TOUCH   Use a wisp of cotton wool twisted into a point and apply light strokes to the skin.

DISCRIMINATIVE SENSATION   With cerebral cortical lesions the primary modalities of sensation may be relatively preserved while discriminatory sensation is affected. The affected sensations include joint position sense, two-point discrimination, complex pattern recognition on skin, tactile localization, and stereognosis. Carry out the examination with the patient's eyes closed or blindfolded. Test joint position sense as described above. Test two-point discrimination using a compass with two blunt tips. Touch the skin of a finger with one tip and then two, and ask how many points touched the skin. Normally two points can be detected 3 mm apart at the tip of the fingers, about 1 cm for the palm of the hand, and about 5 cm on the body. Test complex pattern recognition by drawing on the patient's hand a number such as 3 and ask for the number. This test can be applied to the face, trunk, and legs. Test tactile localization by lightly touching the patient's skin and asking the patient to put an index finger on the site that was just touched. Test stereognosis by placing an object such as a metal screw in the patient's palm and ask the identity of the object. Other common objects that can be used include coins of different sizes, paper clips, and keys.

INTERPRETATION OF THE NEUROLOGIC EXAMINATION

The neurologic examination makes it possible to determine with considerable precision the site or sites in the nervous system responsible for the patient's symptoms and signs. The chapters that follow give detailed information concerning the localization of diseases in the nervous system based on the clinical findings. In serving as an introduction to the many details that follow in this book, this section presents a brief summary of guidelines to localization.

Disorders at the level of the cerebral cortex can cause focal abnormalities or general intellectual disturbances. With focal pathology, the clinical signs vary with the location of the disorder. Since an overwhelming majority of people have left cerebral hemisphere dominance for speech, injury to the pathways involved with language in this hemisphere commonly leads to disorders of language that are termed aphasias. Lesions of the posterior part of the left superior temporal gyrus (Wernicke's area) result in disorders in the comprehension of language, often with fluent, rambling, and incoherent speech; paraphasic errors; neologisms; and poor insight into the presence of the disorder, but usually without limb weakness. With injury to the base of the left frontal convexity (Broca's area), disorders in the execution of speech occur, often with telescoping of sentences into a few words, at times with stammering, hesitation, and frustration in attempts to express well-preserved thoughts, and often in association with paralysis of the right lower face, arm, and leg (right hemiplegia). Interruption of the conduction pathway connecting Wernicke's area with Broca's area results in a combination of difficulties in the comprehension and execution of speech, often with difficulty with repetitions and an associated right hemiplegia.

Injury of a large proportion of the corticospinal projections arising in the left precentral or postcentral cortex, as in lesions of the internal capsule, causes hemiplegia of the right limbs with weakness of the right lower face. Injury of restricted parts of this projection from lesions localized to the cerebral cortex causes focal weakness of the lower portion of the face or the arm or leg, depending on the location of the lesion. Injury along the interhemispheric fissure disturbs leg function whereas lesions of the convexity affect arm or face function. With an acute injury the weakness is hypotonic, and the limbs have diminished resistance to passive manipulation and decreased stretch reflexes, often with an extensor plantar reflex. With time after an acute injury or with chronic lesions such as brain tumors, the weakness is hypertonic (i.e., accompanied by spasticity, hyperreflexia, and an extensor plantar response). With damage to the sensory projection area in the left postcentral region, the primary modalities of sensation (pain, temperature, and touch) are usually intact, but more complex aspects of sensation such as stereognosis and two-point discrimination are impaired on the right side of the body. Lesions of the left occipital region cause loss of vision in the contralateral half of the visual fields of both eyes (right hemianopsia).

Lesions of the right cerebral hemisphere usually do not affect speech or language, but injury to the precentral or postcentral cortex causes weakness of the left side of the body, with paresis of the lower part of the face, arm, or leg, depending on the site of the lesion. With involvement of the postcentral region, disorders of stereognosis and two-point discrimination occur in the left limbs. More extensive lesions of the right parietal lobe cause inattention to the entire left side of space, with lack of recognition of the left side of both personal (the patient's own body) and extrapersonal (the room, including objects and people in the room) space. Patients with acute lesions of the right parietal lobe may have a dense left hemiplegia, but do not acknowledge that these limbs are paralyzed, and may actually deny that the limbs belong to them if the examiner picks up the limbs and places them in the intact (right) visual field. This phenomenon is termed anosognosia and occurs only acutely after the lesion, decreasing with time. Lesions of the right occipital region cause loss of vision in the left visual fields of both eyes (left hemianopsia).

Diseases affecting the premotor parts of both frontal lobes result in preserved motor and sensory function and usually intact speech and language, but disturbances of judgment and insight commonly occur. These disorders are often accompanied by signs of frontal lobe "release," including grasping and sucking reflexes. Injury to large areas of both cerebral hemispheres as in Alzheimer disease results in a disturbance of many aspects of higher intellectual function that constitutes dementia. These disorders include difficulty with learning, memory, calculation, abstract concepts, judgment, and insight.

Unilateral lesions of the thalamus usually cause a contralateral hemiparesis accompanied by loss of the primary modalities of sensation (pinprick, cold, light touch, vibration sense, and position sense). Basal ganglia diseases, which commonly occur bilaterally, lead to hypokinetic or hyperkinetic movement disorders. Parkinson disease is the most common of the hypokinetic movement disorders and is characterized by bradykinesia, masked face, limb rigidity, difficulty walking, and a distal resting tremor. Many hyperkinetic movement disorders occur and are most common in Parkinson disease owing to excessive levodopa treatment, Huntington disease, long exposure to neuroleptic medications, and various dystonias.

Diseases of the cerebellum and its connections are characterized by ataxia, which consists of irregular movements resulting in part from abnormalities of rate, rhythm, and direction of movement. Lesions of the midline parts of the cerebellum (vermis) result in difficulty with standing and walking whereas lesions of the cerebellar hemisphere cause ataxia of the limbs on the ipsilateral side of the body. Unilateral lesions of the brainstem characteristically cause an ipsilateral disturbance of cranial nerve function with a contralateral hemiplegia and often a contralateral hemisensory disturbance.

Bilateral diseases of the spinal cord cause weakness and sensory disturbances below the level of the lesion. When unilateral, spinal cord diseases cause ipsilateral weakness and disturbances of position and vibration sense, with contralateral disorders of pain and temperature sensation, all occurring below the level of the lesion (Brown-Séquard syndrome). Disorders of the spinal nerve roots lead to weakness and sensory loss with diminished stretch reflexes in the innervation pattern of the involved roots. Diseases of peripheral nerves affecting a single nerve cause loss of motor and sensory function in the distribution of that nerve, and more widespread peripheral neuropathies usually cause weakness and sensory disorders of the distal parts of the limbs.

REFERENCES

Brazis PW, Masdeu JC, Biller J: *Localization in Clinical Neurology*, 2d ed. Boston, Little Brown, 1990.

Gelb DJ: *Introduction to Clinical Neurology*. Boston, Butterworth-Heinemann, 1995.

Gilman S, Newman SW: *Manter and Gatz's Essentials of Clinical Neuroanatomy and Neurophysiology*, 9th ed. Philadelphia, FA Davis, 1996.

Haerer AF: *DeJong's The Neurologic Examination*, 5th ed. Philadelphia, Lippincott, 1992.

DAVID KNOPMAN

THE MENTAL STATUS EXAMINATION

CHAPTER 3

The goal of the mental status examination is to define the integrity of the cognitive and affective aspects of brain function. Assessment of mental status is critical for the care of patients with a variety of disorders, not only neurologic. In some disorders such as dementia, delirium, stroke, or craniocerebral injury, the mental status examination may be the most important part of the neurologic assessment. The mental status examination is most useful in diagnosis, but it is a necessary component of the long-term management of cognitive disorders.

The mental status examination should be given under circumstances that minimize distractions. A well-lit, quiet room with no wall clock or calendar is optimal. Family members should leave. Attempt to establish rapport with the patient before beginning the examination, and both before and during the examination, observe the patient's level of alertness, behavior, affect, and speed of response. If the patient has poor arousal or attentiveness, you may not be able to assess cognition.

In patients with altered consciousness, the coma examination should be performed to localize the cause of the disorder. When the cause is known, the coma examination is useful for monitoring the patient and judging prognosis. The coma examination is reviewed at the end of the chapter.

DETERMINING THE CONTENT OF THE MENTAL STATUS EXAMINATION

Many factors affect the content and interpretation of mental status. The patient's age is important, especially in children. Under age 12, different approaches must be used as described in Chap. 9. Between the ages of about 12 to 70 years, age effects on performance are negligible except for knowledge about pop culture or historical events. Over the age of 70, some cognitive functions may decline, especially those involving speed of thinking (Koss et al, 1991; Schaie, 1989). Individuals above age 75 years should be tested in the same way as any other adult patient.

Premorbid intelligence affects the interpretation of the mental status examination. Performance on a number of tasks, for example, arithmetic, varies considerably by educational level. In adults, premorbid intelligence can be estimated by educational and occupational achievement, although the correlation between education and intellect is modest. Some components of the mental status examination should be modified if the patient's premorbid intelligence is exceptionally low or very high. If premorbid intellect is important in the examination, referral to a neuropsychologist may be appropriate. Some neuropsychologic tests can be used to estimate premorbid intellect.

Keep the hierarchical nature of mental status in mind when approaching the patient. Intact arousal and attention are prerequisites for assessing cognition, and disturbances of

TABLE 3-1.   The Mini-Mental State Examination

Function	Score	Method or Query
Arousal		Is the patient responsive to you upon entering the exam room?
Affect		Does the patient look depressed or despondent, admit to being depressed, and demonstrate psychomotor retardation?
Orientation	1	Name of facility
	1	Floor
	1	Town/City
	1	State/Province
	1	County
	1	Day of week (exact)
	1	Month (exact)
	1	Date ($\pm$ 1 day only)
	1	Year (exact)
	1	Calendar season (exact)
Registration	3	Repeat three words "ball, tree, flag"
Sentence repetition	1	Repeat "No ifs, ands, or buts"
Auditory comprehension	3	Follow the three-step command: "Take this paper in your (nondominant) hand, fold it in half, and place it on your lap"
Naming	2	Ask patient to name: pencil, watch
Writing	1	Ask patient to write a sentence
Construction	1	Copy a figure (intersecting pentagons)
Attention/concentration	5	Spell "world" backwards or count backwards from 100 by 7s (take best score)
Read	1	Read and execute "Close your eyes"
Recall	3	Recall the three words

affect and motivation may lower performance. The mental status examination should assess language, visuospatial synthesis, recent memory, and abstract reasoning. Although abstract reasoning and recent memory testing usually require intact language function, these four domains are independent of one another.

The extent of the mental status examination should be appropriate for the patient and the presenting problem. If the chief complaint suggests a cognitive disorder, the examination should be extensive. If the history indicates intact cognition, a cursory examination will suffice. In other patients, only a screening examination is required.

Structured mental status examinations present many advantages over ad hoc collections of questions. You can quantitate performance, and you can readily compare your examination with one performed by other physicians who used the same instrument. For most clinicians, structured mental status examinations provide the best means of achieving familiarity with specific items of the mental status examination.

Structured mental status examinations ensure that you will cover the major areas of cognitive function. They do, however, have some disadvantages. Over-reliance on a particular examination may result in failure to assess clinically important cognitive functions. Focusing on the examination score may cause you to overlook the overall clinical picture. Both floor and ceiling effects may occur. Ceiling effects are seen with patients who perform at high levels but are impaired when tested with challenging examinations. Floor effects occur when patients have very low scores, which can give the false impression on repeat testing that intellectual decline has been arrested. If you are aware of these limitations, you can be prepared to supplement a structured mental status examination with additional tasks.

Several structured mental status examinations are available, including the Mini-Mental State Examination (MMSE) (Folstein et al, 1975), the Modified Mini-Mental State Examination (Teng and Chui, 1987), the Short Test of Mental Status (Kokmen et al, 1991), the Orientation-Memory-Concentration Test (Katzman et al, 1983), and the Neurobehavior Cognitive Status Examination (Kiernan et al, 1987). These instruments utilize many common items for testing but vary in the breadth and depth of coverage of specific cognitive domains. The total score on one mental status examination is highly correlated with the total score on one of the other examinations (see, for example, Salmon et al, 1990).

THE MINI-MENTAL STATE EXAMINATION

The MMSE (Table 3-1) is the most widely used, brief, structured instrument in North America. It has been extensively studied in normal and neurologically impaired populations (Tombaugh and McIntyre, 1992; Crum et al, 1993; Tangalos et al, 1996). The weaknesses of the MMSE include its overemphasis on language functions and underemphasis on recent memory, constructions, concentration, and abstract reasoning. Consequently, it has modest diagnostic accuracy in delirium and dementia (Anthony et al, 1982). Scores are inversely correlated with age and education.

The methodology for administering the MMSE (Table 3-1) is simple and follows certain conventions in order to achieve consistency across examiners.

Orientation. The MMSE has five questions about orientation for time and five for place. Responses to queries of date are reliable and easy to interpret. Allow ±1 day around the date, and ± 1 week for any season. Any other error on temporal orientation should be considered abnormal. Responses about orientation to place are somewhat less reproducible and hence reliable, depending on locale. Ask for the name of your clinic or hospital, the floor of the hospital or clinic (if appropriate), city or town, county, and state or province. Do not give cues or hints. Temporal and place orientation deficits are highly specific but not sensitive for brain disease. Orientation items lack sensitivity for detecting mild cognitive impairment. Incorrect responses are also not localizing. Orientation deficits may reflect disordered language, memory, judgment, spatial orientation, attention, or concentration.

Recite the words that will be used for later recall. Provide a three-word list and request free recall 3 to 5 min later. Recite the words to the patient (e.g., ball, tree, flag) and ask the patient immediately to repeat them. An immediate second repetition should be carried out to ensure that the patient has encoded the material.

Sentence repetition is tested with "No ifs, ands, or buts." Some patients have over-learned the sentence, and their successful performance can be misleading. It contains a number of words that may be difficult for individuals with high-tone hearing loss to perceive. An exact repetition is necessary to score this item as correct.

Naming. Ask the patient to name a pencil and a watch. Exact answers are required. Use of a pencil and not an ink pen avoids ambiguity. Clock is not an acceptable alternative to watch.

Reading. Ask the patient to read the command, "Close your eyes." Ensure that the patient is wearing corrective lenses if needed. Patients with severe cognitive impairment may be able to read aloud the written command, but fail to execute it.

Writing a sentence. Ask the patient to write an entire sentence. Score the sentence correct if it has a subject and verb. Spelling accuracy is not crucial.

Following commands. Ask the patient to take a piece of paper in the nondominant hand, fold it in half, and then return it to the examiner. For scoring, any level of performance less than 3 commands executed is considered abnormal. State the commands clearly and do not repeat them or prompt the patient.

Drawing of the intersecting pentagons. Show the patient the drawing of intersecting pentagons and ask the patient to copy the figure. Interpret the patient's performance in light of the integrity of limb-motor function and basic visual function. Score as an error any deviation from an exact copy of two 5-sided figures that overlap in a 4-sided figure (Fig. 3-1).

Spell "world" backwards or count backwards from 100 by 7s. Ask the subject to spell the word "world" backwards. This task requires a certain minimum literacy. There are several methods for scoring performance, but one straightforward one involves counting the number of letters given in correct order prior to an error. For example, the response "D-L-O-R-W" would be scored as 2 correct. For serial 7 subtraction ask the subject to start at 100 and then subtract down by 7s. For serial 7s, stop after five responses (93-86-79-72-65). If the subject has a memory disorder, it is necessary and acceptable to repeat the instructions after each subtraction. Take the highest score of the two tasks.

Recall the three words that had been previously presented. At a point 3 to 5 min after initial exposure to the words, ask the patient to recall the words presented previously. Provide no clues. The delay interval is filled with other activities of the MMSE so that the patient is not able to rehearse the list overtly.

The total correct score on the MMSE is 30. No single score level separates cognitively normal individuals from those with impairment. In some patients with low education or

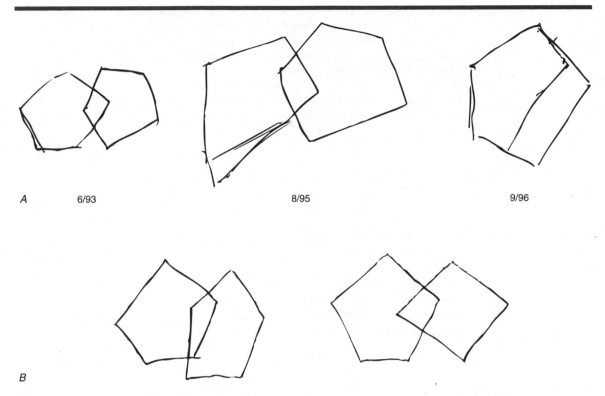

A   6/93   8/95   9/96

B

Figure 3-1 Examples of disturbed performance on drawing of intersecting pentagons, from the MMSE. (A) Three examples of performance from one patient with Alzheimer disease over a 3-year period, showing the dissolution of constructional ability. While the 8/95 *(middle)* drawing is nominally correct in that the patient spontaneously added the extra line in the left hand figure to make it into a pentagon, her prior performance clearly illustrates the deterioration she had experienced. (B) Two examples of subtle errors that patients with mild constructional difficulty are likely to commit: failure to overlap the figures correctly *(left)* or simplification of one figure into a rectangle *(right).*

occupational achievement, a score of 24 may indicate normal cognitive function. Other patients with serious recent memory impairment or visuospatial synthesis impairment, for example, might achieve scores of 28 or 29. Scores on the mental status examination should be related to the patient's chief complaint and history. Do not make diagnoses based on mental status examination scores in isolation.

BACKGROUND AND METHODOLOGY FOR MORE DETAILED ASSESSMENT OF MENTAL STATUS

Upon completion of the MMSE or another structured mental status examination, you may wish to examine certain aspects of mental status in further detail including the

TABLE 3-2.   Observational Aspects of Affect, Behavior, Comportment

Appearance: neat, slovenly, clothing soiled, dressed appropriately, dressed inappropriately
Posture, motor activity: calm, bradykinetic, psychomotorically retarded, pacing, fidgety,
  hyperactive, stooped, slouched, erect
Facial expression: cheerful, sad, angry, anxious, withdrawn
Socially appropriate response to physician greeting and initiation of interview
Mood during interview: cooperative, hostile, irritable, angry, attentive, tangential, euphoric,
  manic, tearful, suspicious, forthright
Eye contact

following:

- Affect, comportment, and insight
- Attention and concentration
- Speech and language
- Learning and memory
- Constructional ability, visuospatial function, and neglect
- Executive functions, abstract reasoning, calculations, and the frontal lobes
- Ideomotor praxis

Affect, Comportment, and Insight

Affect, comportment, and insight must be assessed separately from a structured examination. Assessment of affect begins with observation (Table 3-2). Table 3-3 lists affective states and their synonyms.

Assess depression by using several different terms (melancholia, feeling blue, sadness, as well as related terms like nervousness and anxiety) since patients may respond to one term but not another. Standardized questionnaires are helpful, particularly the Geriatric Depression Scale (Sheikh and Yesavage, 1986) (Table 3-4), which is self-administered, and the Hamilton Depression scale (Hamilton, 1960) (Table 3-5), which a clinician administers. The questions in Tables 3-4 and 3-5 probe symptoms of depression from different angles.

TABLE 3-3.   Affective States and Their Synonyms

Euthymic	Calm, comfortable, appropriate
Angry	Confrontational, hostile, impatient, irascible, sullen
Euphoric	Elated, excessively or incongruently cheerful
Apathetic	Flat, dull, bland, abulic
Depressed	Dysphoric, despondent, sad, remorseful, blue
Anxious	Apprehensive, fearful, tense, worried, panicked

SOURCE: From Trzepacz and Baker, 1993 (Table 3-1), with permission.

TABLE 3-4. Geriatric Depression Scale

Items (and answers if mood were ideal)
    Are you basically satisfied with your life? (yes)
    Have you dropped many of your activities and interests? (no)
    Do you feel that your life is empty? (no)
    Do you often get bored? (no)
    Are you in good spirits most of the time? (yes)
    Are you afraid that something bad is going to happen to you? (no)
    Do you feel happy most of the time? (yes)
    Do you often feel helpless? (no)
    Do you prefer to stay home, rather than going out and doing new things? (no)
    Do you feel you have more problems with memory than most? (no)
    Do you think it is wonderful to be alive now? (yes)
    Do you feel pretty worthless the way you are now? (no)
    Do you feel full of energy? (yes)
    Do you feel that your situation is hopeless? (no)
    Do you think that most people are better off than you are? (no)
A score of five or more "wrong" responses suggests depression.

SOURCE: From Sheikh and Yesavage, 1986, with permission.

Insight refers to the ability to assess and monitor one's own cognitive, motor, or sensory function. Orientation for circumstance is another term that expresses the concept of awareness of one's health. Insight and contact with reality are frequently impaired in neurologic and psychiatric diseases. Begin an interview with the query, "Why are you seeing

TABLE 3-5. Hamilton Depression Scale

Depressed mood
Feelings of guilt
Suicidal ideation
Insomnia
Difficulties with work and loss of interests
Psychomotor retardation
Restlessness associated with anxiety
Anxiety, psychic and somatic
Somatic symptoms: gastrointestinal, general
Sexual dysfunction
Hypochondriasis
Weight loss
Impaired insight
Depersonalization and derealization
Paranoid ideation, including suspiciousness, delusions, and hallucinations
Obsessional symptoms

SOURCE: Adapted from Hamilton, 1960, with permission.

a doctor?" or "Why are you here in the hospital?" Patients with impaired insight may express indifference, offer extraneous reasons, or blame others for their problems. Impaired insight is pervasive in cognitive disorders, and responses of the cognitively impaired can be unreliable.

Impaired thought content can occur in neurologic as well as psychiatric disorders. In conversation and history-taking, you should gauge the presence and severity of circumstantiality, flight of ideas, loose associations, tangential thinking, and neologisms. Depending on the context of the assessment and the patient's history, you should inquire about hallucinations (false perceptions) or delusions (false beliefs).

Comportment refers to the manner in which patients conduct themselves in relation to others. You can draw some conclusions about the patient's comportment and social conduct from the patient's behavior toward you. You will also need input from a knowledgeable informant.

Attention and Concentration

DEFINITIONS   Attention refers to the ability to focus on a particular stimulus, task, or situation. Intact attention implies resistance to distraction from extraneous stimuli or internal phenomena (e.g., thoughts, delusions). Concentration is a related concept that refers to the ability to sustain attention. Alteration in attention and concentration are the earliest indicators of delirium and coma. Concentration is necessary but not sufficient to perform more complex mental activities such as abstract reasoning.

EXAMINATION   The MMSE does not assess attention and concentration well. The preferred approach to testing attention is as follows:

1.   Reciting the months of the year backwards. Ask the patient to "start with December and recite the months backwards to January." This task requires sufficient mental agility to state the prior month's name while thinking of the sequence of months in the forward order. People tend automatically to recite the months in the highly overlearned direction, and require considerable mental effort to suppress that tendency. This task is nearly independent of cultural and educational factors. Patients with mild deficits may leave out only one month or reverse a pair. As concentration deficits worsen, as in both delirium and dementia, patients will leave out several months, quit half-way through, or be unable even to initiate the task.

2.   Counting backwards from 20. Ask the subject to "start at 20, and count backwards down to 10 (or 1)." Any errors should be considered as impaired performance. This task is useful for more impaired individuals, especially those who fail the months-backwards test. This task requires less concentration and attention than the months backwards task, perhaps because counting backwards is more familiar.

3.   Digit span forward. After explaining the task, recite a series of digits at a rate of 1 per second, and immediately upon finishing, ask the subject to repeat them back in the exact order that you used. Avoid emphasizing any cluster and avoid well-known sequences, e.g., 1492. Begin the test with a three-digit length, and proceed by increasing the length of the list of digits up to seven digits. A patient's digit span is the longest number of digits repeated in exact order on at least one of two attempts at that length. Normal subjects complete 7 ± 2 digits.

4. Digit span backwards. After explaining the task, recite a sequence of digits (just as in digits forward) and then ask the patient to repeat them in backwards order. In addition to attention and concentration, this task assesses mental agility but it places a high short-term memory demand on patients. In contrast to reciting the months backwards, which are highly overlearned, the digit span backwards task involves rearranging novel information. Patients with anterograde amnesia may not be able to recite more than two or three digits backwards even if their attention is otherwise intact because of the memory load that four digits forward imposed.

Speech and Language

DEFINITIONS   Aphasia is a disorder of speech and language due to cerebral dysfunction. The three primary aphasic deficits are in expressive language, comprehension of spoken language, and naming. Aphasic deficits have localizing value. Approximately 90 percent of the population is right-handed and left hemisphere dominant for language. Among left-handers, about two-thirds probably also have left hemisphere language dominance (Lezak, 1995, p 302), while the remainder have varying degrees of mixed or right hemisphere dominance. In any left-hander, mixed dominance should be assumed.

Expressive language deficits (see Table 3-6 for definitions), including dysfluency and agrammatism, are localized to the operculum of the dominant frontocentral cortex. Dysfluent speech has a labored quality, is often dysarthric, has numerous paraphasic errors, and lacks prosody. Broca's aphasia, a specific variant of nonfluent aphasia characterized by agrammatic speech and nonfluency is localized anterior to the motor strip in the same region (Fig. 3-2). Dysarthria (impaired articulation or phonation) may occur with neocortical lesions, but it is more commonly due to lesions in subcortical sites.

Wernicke's aphasia principally involves impaired auditory comprehension and severe anomia. Spontaneous speech sounds normal melodically, but it is empty of content or filled with nonsense syllables or words, known as jargon aphasia. Lesions that cause impaired comprehension involve the dominant inferior parietal and posterior temporal lobes (Fig. 3-2).

Naming deficits, or anomia, are the least localizing but most sensitive measure of dysfunction in the dominant perisylvian region. Naming is impaired in almost all forms

TABLE 3-6.   Characteristics of Aphasic Speech

Aphasic speech may exhibit one or more of the following abnormalities:	
Agrammatic	Missing small grammatical words, telegraphic
Anomic	Word-finding pauses or failures
Dysfluent	Reduced number of words per utterance
Dysprosodic	Flat intonation, loss of melodic variation in running speech
Paraphasias	Phoneme or word substitutions
Dysarthria	Altered articulation

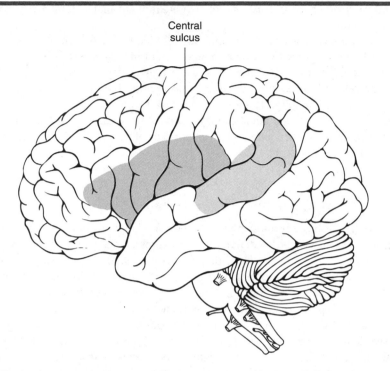

Figure 3-2   The lateral cerebral hemisphere demonstrating the regions most likely to be lesioned in disorders of verbal expression (the anterior regions) and auditory comprehension (the posterior regions). Subcortical white matter lesions underlying either one may replicate the cortical pathology. The anterior region spans the inferior portion of the pre- and postcentral gyri as well as the posterior portion of the inferior frontal gyrus. The posterior region includes the posterior superior temporal gyrus and the supramarginal gyrus.

of aphasia and in many instances of other cognitive disorders (e.g., delirium, dementia, craniocerebral trauma).

Lesions of the dominant cerebral hemisphere in the distribution of the anterior cerebral artery produce a language deficit characterized by marked reductions in spontaneous speech, probably secondary to impaired function in motor association cortices. Intact repetition in the setting of very laconic speech is an important diagnostic clue that the responsible lesion is in the anterior cerebral artery distribution. This syndrome is referred to as transcortical motor aphasia. A pattern of impaired comprehension with spared repetition referred to as transcortical sensory aphasia is usually due to lesions in the dominant superior parietal region that spare the perisylvian temporal-parietal cortex.

EXAMINATION   Examine spontaneous speech, auditory comprehension, naming, repetition, reading, and writing. The MMSE covers most aspects of language except for spontaneous speech.

Spontaneous speech. You can assess the patient's spontaneous speech in the course of history-taking or open-ended conversation. An alternative approach is to ask the patient to describe a complex scene. The Boston Diagnostic Aphasia Examination (BDAE) (Goodglass and Kaplan, 1983) uses a picture of a child trying to steal a cookie from a jar while his mother looks on. Spontaneous speech is rated for the amount of words per utterance, the semantic content, the melody and prosody, and the quality of articulation and phonation.

In an aphasic patient, dysarthria (incorrect articulation or phonation) can be difficult to distinguish from phonologic paraphasias (substitution of one phoneme for another). Paraphasic errors with one speech sound are often followed or preceded by perfect pronunciation of the same sound. Dysarthric errors tend to result in a more consistent pattern of mispronunciations of particular phonemes. A summary of alterations in expressive speech is given in Table 3-6.

Auditory comprehension. You can assess the patient's comprehension of spoken speech during history-taking or open-ended conversation. However, conversational assessment may fail to detect subtle comprehension deficits. To focus on comprehension, structured assessment of auditory comprehension requires a setting in which nonverbal cues are minimized, visual processing is not taxed, and memory demands are minimized. The MMSE employs a three-part spoken command.

As an alternative to the MMSE paper-folding test, place three objects (e.g., watch, pencil, keys) in front of the patient. Ask the patient to point to the three items in a sequence other than their left to right order. If the patient succeeds, add a relational component to the three-step command, such as "put the pencil *next* to the keys and then pick up the watch." If the patient fails at the three-step pointing level, try a two-step pointing task, and if failure occurs, utilize a one-step command.

In patients with impaired limb movement, you may need to use yes/no questions. In severely demented or aphasic patients, you can use axial commands. Axial commands include "stand up," "sit down," "roll over," "close your eyes," or "stick out your tongue."

Naming to confrontation. The MMSE uses two words only, but a minimum of four or five objects is desirable for testing naming in cognitive dysfunction. Be careful to minimize auditory or somesthetic cues when testing naming. Table 3-7 contains several series of items that may be found in the examination room that are suitable to test naming. Listen for paraphasic errors and circumlocutions.

TABLE 3-7. Items Available at Bedside for Use in Testing of Naming[a]

Colors	Body Parts	Objects in Room	Parts of Objects
Red	Shoulder	Door	Watch stem (winder)
Blue	Chin	Watch	Coat lapel
Yellow	Forehead	Shoe	Watch crystal
Pink	Elbow	Shirt	Sole of shoe
Purple	Knuckles	Ceiling	Buckle of belt

[a] In ascending order of difficulty.

SOURCE: With permission, from Strub and Black, 1993; body parts from Modified Mini-Mental State Exam, Teng and Chui, 1987.

TABLE 3-8. Memory Nomenclature

	Immediate Recall	Recent Memory	Remote Memory
Synonyms	Primary Short-term	Secondary Intermediate	
Method of bedside assessment	Auditory attention span (repeating after 0-s delay)	Memory for 3–5 items after 5 min	Personal history, current events
Prototypical disorders	Delirium, "conduction" aphasia	Anterograde amnesias	Advanced dementias aphasia
Presumed anatomic locus	Auditory association cortex	Hippocampal system and heteromodal association cortices	Dominant temporo-parietal cortex

Sentence repetition. An alternative approach to the MMSE sentence is to ask the patient to repeat a simple sentence such as, "The boy jumped over the fence" and then go on to a longer one such as, "The ship sailed into port to escape the storm."

To test reading, ask the subject to read a simple command, such as the one in the MMSE. A more detailed assessment of reading, as in a patient with developmental dyslexia, may require neuropsychologic referral.

Learning and Memory

DEFINITIONS In Table 3-8, the terms immediate recall, recent memory, and remote memory are used to distinguish the three categories of memory retrieval that are assessed in a clinical setting.

Immediate recall involves a memory function that is measured in seconds. It is nearly equivalent to attention. Immediate recall has limited capacity and is highly susceptible to interference. The anatomic loci of immediate recall are the prefrontal cortex and either the auditory or visual association cortex, depending on the modality.

Recent memory involves new learning that persists for minutes to hours. A deficit in recent memory defines anterograde amnesia. Some of the features of the recent memory system are highlighted in Table 3-9. Its anatomic basis involves the hippocampal formation, the entorhinal cortex nearby, medial thalamic structures, and their associated pathways (Squire, 1992) (Fig. 3-3). Anterograde amnesia is a key deficit in Alzheimer disease (Welsh et al, 1991).

Retrieval from remote memory allows access to the vast store of personal knowledge, information about current events, and vocabulary. In contrast to the other two memory systems, you assess retrieval alone when testing remote memory. Remote memories are represented diffusely in the cerebral cortex, with linguistically related material preferentially localized to the dominant hemisphere.

EXAMINATION Test immediate verbal recall with digit span, which was discussed previously. Testing recent verbal memory requires that the patient recall newly learned

TABLE 3-9. Features of Recent Memory Function and Its Assessment

Feature	Contrast	Methodology	Comment
Types of learning (encoding)	Incidental versus intentional	Examiner doesn't tell patient that memory will be checked at a later point	Retrieval following incidental learning is less successful
Learning (encoding) strategy	Nonelaborative versus elaborative	Elaborate encoding methods include making a sentence, pointing to a picture of item, making a judgment about the item	Retrieval is almost always better after elaborative encoding
Delay between learning and retrieval	Zero versus distraction-filled delay of >1 min to days	Distractor-filled delay prevents rehearsal	Retrieval decreases as soon as a distractor-filled delay is interposed after learning Rate of decline of retrieval performance after 1–5 min up to 24 h is slight
Amount of material	Subspan versus supraspan (span refers to digit span forward capacity)	Presented in same way	Supraspan length to be learned material prevents short-term memory and rehearsal from compensating for impaired long-term memory
Type of retrieval	Recognition Free recall Cued recall (implicit)	Recognition task may be "yes-no" or forced-choice; cued recall may involve studied word pair as cue or semantic category cue	Recognition > cued recall > free recall in almost all clinical situations. Implicit methods of retrieval are not used at the bedside.

material after a delay. The three-word recall test on the MMSE is crucial for screening purposes, but this test lacks sufficient range to separate normal from abnormal performance (Cullum et al, 1993). The delayed word recall test is superior to the three-word recall test (Knopman and Ryberg, 1989). You need a set of 3×5 cards containing the 10 test words: "chimney, button, finger, salt, harp, sister, train, rug, book, flower." Ask the patient to read the words aloud one at a time. Next, show each card and ask the patient to make a sentence out of the word. Go through all 10 cards. Repeat the process. Tell the patient to use the word in the same sentence you gave or produce another sentence. After 5 min of administering other tasks, ask for recall of the words (not the sentences). Provide no cues. Recall of four or more words is normal. The test has a wider range of performance than the three-word test, and you can better separate normal and abnormal performance. Extensive normative data are available on this task, and it varies only modestly with age and education (Cerhan et al, 1998). If performance during recent memory

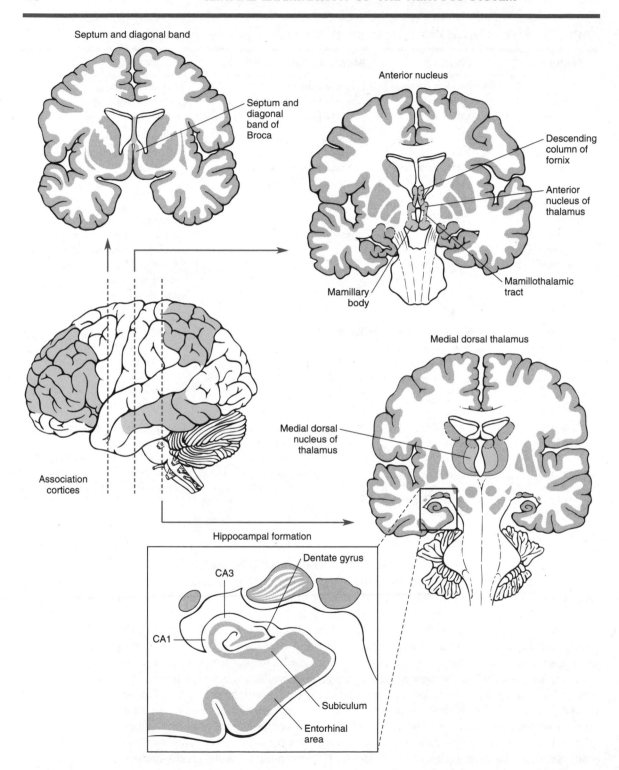

Septum and diagonal band

Septum and diagonal band of Broca

Anterior nucleus

Descending column of fornix

Anterior nucleus of thalamus

Mamillothalamic tract

Mamillary body

Association cortices

Medial dorsal thalamus

Medial dorsal nucleus of thalamus

Hippocampal formation

Dentate gyrus

CA3

CA1

Subiculum

Entorhinal area

testing is inconsistent or difficult to interpret, consider a referral for neuropsychologic assessment. The neuropsychologic assessment of memory offers greater precision for quantitating deficits.

Assess both recent and remote memory by asking patients to tell you about themselves or what they think of current events. Ask about current and past presidents or other elected officials. Events such as John Kennedy's assassination or dates of World War II may be memorable to most patients. For others, incorrect responses may be difficult to interpret due to educational, cultural, or ethnic diversity. Responses to typical questions for private life must be verified by an alternative informant. Questions include recent family gatherings, date of birth, place of birth, high school, college, profession, employers, (spouse's employers), and children's and siblings' names. The diagnostic value of failures in knowledge of current/past events is limited, because deficits could arise due to problems with language, memory, and frontal lobe/executive functions. Successful performance on queries of recent events does not rule out mild cognitive impairment. Recall of more recent events might fail due to anterograde amnesia, while loss of more distant events might be due to anomia.

Constructional Ability, Visuospatial Function, and Neglect

The assessment of visuospatial function requires that elementary visual function be intact. Elementary visuospatial function depends on the integrity of the visual pathway from the cornea to the primary visual areas and adjacent first-order association cortices. Testing of this pathway is discussed in Chap. 4. In the mental status examination, you are trying to capture the higher, more integrative aspects of visuospatial function, hence the term visuospatial synthesis.

DEFINITIONS Visuospatial synthesis involves two fundamental processes, recognition ("what") and localization ("where") (Coslett and Saffran, 1992). These two processes are mediated by different brain regions (Fig. 3-4). Distinct deficits arise depending on which pathway is involved. Visual agnosia, in which patients lose the meaning of objects in the visual world, and prosopagnosia, the inability to recognize familiar faces, are two prototypical disorders of visuospatial synthesis due to lesions in the temporo-occipital re-

Figure 3-3 The anatomic regions that play a role in recent memory. At the center left are the heteromodal association areas of the frontal, temporal, and parietal lobes. In the top left hand corner, the coronal section is at the level of the septum and diagonal band of Broca, the source of cholinergic input to the hippocampus. In the lower right hand is a coronal section at the level of the medial dorsal nucleus of the thalamus and the hippocampus. The hippocampus itself is shown in detail in the insert at the bottom. The entorhinal cortex is a major target for inputs from the association cortices. The key intrinsic circuit of the hippocampus begins at the entorhinal cortex, which sends fibers to the dentate gyrus. From there, the pathway goes to CA3, CA1, and subiculum and back to association cortices. In the upper right corner, the coronal section blow-up is at the level of the descending columns of the fornix, the mamillary bodies, the mamillothalamic tract, anterior nucleus of the thalamus. The CA1 region of the hippocampus sends a pathway, via the fornix, to the mamillary bodies and from there, via the mamillothalamic tract, to the anterior nucleus of the thalamus, and then on to the cingulate gyrus. The relationships between the entorhinal–association cortices pathway and the hippocampal–fornix–thalamic pathway are not known, but the recent memory disorder that occurs with both is clinically indistinguishable.

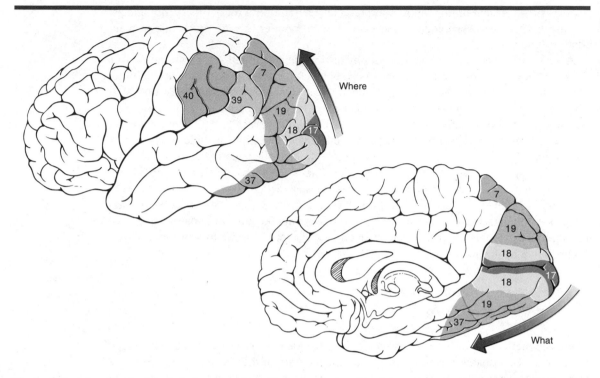

Figure 3-4 A lateral and midsagittal view of the brain illustrating the location of the major areas involved in visual processing. These regions include area 17 (primary visual area); areas 18 and 19 (first-order association areas); areas 7, 39, and 40 (heteromodal association areas thought to be involved in aspects of visual processing relating to "where" an object is in space, part of the dorsal pathway of visual processing); and area 37 (also known as IT, a region critically involved in the "what" the object is, part of the ventral pathway of visual processing).

gions (Damasio, 1985). Simultanagnosia, an inability to process complex visual scenes, is due to parietal lobe lesions (Damasio, 1985). Patients with simultanagnosia have impoverished ocular exploration of visual scenes. These syndromes, usually due to stroke, are rare in isolation but may occur with dementia, delirium, or craniocerebral trauma.

EXAMINATION Screen for disorders of complex visual processing with constructional tasks and naming tasks, but comprehension deficits, refractive deficits, hemiparesis, ataxia, or limb apraxia may interfere with performance. Measurement of visuospatial function without the confounding effects of language or motor function requires referral to a neuropsychology laboratory.

The MMSE utilizes copying of a pair of intersecting pentagons as the construction task. Copying a cube is used in other mental status examinations. Copying involves both figure-ground discriminations and object recognition.

Drawing a clock is a constructional task that requires the patient to access a "mind's eye" view of the object. Clock drawing also involves planning and foresight and has broad applicability across educational and cultural groups. There are formal scoring methods (Mendez et al, 1992), but for clinical use, a qualitative assessment usually suf-

Clock Drawings

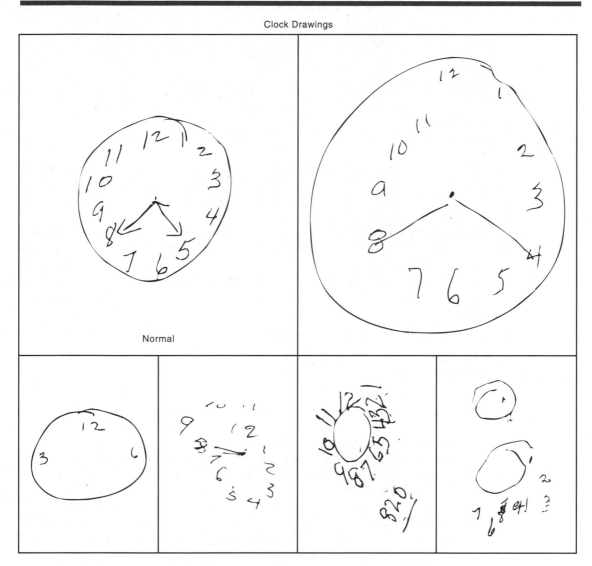

Normal

Figure 3-5 Examples of disturbed performance on drawing of a clock. Mild impairment may be characterized by irregularity of situating the numbers around the perimeter of the circle. Hand placement will also be impaired. More impaired individuals will leave out numbers or grossly misplace most of the numbers.

fices (Fig. 3-5). Ask the patient to draw a clock, place the numbers on the face, and set the hands to 8:20. Clock drawing should be considered abnormal if the numbering is unevenly distributed or the hands are more than a few minutes off in placement.

The methods described above are only for screening of visuospatial synthesis function. If performance on your testing of visuospatial synthesis is inconsistent or difficult to interpret, consider a referral to a neuropsychologist, who will have more elaborate testing materials available.

Testing of recognition of familiar or famous faces, such as political leaders or movie stars, is necessary in only rare instances when you suspect prosopagnosia. Recognition of famous faces relies on long-term memory and language function in addition to visuospatial synthesis abilities. A useful way to assess recognition of faces is to develop a notebook of photos of famous faces from magazines.

Hemispatial neglect results from lesions in the nondominant cerebral hemisphere, though neglect does occur with lesions of the dominant hemisphere. The disorder involves impairment of both visual orientation and visuospatial synthesis. Hemispatial neglect can be detected from observation. The patient consistently fails to attend to stimuli in one hemispace or will not use the affected limbs. In hemispatial neglect immediately following acute stroke, patients may show striking unawareness of the affected limb even when you point out to them that they are not using it. These patients even deny that the limb belongs to them. Examine additional aspects of neglect when testing visual fields, somesthetic sensation, and motor function.

Use graphesthesia and stereognosis to assess "cortical" sensory functions of shape and form recognition (see Chap. 7, Examination of Sensory Function). With the patient's eyes closed, test graphesthesia by drawing numbers in the palm of the patient's hand and stereognosis by placing objects such as coins into the patient's hand and asking for object identification. If the patient has sensory deficits due to spinal cord or peripheral nerve disease, these assessments may not be feasible.

Executive Functions, Abstract Reasoning, Calculations, and the Frontal Lobes

DEFINITIONS   Executive cognitive function refers to the ability to

- Exhibit concentration, mental flexibility, and agility
- Shift attention and mental effort from one task to another with the least inertia
- Focus on, and sustain attention to, a particular task
- Remain free of distraction

Related features include the ability to carry on two mental activities at once and to demonstrate foresight and planning. Executive abilities are necessary to perform challenging abstract reasoning tasks such as arithmetic or verbal similarities. Executive function is localizable to the frontal lobe systems (Fuster, 1989; Mesulam, 1985; Damasio and Anderson, 1993; Cummings, 1993). The prefrontal cortex has powerful interconnections with other cortical regions and several subcortical regions, especially the medial thalamus and neostriatum (Fig. 3-6). Consequently, either focal frontal disease or diffuse cerebral disease can produce executive deficits in addition to other types of dysfunction. The dorsolateral portions of frontal lobe are thought to subserve the major cognitive functions, while orbital and medial frontal regions are more involved in affect and behavior.

Abstract reasoning refers to the capacity to manipulate complex concepts and involves a combination of executive mental ability and previously acquired knowledge. Deficits in abstract reasoning cannot be localized to a single region.

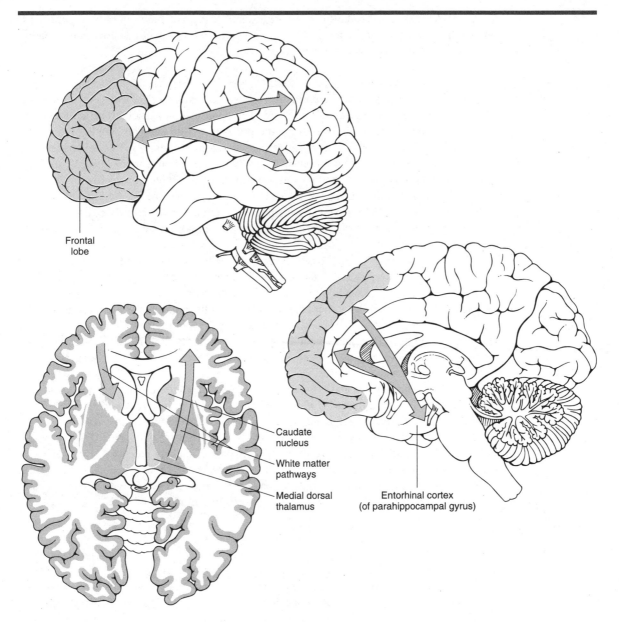

Figure 3-6 Diagram of key portions of the frontal lobe and major afferent and efferent structures. These include other heteromodal association areas, the entorhinal cortex, the medial dorsal thalamus (that sends afferent fibers to the lateral prefrontal region), the caudate nucleus (the destination of a major outflow pathway from the prefrontal cortex), and the white matter pathways responsible for the linkage. Lesions in these other regions may produce executive cognitive and behavioral deficits that mimic "pure" involvement of the prefrontal neocortex. Other regions not shown on the figure with important connections to the prefrontal region include the amygdala, hypothalamus, mesencephalic tegmentum, and locus ceruleus.

EXAMINATION   Assess abstract reasoning and executive function only after you ascertain that attention and language function are sufficiently intact to allow interpretation of the patient's performance of higher level tasks.

1.   Give the patient arithmetic problems to solve, but tailor the test to the patient's educational level. Test with serial 7 subtraction and serial 3 subtraction and ask for the number of nickels in $0.35 and quarters in $6.75. The latter task is particularly illuminating in that highly functioning individuals solve the problem within seconds, while others must break the problem into two parts, the $6 and the $0.75 parts. Patients with executive deficits sometimes compute correct answers to the two parts but cannot integrate their responses into the final answer. You can also use ordinary arithmetic problems. In the Short Test of Mental Status (Kokmen et al, 1991), for example, the problems are: 5×13, $65 - 7$, $58 \div 2$, and $29 + 11$. In a patient with prior educational and occupational achievement deemed adequate to have performed calculations in a premorbid state, any errors should be considered abnormal.

2.   Give the patient problems to solve such as, "What would you do if you saw from your window your neighbor's house on fire?" Acceptable responses are "Call 911," or "Call the fire department," while unacceptable answers are, "Don't know," "Nothing," or "Try to put it out myself." Another example is used in the Clinical Dementia Rating Scale examination (Hughes et al, 1982). "If you were in an unfamiliar city and wanted to look up a friend who lived there, how would you go about finding that friend if you didn't have his/her address?" Acceptable answers are "Look the person up in the phone book," or "Contact a common acquaintance."

3.   Test verbal similarities and differences by asking the patient, "Tell me how these two words are similar (or different.)" Commonly used word pairs are given in Table 3-10. Seek answers that are abstract; concrete responses should be considered errors.

4.   Examine verbal fluency by asking for words that begin with a particular letter of the alphabet: (*F*, *A*, and *S* are commonly used) or words from one category (e.g., names of animals). Ask that the patient produce as many words as rapidly as possible within 1 min. Do not allow the patient to use names or places. Performance varies with age and education, but most patients produce more than 10 words in 1 min.

TABLE 3-10.   Items for Verbal Similarities and Differences

Item Pair	Acceptable Answer	Typical Incorrect Answer
Similarities		
Orange–banana	Fruit	Round
Poem–statue	Art	Describes only one
Turnip–cauliflower	Vegetables	Green
Desk–bookcase	Hold books, office furniture	Describes only one
Differences		
Lie–mistake	Intentional–accidental	Describes only one
River–canal	Natural–synthetic	Size differences

Other tasks can be used but are less quantitative:

1. Assess proverb interpretation, which is a better indicator of psychotic thinking than it is of abstract reasoning. The problems with this test are that determination of the differences between "concrete" versus "abstract" responses is difficult, and proverbs are highly overlearned by some individuals.

2. Test motor sequencing and the ability to suppress perseverative responses by asking the patient to write in script an alternating series of *n*s and *m*s. Alternatively, ask the patient to draw a line with alternating square and triangular deviations without lifting the pencil point from the paper.

3. Use the Luria hand posture sequence by asking the patient to perform a series of hand movements (slap, fist, cut) that you demonstrate. The task involves comprehending the commands and the ability to execute volitionally a motor act (praxis). The sequencing of several actions is the executive aspect of the task. Deficits in sequencing are probably correlated with deficits in ideomotor praxis (see below).

4. Provide anomalous commands to assess how well patients shift their mental set by disregarding a visual cue in favor of a countermanding verbal cue. Two examples are: you touch your own ear, and then tell the patient to raise his/her finger, or you raise your finger, but tell the patient to touch his/her ear (from Royall, Mahurin, and Gray 1992).

Supplement your tests of executive function and abstract reasoning with information obtained from observation and the history. Look for perseveration, motor impersistence, aspontaneity, echolalia, impulsiveness, disinhibition, comportment, and insight.

If performance on your testing of executive function and abstract reasoning is inconsistent or difficult to interpret, consider a referral to a neuropsychologist. There are a number of extensive test procedures for executive function and abstract reasoning that a neuropsychologist can use to quantify these domains more precisely than can be done at the bedside.

Primitive or "release signs" such as snout, suck, or palmomental signs are not specific for frontal lobe disease, although they are seen frequently in diseases in which frontal lobes are involved. The grasp reflex is the only primitive reflex that has localizing value to the frontal lobes.

Ideomotor Praxis

DEFINITIONS Ideomotor praxis refers to the ability to execute motor actions volitionally. The pathways involved are between the motor cortex, supplementary (premotor) areas, caudate nucleus, and the dominant-hemisphere posterior temporal–inferior parietal regions. Apraxia, the inability to perform specific motor actions in the absence of limb paralysis, can result from cortical or subcortical lesions that disrupt this pathway. Patients with nonfluent aphasia often have buccal apraxia without necessarily having limb ideomotor apraxia.

EXAMINATION To assess praxis, ensure that the patient's auditory comprehension and elementary motor functions are intact. Proximal arm muscle weakness may prevent execution of the limb praxis commands since the actions involve shoulder movements.

TABLE 3-11. Assessment of Ideomotor Praxis

1. Facial (kiss, blow out a match, sip through a straw, stick out tongue, cough)
2. Limb intransitive (wave, salute, hitchhike, motion to "come here")
3. Limb transitive (use a key, comb, toothbrush, hammer, screwdriver, scissors, eraser; throw a ball, flip a coin, stir with a spoon)
4. Whole body (stand up, sit down, roll over in bed, turn head)

SOURCE: From Shelton and Knopman, 1991, with permission.

Distal weakness can also interfere with execution of limb-object actions. There are four categories for assessment of ideomotor praxis (Table 3-11). Ask the patient to perform these actions one at a time. Do not pantomime the task while saying it to the patient. With the facial commands, affected patients may verbalize the action rather than doing it, that is, saying "cough" instead of actually coughing. For limb transitive actions, the earliest failures take the form of using the hand as the object. For example, when showing the examiner how to use a comb, patients will run their fingers through their hair rather than pretend to grip a comb. Performance will be improved with the actual object in hand, but that is a different task because of the extra visual and tactile cues. Truncal or whole-body commands are the most resistant to dysfunction even in severely demented individuals.

AROUSAL, LEVEL OF CONSCIOUSNESS, AND THE EXAMINATION OF COMATOSE PATIENTS

ANATOMIC BASIS AND CLINICAL-PATHOLOGIC CORRELATION Consciousness requires the integrity of the reticular formation located in the rostral pons and the midbrain (Fig. 3-7) and at least one cerebral hemisphere. The reticular formation sends fibers to the forebrain, including the thalamus, hypothalamus, limbic structures, and neocortex. Small lesions in the tegmentum of the rostral pons and midbrain can cause altered consciousness, but lesions in the cerebrum must be bilateral and, therefore, large to produce coma. Coma is caused by one of four pathophysiologic mechanisms (Table 3-12) (Plum and Posner, 1980).

EXAMINATION The most commonly used standardized examination of comatose patients is the Glasgow coma scale (Table 3-13). The scale is intended for grading coma

TABLE 3-12. Mechanisms of Coma

Supratentorial mass lesions with "herniation"
Primary lesions of brainstem
Brainstem compression secondary to lesions in the cerebellum
Diffuse encephalopathies

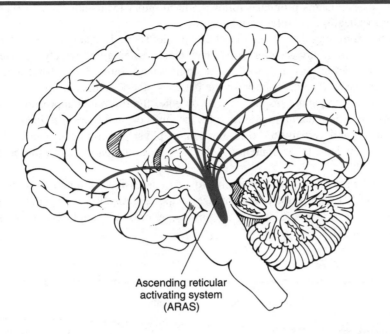

Figure 3-7   Midsagittal section of brain with superimposed location of consciousness maintenance systems. The ascending reticular activating system (ARAS) is not a discrete collection of neurons but rather a functionally defined region extending from the midpons (the lowest location where a lesion will produce impaired consciousness) into the diencephalon. The projections from the ARAS probably include the well-described dopaminergic and serotonergic pathways, as well as less well-known pathways to nonspecific nuclei of the thalamus, limbic system, hypothalamus, and ultimately neocortex.

TABLE 3-13.   Glasgow Coma Scale

	Test	**Patient Response**	**Score**
Eye opening	Spontaneous	Opens eyes	4
	To speech	Opens eyes	3
	To pain	Opens eyes	2
	To pain	Doesn't open	1
Best verbal response	Speech	Conversation carried out correctly	5
		Confused, disoriented	4
		Inappropriate words	3
		Unintelligible sounds only	2
		Mute	1
Best motor response	Commands	Follows simple commands	6
	To pain	Pulls examiner's hand away	5
	To pain	Pulls part of body away	4
	To pain	Flexes body to pain	3
	To pain	Decerebrates	2
	To pain	No motor response	1

SOURCE: From Teasdale and Jennett, 1976, with permission.

severity and establishing prognosis following head injury (Marshall et al, 1991) but is not useful for localization and differential diagnosis.

Begin by examining the patient's level of consciousness. Lethargy, stupor, obtundation, and coma are commonly used terms that lack clear meaning and widely accepted definitions. Use the definitions in the Glasgow coma scale (Table 3-13). Next, describe the patient's responses. The description of the patient is the key in assessing and documenting coma. Does the patient respond when you enter the room and approach the bedside? If so, does the patient attend to you for a few seconds or on a more sustained basis? Does the patient respond verbally to voice, nonpainful physical stimuli, or painful stimuli? If the patient verbalizes, is the content appropriate? Does the patient have motor responses to these stimuli?

Examine the pupils and eye movements to aid in assessing the function of the midbrain and rostral pons. Examine the pupils for size, shape, and reaction to direct and consensual light stimuli. Several diagnostically important patterns of pupillary abnormalities are illustrated in Fig. 3-8.

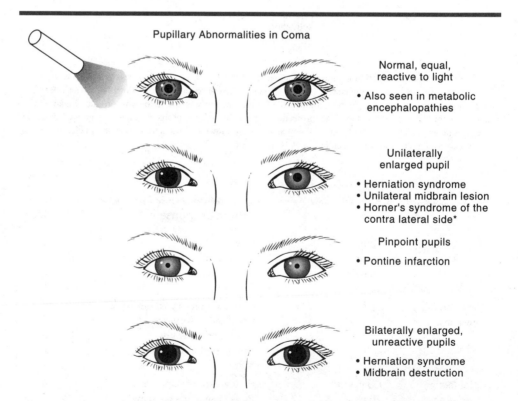

Pupillary Abnormalities in Coma

Normal, equal, reactive to light
- Also seen in metabolic encephalopathies

Unilaterally enlarged pupil
- Herniation syndrome
- Unilateral midbrain lesion
- Horner's syndrome of the contra lateral side*

Pinpoint pupils
- Pontine infarction

Bilaterally enlarged, unreactive pupils
- Herniation syndrome
- Midbrain destruction

Figure 3-8 Pupillary abnormalities that may be seen in coma. The anatomic separation of the parasympathetic and sympathetic pupillary control pathways allows different patterns of pupil size and symmetry to occur with involvement at different levels in the nervous system and with differing etiologies of coma. Several pupillary abnormalities that are useful for localization are shown.

*In Horner's syndrome the "enlarged" pupil is normal in size, and the abnormal pupil miotic.

Describe the position of the eyelids. A unilaterally drooping eyelid might indicate either a Horner syndrome or a third cranial nerve lesion. Look for abnormalities in primary gaze such as skew deviations. Use the doll's-eye maneuver (oculocephalic reflex) and caloric testing (oculovestibular reflex) to assess the integrity of the reflex pathway from the vestibular receptors in the semicircular canals to the pons and midbrain.

Use the doll's-eye maneuver in unresponsive patients only after you have established that there are no cervical fractures. With the patient supine, turn the patient's head to one side and observe the movement of the eyes. Because the fast phase of nystagmus is abolished with altered consciousness, you will observe the slow phase of nystagmus. Deviation of the eyes horizontally opposite the direction of head turning indicates an intact response.

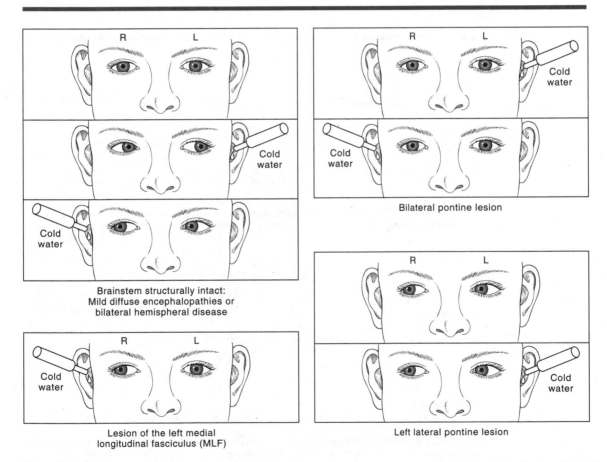

Figure 3-9 Patterns of abnormalities in the extraocular muscles that may be seen in coma. The anatomic localization of cranial nerve nuclei III, IV, and VI is immediately dorsal to the reticular formation of the midbrain and pons, where the ascending reticular activating system (ARAS) resides. Dysfunction at different levels of the ARAS is mirrored in differing patterns of extraocular dysfunction. Several extraocular abnormalities that are useful for localization are shown.

Test caloric responses in unresponsive patients only after establishing that there is no basilar skull fracture, the tympanic membranes are intact, and cerumen is not obstructing the canals. Draw ice-cold water into a 30- to 50-cc syringe, and with the aid of a small catheter, instill the water into the external canal. Deviation of both eyes toward the ear in which the cold water is being instilled indicates an intact response. Caloric testing is more sensitive than the doll's-eye maneuver in assessing function of the extraocular system. Patterns of abnormalities on caloric testing help to localize lesions responsible for coma (Fig. 3-9).

The motor examination in an unresponsive patient is focused on the type of movement evoked by pain (Fig. 3-10) but also involves assessment of resistance to passive manipulation of the limbs ("tone"), posturing and muscle stretch reflexes and plantar responses. Possible findings include asymmetries in motor postures and responses and different automatic responses to painful stimuli such as decorticate, decerebrate, or absence of motor posturing. Motor system findings in comatose patients allow inferences about the

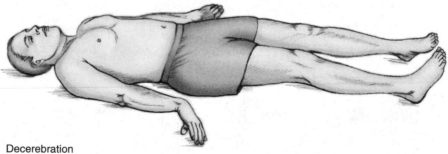

Posturing in Comatose States

Decortication
The arm, wrist, fingers are flexed with thumb trapped in palm. The arms are adducted and in position resting on chest. Legs are extended pronated. Seen in lesions of the thalamus.

Decerebration
The arms are extended, pronated. Legs extended. Seen in lesions of the midbrain.

Figure 3-10 The appearance of decorticate and decerebrate posturing. *(Top)* Decorticate posturing is demonstrated: The arms, wrist, and fingers are flexed with thumbs trapped in palm. The arms are adducted and in a pronated posture resting on chest. The legs are extended. Lesions at the level of the thalamus, with sparing of more caudal structures, is the most frequent anatomic correlate of this posture. *(Bottom)* Decerebration is demonstrated. The arms and legs are both extended. The arms are internally rotated. Lesions at the level of the midbrain with sparing of caudal structures are the most frequent structural lesions associated with this posture.

longitudinal localization of lesions in the cerebral hemispheres and brainstem. The Glasgow coma scale provides a simple set of sequentially more dysfunctional motor responses (Table 3-13).

Observation of respiration is pertinent because the neuronal systems for automatic respiration are in the brainstem. Three clinically common patterns of abnormal breathing occur in comatose patients. Cheyne-Stokes respirations are characterized by a periodic crescendo and decrescendo amplitude of respiration. Cheyne-Stokes respirations are associated with pathology in the cerebral hemispheres. Central neurogenic hyperventilation, a sustained hyperventilation, is associated with lesions in the midbrain and pons. Ataxic respirations are irregular and arrhythmic, resulting in inadequate ventilatory effort. Ataxic respirations are associated with lesions of the medulla.

BRAIN DEATH

Brain death is defined by the absence of both cerebral function and brainstem reflexes. Several requirements must be met before undertaking a brain death examination: "(1) There must be definite clinical or neuroimaging evidence of an acute CNS catastrophe that is compatible with brain death; (2) complicating medical conditions that may confound clinical assessment should be excluded; (3) drug intoxication or poisoning must be absent; and (4) core temperature must be at least 32°C" (Wijdicks, 1995).

The clinical diagnosis of brain death must include absence of response to painful stimuli (scores of 1 on each item of the Glasgow Coma Scale), absence of pupillary light reflexes, absent oculocephalic and oculovestibular reflexes, absent corneal reflexes, absent pharyngeal and tracheal reflexes, and apnea. To test for apnea, disconnect the patient from the ventilator and place an oxygen cannula (100% O_2 at 6 L/min) at the level of the carina. Observe the patient for 8 min for signs of respiration. Most hospitals have specific policies governing the performance of the brain death examination. Those policies may contain additional requirements for the diagnosis.

REFERENCES

Anthony JC, LeResche L, Niaz U, et al: Limits of the "Mini-Mental State" as a screening test for dementia and delirium among hospital patients. *Psychol Med* 12:397–408, 1982.

Benson DF, Geschwind N: Aphasia and related disorders: A clinical approach, in Mesulam M-M (ed): *Principles of Behavioral Neurology*. Philadelphia, FA Davis, 1985, pp 193–258.

Cerhan JR, Folsom AR, Mortimer JA, et al: Correlates of cognitive function in middle-aged adults. *Gerontology* 44:95–105, 1998.

Coslett HB, Saffran EM: Disorders of higher visual processing: Theoretical and clinical perspectives, in Margolin D (ed): *Cognitive Neuropsychology in Clinical Practice*. New York, Oxford University Press, 1992, pp 353–404.

Crum RM, Anthony JC, Basssett SS, Folstein MF: Population-based norms for the mini-mental state examination by age and educational level. *JAMA* 269:2386–2391, 1993.

Cullum CM, Thompson LL, Smernoff EN: Three-word recall as a measure of memory. *J Clin Exp Neuropsychol* 15:321–329, 1993.

Cummings JL: Frontal-subcortical circuits and human behavior. *Arch Neurol* 50:873–880, 1993.

Damasio AR: Disorders of complex visual processing: Agnosias, achromatopsia, Balint's syndrome, and related difficulties of orientation and construction, in Mesulam M-M (ed): *Principles of Behavioral Neurology*. Philadelphia, FA Davis, 1985, pp 259–288.

Damasio AR, Anderson SW: The frontal lobes, in Heilman KM, Valenstein E (eds): *Clinical Neuropsychology*, 3d ed. New York, Oxford University Press, 1993, pp 409–460.

Folstein MF, Folstein SE, McHugh PR: "Mini-mental state": A practical method for grading the cognitive status of patients for the clinician. *J Psychiatr Res* 12:189–198, 1975.

Fuster J: *The Prefrontal Cortex: Anatomy, Physiology, and Neuropsychology of the Frontal Lobe*. New York, Raven Press, 1989.

Goodglass H, Kaplan E: *Boston Diagnostic Aphasia Examination*. Philadelphia, Lea & Febiger, 1983.

Hamilton M: A rating scale for depression. *J Neurol Neurosurg Psychiatr* 23:56–62, 1960.

Hughes CP, Berg L, Danziger W, et al: A new clinical scale for the staging of dementia. *Br J Psychiatr* 140:566–572, 1982.

Katzman R, Brown T, Fuld P, et al: Validation of a short orientation-memory-concentration test of cognitive impairment. *Am J Psychiatr* 140:734–739, 1983.

Kiernan RJ, Mueller J, Langston JW, Van Dyke C: The neurobehavioral cognitive status examination: A brief but differentiated approach to cognitive assessment. *Ann Intern Med* 107:481–485, 1987.

Knopman DS, Ryberg S: A verbal memory test with high predictive accuracy for dementia of the Alzheimer type. *Arch Neurol* 46:141–145, 1989.

Kokmen E, Smith GE, Petersen RC, et al: The short test of mental status. Correlations with standardized psychometric testing. *Arch Neurol* 48:725–728, 1991.

Koss E, Haxby J, DeCarli C, et al: Patterns of performance preservation and loss in healthy aging. *Dev Neuropsychol* 7:99–113, 1991.

Lezak MD: Neuropsychological Assessment, 3rd ed. New York, Oxford University Press, 1995.

Marshall LF, Gautille T, Klauber MR, et al: The outcome of severe closed head injury. *J Neurosurg* 75 (suppl):s28–s36, 1991.

Mendez MF, Ala T, Underwood KL: Development of scoring criteria for the clock drawing task in Alzheimer's disease. *J Am Geriatr Soc* 40:1095–1099, 1992.

Mesulam M-M: Patterns in behavioral neuroanatomy: Association areas, the limbic system, and hemispheric specialization, in Mesulam M-M (ed): *Principles of Behavioral Neurology*. Philadelphia, FA Davis, 1985, pp 1–70.

Petersen RC, Smith G, Kokmen E, et al: Memory function in normal aging. *Neurology* 42:396–401, 1992.

Plum F, Posner JB: *The Diagnosis of Stupor and Coma*, 3d ed. Philadelphia, FA Davis, 1980.

Royall DR, Mahurin RK, Gray KF: Bedside assessment of executive cognitive impairment: The executive interview. *J Am Geriatr Soc* 40:1221–1226, 1992.

Salmon DP, Thal LJ, Butters N, Heindel WC: Longitudinal evaluation of dementia of the Alzheimer type: A comparison of 3 standardized mental status examinations. *Neurology* 40:1225–1230, 1990.

Schaie KW: The hazards of cognitive aging. *Gerontologist* 29:484–493, 1989.

Sheikh JI, Yesavage JA: Geriatric depression scale: Recent evidence and development of a shorter version. *Clin Gerontol* 5:165–172, 1986.

Shelton PA, Knopman DS: Ideomotor apraxia in Huntington's disease. *Arch Neurol* 48:35–41, 1991.

Squire LR: Memory and the hippocampus: A synthesis from findings with rats, monkeys and humans. *Psychol Rev* 99:195–321, 1992.

Strub RL, Black EW: *The Mental Status Examination in Neurology*, 3d ed. Philadelphia, FA Davis, 1993.

Tangalos EG, Smith GE, Ivnik RJ, et al: The Mini-Mental State Examination in general medical practice: Clinical utility and acceptance. *Mayo Clin Proc* 71:829–837, 1996.

Teasdale G, Jennett B: Assessment and prognosis of coma after head injury. *Acta Neurochirurgica* 34:45–55, 1976.

Teng EL, Chui HC: The modified mini-mental state (3MS) examination. *J Clin Psychiatr* 48:314–318, 1987.

Tombaugh TN, McIntyre NJ: The mini-mental state examination: A comprehensive review. *J Am Geriatr Soc* 40:922–935, 1992.

Trzepacz PT, Baker RW: *The Psychiatric Mental Status Examination*. New York, Oxford University Press, 1993, pp 13–52, 82–120.

Welsh K, Butters N, Hughes J, et al: Detection of abnormal memory decline in mild cases of Alzheimer's disease using CERAD neuropsychological measure. *Arch Neurol* 48:278–281, 1991.

Wijdicks EFM: Determining brain death in adults. *Neurology* 45:1003–1011, 1995.

ADRIANA A. KORI / R. JOHN LEIGH **CHAPTER**

THE CRANIAL NERVE EXAMINATION

4

Examination of the cranial nerves presents an unparalleled opportunity to apply knowledge of anatomy and physiology to a clinical evaluation. Although a systematic examination is essential, the distinctive features of each cranial nerve mean that testing of some functions is more sensitive and informative than is testing of others. Figure 4-1 provides an overview of the location of the cranial nerve nuclei.

THE OLFACTORY NERVE (CRANIAL NERVE I)

Anatomy and Physiology

The sense of smell depends on chemoreceptors in ciliated cells on the superior nasal concha and the facing nasal septum. Recent work has identified different types of receptors that recognize specific molecules and has shown that transduction of olfactory stimuli may involve cyclic nucleotide second messengers (Dodd and Castellucci, 1991). The central processes of these cells form bundles of axons that project through the cribriform plate of the ethmoid bone to the ipsilateral olfactory bulb on the undersurface of the frontal lobe. Here they synapse with second-order neurons that are called mitral and tufted cells to form dense aggregates of neuropils called glomeruli. The glomeruli project posteriorly as the olfactory tract, running beneath the orbital surface of the frontal lobe in the olfactory groove. The olfactory tract divides into medial and lateral olfactory stria, which pass on either side of the anterior perforated substance, and some of these fibers decussate in the anterior commissure before terminating in the piriform cortex of the medial temporal lobe (primary olfactory cortex), the amygdala, and the septal nuclei. Projections from the piriform cortex to the orbitofrontal cortex also contribute to olfactory discrimination (Zattore and Jones-Gotman, 1991).

Clinical Examination

Patients may not be aware of loss of smell, and so it is worth performing a simple screening test using coffee, vanilla, or lavender. Avoid irritant odors that also stimulate the

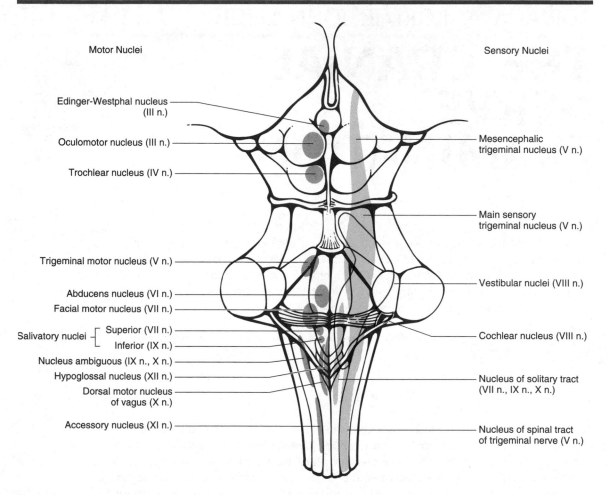

Motor Nuclei

Sensory Nuclei

Edinger-Westphal nucleus
(III n.)

Oculomotor nucleus (III n.)

Trochlear nucleus (IV n.)

Mesencephalic
trigeminal nucleus (V n.)

Main sensory
trigeminal nucleus (V n.)

Trigeminal motor nucleus (V n.)

Abducens nucleus (VI n.)
Facial motor nucleus (VII n.)

Vestibular nuclei (VIII n.)

Salivatory nuclei — Superior (VII n.)
Inferior (IX n.)

Nucleus ambiguous (IX n., X n.)

Hypoglossal nucleus (XII n.)

Dorsal motor nucleus
of vagus (X n.)

Accessory nucleus (XI n.)

Cochlear nucleus (VIII n.)

Nucleus of solitary tract
(VII n., IX n., X n.)

Nucleus of spinal tract
of trigeminal nerve (V n.)

Figure 4-1   Columnar arrangement of the motor *(left)* and sensory *(right)* cranial nerve nuclei from the dorsal aspect of the brainstem. (Adapted from Kandel, Schwarz, and Jessell, 1991.)

trigeminal nerve. Test each nostril separately, occluding the other one. Olfactory acuity varies enormously in normal subjects. When called for, more quantitative tests are available (Mott and Leopold, 1991). If smell is abnormal, determine whether the defect is one of detection or identification. Distinguish between total anosmia, partial loss of smell (hyposmia), perversion of small (parosmia), and the hallucination of an unpleasant odor (cacosmia).

Disorders of Function

Loss of smell most commonly results from local nasal disease such as the common cold. Anosmia after head injury is common and usually results from tearing of the olfactory fibers as they perforate the cribriform plate. Rarely, loss of smell occurs with meningiomas arising from the olfactory groove; such tumors also may compress the optic nerve. Impaired perception of odors despite preserved detection reflects disturbance of the temporal or orbitofrontal cortex. Olfactory defects caused by temporal lobe lesions affect the ipsilateral nostril, but with the right orbitofrontal cortex the disturbance affects both nostrils (Zattore and Jones-Gotman, 1991). Persistent parosmia and cacosmia are rare and usually are encountered in patients who have suffered a head injury or have a psychiatric disease such as depression. Episodic cacosmia (classically, the smell of burned rubber) is a common manifestation of complex partial seizures.

THE OPTIC NERVE (CRANIAL NERVE II)

Anatomy and Physiology

The photodetectors—rods and cones—lie in the deepest part of the retina and project to the retinal ganglion cells via bipolar and amacrine cells. The optic nerve is formed by the central processes of the retinal ganglion cells, which converge toward the optic disc. Thus, the optic nerve constitutes a tract of the brain, and its axons are sheathed by central myelin. The four portions of the optic nerve are (1) intraocular, or the optic nerve head (1 mm), (2) intraorbital, surrounded by fat, the extraocular muscles and their nerves, and the ophthalmic artery (25 mm), (3) intracanalicular, running posteriorly, medially, and superiorly with the ophthalmic artery (9 mm), and (4) intracranial, between the optic foramen and the chiasm, lying above the carotid artery where that artery gives off the ophthalmic branch (4 to 16 mm, depending on the position of the artery with respect to the sella turcica). The optic chiasm lies above the pituitary gland, below the suprachiasmatic recess of the third ventricle and the hypothalamus, and anterior (in most cases) to the pituitary stalk. In the optic nerve, fibers from the upper retinal quadrants occur in the upper parts of the nerve, fibers from the lower retina in the lower parts, and macular fibers in the center. At the chiasm the fibers undergo a partial decussation: Fibers emanating from the temporal halves of the retina continue without crossing, while fibers from the nasal halves cross in the chiasm to the optic tract of the opposite side. Some of the decussating fibers from the lower nasal retinal quadrant do not cross directly but after passing the midline project forward a short distance into the opposite optic nerve (Wilbrand's knee) (Fig. 4-2).

From the optic chiasm, most axons continue as the optic tract to reach the lateral geniculate body; some fibers pass to the midbrain to synapse in the superior colliculus and the pretectal region. The optic tracts lie close to the posterior cerebral and posterior communicating arteries. The lateral geniculate nucleus—the visual thalamus—consists of six sharply laminated layers: fibers from the contralateral retina synapse in layers 1, 4, and 6, and fibers from the ipsilateral retina synapse into layers 2, 3, and 5. As fibers pass from the optic tract to synapse in the lateral geniculate nucleus, they rotate 90 degrees so that the upper retinal fibers terminate in the medial segment and the lower retinal fibers terminate in the lateral portion; macular fibers synapse in a central wedge-shaped segment of layers 3 through 6. Another important division of the lateral geniculate nucleus is into magnocellular (1 and 2) and parvocellular (3 through 6) layers; the former are mostly concerned with coarse motion vision, and the latter with fine features and color.

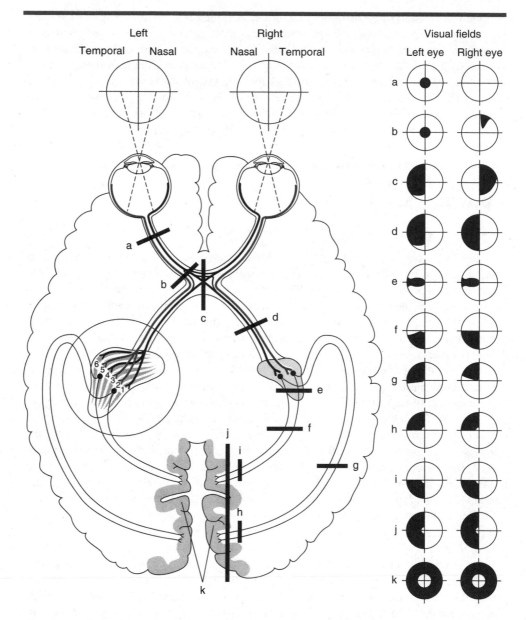

Figure 4-2　Some characteristic defects of the visual field produced by lesions at various points along the visual pathways (see text for discussion).

From the lateral geniculate nucleus, axons sweep posteriorly around the lateral aspects of the lateral ventricles as the optic radiation, which projects to the striate cortex (primary visual cortex, V1) of the occipital lobe. Fibers representing the superior retina turn posteriorly and run through the deep parietal white matter, but fibers representing the lower retina loop forward around the temporal horn of the lateral ventricles, forming "Meyer's loop." Fibers carrying vision from the upper and lower retinae terminate in the upper and lower banks of the calcarine fissure, respectively, with the horizontal meridian running along the base of the fissure. Peripheral vision is represented anteriorly, and central vision posteriorly; recent maps assign a larger portion to the representation of the fovea (macula), which is located where the striate cortex wraps around onto the lateral convexity of the occipital pole (Horton and Hoyt, 1991).

Clinical Examination

Before proceeding to the examination, ask the patient about impairment of vision, the duration of any impairment, and whether it is monocular or affects one part of the visual field. Characterize transient disturbance of vision in terms of onset and development, severity, extent of visual field loss, manner or resolution, the presence of positive symptoms (e.g., flashing lights or formed visual hallucinations), and any symptoms that accompany (e.g., hemiparesis) or follow (e.g., headache) the visual disturbance. Even in patients with no visual complaints, it is wise to test visual acuity and the visual fields.

Test the visual acuity of each eye separately with refractive correction. If the patient lacks spectacles, use a pinhole to correct refractive errors. Use a Snellen chart at 20 ft (6 m) to test distance vision and a Jaeger chart to test near vision; record the smallest type

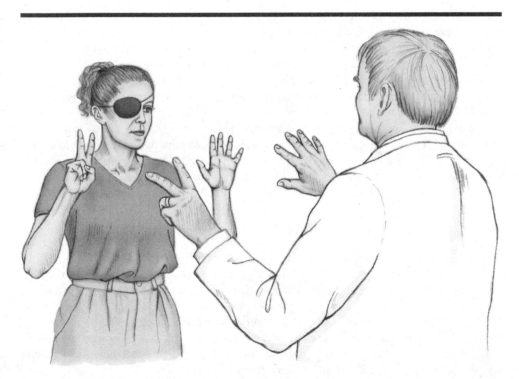

Figure 4-3   Visual field testing by confrontation (see text for details). The patient may respond by naming the number of fingers that have been presented or by imitating.

the patient can read. If vision is poor, ask the patient to count your fingers or detect a flashlight presented centrally and in the four quadrants of the visual field.

Screen for visual field defects by confrontation (Fig. 4-3). Sit facing the patient, at the same level. Test each eye separately, using yourself as a control. First, cover the patient's left eye while the patient fixes on your left eye; close your right eye shut. Start by holding up two fingers on each hand and ask the patient to report the number of fingers on each hand. Then present briefly (for about 0.5 s) zero to five fingers from each hand simultaneously in opposite quadrants of the visual field (e.g., upper nasal and lower temporal). During each presentation, ensure that the patient is fixed on the pupil of your left eye. After a few practice runs, most patients will understand the nature of the test and be ready to make responses either verbally or by holding up the same number of fingers. This technique is superior to the presentation of a moving stimulus (e.g., wagging finger) in one visual field and also will pick up hemineglect as well as visual field defects. In patients who have a visual field defect, map out the extent of the field defect by using a red test object such as a match; this technique is especially helpful with central field defects and in comparing the size of the patient's blind spot with your own. Patients with visual field defects may require quantitative perimetry (Glaser, 1990). Visual field testing requires attention and cooperation and may not be possible in some subjects, such as confused patients and some children. In such individuals, presentation of an attractive object (e.g., a photograph or toy) in one visual hemifield may induce the patient to shift the gaze toward the object, suggesting preservation of that hemifield.

Comparing the hue of a red test object by the two eyes is a useful means of detecting subtle defects of vision. Formal testing of color vision using Ishihara plates is not a routine part of the examination but may be valuable in detecting subtle asymmetries of visual acuity caused by optic nerve disease. (Note, however, that some normal males have red-green color blindness.) Similarly, testing contrast sensitivity sometimes reveals an impaired ability to detect sinusoidal gratings with lower spatial frequencies than are represented by Snellen optotypes (Glaser, 1990).

Ophthalmoscopy is best performed after pharmacologic dilatation of the pupil with tropicamide 1%. Note the color of the disc (normally more pink on the temporal half), its edges (the nasal border may normally be less distinct), and whether it appears elevated. Systematically follow the arteries and veins, noting their thickness and caliber and any emboli within them. Look in the retinal periphery for hemorrhages and exudates.

Disorders of Function

Vascular insufficiency in the distribution of the ophthalmic artery and its branches typically causes monocular visual loss and altitudinal defects (above or below the horizontal meridian) of the visual field. Transient monocular visual loss that is often reported to be "like a shutter" coming down or going up is called *amaurosis fugax* and may be associated with atherosclerosis of the cerebral and coronary arteries. Disease affecting the nerve fiber layer of the retina, such as a lesion of the retinal arteriolar supply or the optic nerve before it leaves the eyes, causes an arcuate defect in the visual field; however, arcuate field defects in the nasal field of vision often result from glaucoma.

Acute demyelination of the optic nerve—optic neuritis—causes monocular visual loss, impaired color vision, and visual field defects. Classically, a central scotoma ("an island of blindness in a sea of vision") has been attributed to optic neuritis, although recent studies indicate that diffuse field defects are more common (Keltner et al, 1993). Only when the plaque of demyelination is in the more anterior portion of the nerve will optic disc swelling be evident. Affected patients often complain of pain when they move the affected eye.

Lesions in the region of the optic chiasm cause bitemporal hemianopia (Fig. 4-2). Pituitary tumors, which compress the chiasm from below, tend to produce bitemporal superior quadrantanopia, whereas tumors that press down on the chiasm, such as craniopharyngioma, cause bitemporal inferior quadrantanopia. Injury to the anterior angle of the chiasm may involve Wilbrand's knee, leading to a "junctional scotoma" with a central field defect in the eye on the affected side and a superior quadrantanopia in the opposite side (Fig. 4-2).

Behind the chiasm, lesions cause homonymous hemianopia (Fig. 4-2). Optic tract lesions tend to be incongruous, so that although the visual defects in each eye are confined to the same hemifield, they differ in shape and extent. This is the case because the fibers are not in precise retinotopic register. Visual field defects resulting from ischemia of the lateral geniculate body depend on the vascular territory that is involved. The posterior choroidal artery supplies the central portion of the lateral geniculate body, and its occlusion may result in a horizontal homonymous sector defect (Fig. 4-2). The anterior choroidal artery supplies the hilum and the anterolateral portion of the lateral geniculate body, and its occlusion leads to loss of vision except for the preserved horizontal sector — a "keyhole" field of vision. Lesions affecting the temporal fibers of the optic radiation (Meyer's loop) produce a superior homonymous quadrantanopia, whereas involvement of the parietal fibers produces an inferior homonymous quadrantanopia. Lesions affecting striate cortex produce very congruous homonymous defects, usually sparing the macula. Macular sparing is now thought to reflect the magnified representation of central vision and the blood supply, which comes from branches of both the posterior and the middle cerebral arteries (Horton and Hoyt, 1991). Thus, bilateral visual loss resulting from occipital lobe infarction is rare, requiring bilateral involvement of branches of the posterior and middle cerebral arteries; it presents with a characteristic denial of blindness with confabulation (Anton syndrome). Occasionally with bilateral medial occipital lobe lesions there is macular sparing which produces a ring scotoma (Fig. 4-2). Analysis of the various features of vision depends on parallel processing in secondary visual areas to which striate cortex projects (Zeki, 1993). Thus, disease affecting such secondary visual areas may produce selective defects of color vision, motion vision, and face recognition (prosopagnosia) as well as distortions or persistence of visual images (palinopsia).

Swelling of the optic disc may be due to inflammation such as optic neuritis or anterior ischemic optic neuropathy; these processes impair visual acuity. When passive congestion caused by increased intracranial pressure results in optic disc swelling (papilledema), visual acuity is preserved. In classic papilledema, the disc margins are blurred, the veins are engorged, and exudates and hemorrhages may surround the disk. Visual field testing may reveal enlargement of the blind spot.

Optic atrophy is characterized by a pale, small disc; usually, visual acuity is impaired and there is a concentric contraction of the visual field. Optic atrophy may follow optic neuritis or anterior ischemic optic neuropathy. The latter is due to interruption of the blood supply from the posterior ciliary vessels and is associated with hypertension, diabetes, and giant-cell arteritis. A special case of anterior ischemic optic neuropathy is central retinal artery occlusion, in which the fundus is pale, arteries are thin, and there is a cherry-red spot corresponding to the fovea. Optic atrophy also may follow compression of the optic nerve. In the Foster Kennedy syndrome, optic atrophy is present on the side of the lesion and papilledema is present on the contralateral side; the cause is usually a frontal lobe tumor. Optic atrophy also occurs after long-standing papilledema and is presumed to be due to nutritional and toxic factors in individuals who smoke and drink alcohol to excess.

THE OCULOMOTOR (CRANIAL NERVE III), TROCHLEAR (CRANIAL NERVE IV), AND ABDUCENS (CRANIAL NERVE VI) NERVES

Anatomy and Physiology

These three cranial nerves supply the extraocular muscles, pupils, and eyelids. Eye movements guarantee that people have a clear and stable view of the world. It is useful to think about eye movements in terms of the functions they serve (Table 4-1). Each class of eye movement has a distinctive set of properties that suit it to its purpose and a separate neural substrate. An understanding of the properties of each class of eye movements guides the examination; knowledge of the anatomic substrate aids in topologic diagnosis.

TABLE 4-1.   Functional Classes of Eye Movements

CLASS OF EYE MOVEMENT	MAIN FUNCTION
Visual fixation	Holds the image of a stationary object on the fovea
Vestibulo-ocular reflex	Holds images of the seen world steady on the retina during brief head rotations
Optokinetic	Holds images of the seen world steady on the retina during sustained and low-frequency head rotations
Smooth pursuit	Holds the image of a moving target close to the fovea
Nystagmus quick phases	Reset the eyes during prolonged rotation and direct gaze toward the oncoming visual scene
Saccades	Bring images of eccentrically located objects of interest onto the fovea
Vergence	Moves the eyes in opposite directions so that images of a single object are placed simultaneously on both foveas during gaze shifts in depth

SOURCE: Adapted from Leigh RJ, Zee DS: *The Neurology of Eye Movements*, 2d ed. Philadelphia, Davis, 1991.

The *abducens nucleus* lies under the floor of the fourth ventricle in the lower pons, just lateral to the medial longitudinal fasciculus (MLF), where it is capped by the genu of the facial nerve. The abducens nucleus houses two populations of neurons (Fig. 4-4). The first population consists of abducens motorneurons, which innervate the ipsilateral lateral rectus muscle. The second consists of abducens internuclear neurons, which cross the midline and ascend in the MLF to innervate medial rectus motorneurons in contralateral cranial nerve III. In this way, conjugate horizontal eye movements are coordinated so that the eyes move together. In the brainstem, the MLF is the key pathway for coordinating activity of the medial rectus of one eye with the lateral rectus of the other. Fibers from the abducens motorneurons exit from the medial aspect of the nucleus, coursing ventrally, laterally, and caudally through the pontine tegmentum and medical lemniscus and lateral to the corticospinal tract to emerge at the caudal border of the pons. The abducens nerve then ascends nearly vertically along the clivus, through the prepontine cistern, to the petrous crest, where it bends forward to penetrate the dura, medial to the trigeminal nerve, and passes under the petroclinoid ligament (Fig. 4-5). The nerve continues by coursing forward in the body of the cavernous sinus, where it lies lateral to the internal carotid artery and medial to the ophthalmic division of the trigeminal nerve. The nerve then enters the orbit through the superior orbital fissure to innervate the lateral rectus muscle on the inner surface.

The *trochlear nucleus* lies at the ventral border of the periaqueductal gray matter, dorsal to the MLF, at the level of the inferior colliculus. Its fibers pass dorsolaterally and caudally to decussate in the roof of the aqueduct and emerge from the dorsal aspect of the brainstem, close to the tentorium cerebelli (Fig. 4-5). The trochlear nerve passes laterally around the upper pons, lying between the superior cerebellar and posterior cerebral arteries, and then runs forward on the free edge of the tentorium before penetrating the dura to enter the cavernous sinus. Within the lateral wall of the sinus, the fourth nerve lies below the third nerve and above the ophthalmic division of the fifth nerve, with which it shares a connective tissue coat. It then passes through the superior orbital fissure to reach the medial aspect of the orbit and supply the superior oblique muscle.

The *oculomotor nucleus* is a paired structure that lies at the ventral border of the periaqueductal gray matter, extending rostrally to the level of the posterior commissure and caudally to the trochlear nucleus. The oculomotor nerve innervates the medial rectus, superior rectus, inferior rectus, and inferior oblique muscles; the levator palpebrae superioris; the pupillary constrictor muscle; and the ciliary body. The classic anatomic scheme for the oculomotor nucleus (Warwick, 1953) has been revised with the demonstration that the neurons supplying the medial rectus muscle are distributed into three separate areas, although all three receive inputs from the contralateral abducens nucleus via the medial longitudinal fasciculus (Büttner-Ennever and Akert, 1981). The neurons innervating each superior rectus muscle lie next to each other, and their axons decussate in the caudal portion of this nucleus. The caudal nucleus, which supplies both levator palpebrae superioris muscles, is a single structure. All projections from the oculomotor nucleus are ipsilateral except those to the superior rectus, which are totally crossed, and those to the levator palpebrae superioris, which are both crossed and uncrossed.

The fascicles of the oculomotor nerve pass ventrally through the MLF, the red nucleus, the substantia nigra, and the medial part of the cerebral peduncle. From lateral to medial, the order of fascicles is thought to be inferior oblique, superior rectus, medial rectus and

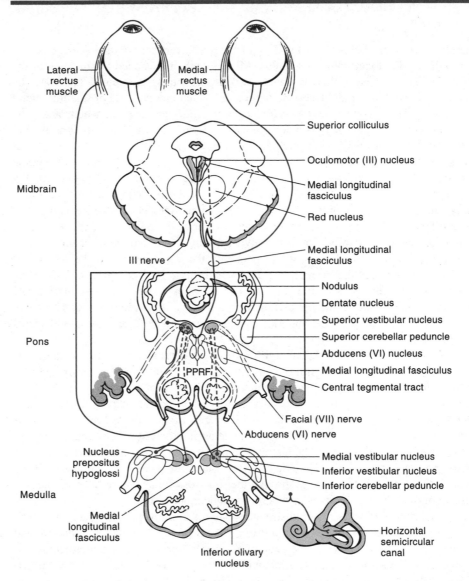

Figure 4-4 Anatomic pathways important in the synthesis of horizontal versional eye movements. The abducens nucleus (VI) contains abducens motorneurons that innervate the ipsilateral lateral rectus muscle (LR) and abducens internuclear neurons with axons that ascend in the contralateral medial longitudinal fasciculus (MLF) to contact medial rectus (MR) motorneurons in the contralateral third nerve nucleus (III). From the horizontal semicircular canal, primary vestibular afferents project mainly to the medial vestibular nucleus (MVN), where they synapse and then send an excitatory connection to the contralateral abducens nucleus and an inhibitory projection to the ipsilateral abducens nucleus. (An ipsilateral projection, via the ascending tract of Deiters, is not shown.) Saccadic inputs reach the abducens nucleus from ipsilateral excitatory burst neurons in the paramedian pontine reticular formation (PPRF) and contralateral inhibitory burst neurons. Eye position information (the output of the neural integrator) reaches the abducens nucleus from neurons within the nucleus prepositus hypoglossi (NPH) and the adjacent MVN. (Adapted from Leigh and Zee, 1991.)

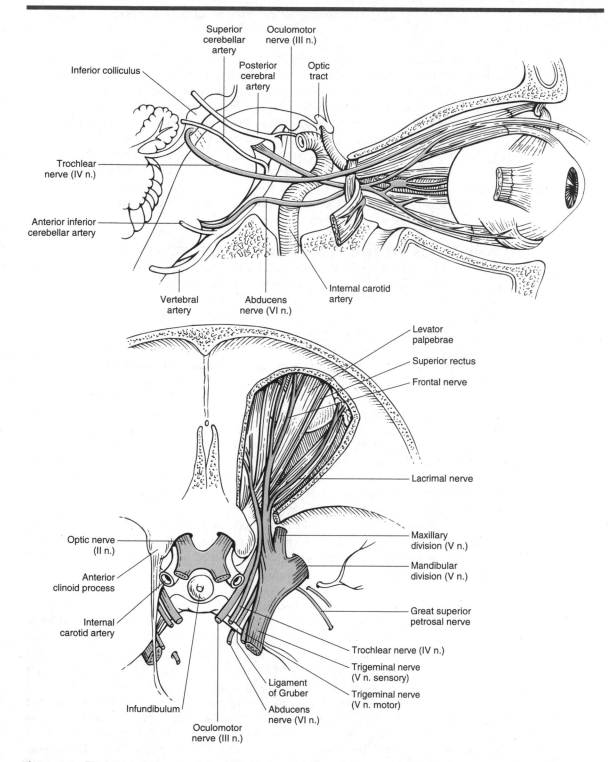

Figure 4-5 The intracranial courses of the third, fourth, and sixth cranial nerves. *(Top)* Parasagittal view. *(Bottom)* Superior view. Lig. of Gruber = petroclinoid ligament. (Adapted from Warwick R: *Wolff's Anatomy of the Eye and Orbit*, 7th ed.) Philadelphia, Saunders, 1976, pp 281, 295.)

levator palpebrae, inferior rectus, and pupil (Castro et al, 1990). The third nerve emerges from the interpeduncular fossa and then runs between the posterior cerebral artery and the superior cerebellar artery, lateral to the posterior communicating artery and below the temporal lobe uncus, just lateral to the posterior clinoid process (Fig. 4-5). During this subarachnoid course, parasympathetic pupillary fibers lie peripherally in the dorsomedial part of the nerve. The oculomotor nerve then enters the cavernous sinus, lying above the trochlear nerve, where it receives sympathetic fibers from the carotid artery. As it leaves the cavernous sinus, cranial nerve III divides into superior and inferior rami, which pass through the superior orbital fissure to enter the orbit. The superior ramus supplies the superior rectus and levator palpebrae muscles. The large inferior ramus supplies the medial rectus, inferior rectus, and inferior oblique muscles and the ciliary ganglion.

PROJECTIONS TO THE NUCLEI OF CRANIAL NERVES III, IV, AND VI

For *conjugate horizontal gaze*, the abducens nucleus receives vestibular inputs from the medial vestibular nucleus, saccadic commands from burst neurons in the paramedian pontine reticular formation (PPRF), pursuit signals from vestibular nuclei and cerebellar fastigial nuclei, and the signal required to hold the eye in steady eccentric gaze from the nucleus prepositus hypoglossi and the medial vestibular nuclei (Fig. 4-4). The premotor commands for vergence eye movements project to medial rectus motorneurons from cells in the mesencephalic reticular formation, dorsolateral to the oculomotor nucleus.

For *conjugate vertical gaze*, the oculomotor and trochlear nuclei receive saccadic commands from a nucleus lying in the prerubral fields of the rostral mesencephalon which is called the rostral interstitial nucleus of the medial longitudinal fasciculus (riMLF) (Fig. 4-6). The riMLF projects to motorneurons that supply yoke muscle pairs (e.g., superior rectus and inferior oblique); in this way, conjugate vertical eye movements are coordinated so that the eyes move together (Moschovakis et al, 1990). The signals required to hold the eye in steady eccentric vertical gaze arise from the interstitial nucleus of Cajal. The signals for vestibular and smooth pursuit eye movements ascend to the midbrain from the lower brainstem, partly in the MLF.

The *cerebellum* calibrates eye movements so that they provide the clearest vision. Two separate parts of the cerebellum participate in the control of eye movements. The dorsal vermis and its projections to the fastigial nucleus are concerned with the accuracy of saccades. The vestibulocerebellum (flocculus, paraflocculus, nodulus, and ventral uvula) influences vestibular pursuit and the mechanism for steady gaze holding. Several areas in *cerebral cortex* that project to the brainstem are important in the control of eye movements (Fig. 4-7). At the temporal-occipital-parietal junction lies visual area V5, which is important for "motion vision" and the programming of pursuit and optokinetic eye movements via an ipsilateral pathway running through the pons and cerebellum. The parietal eye fields lie in the superior part of the angular gyrus and are important for programming saccades concerned with reflexive exploration of the visual environment. The frontal eye fields lie at the confluence of the lateral part of the precentral sulcus, part of the posterior extermity of the middle frontal gyrus and the adjacent precentral sulcus and gyrus, just anterior to the motor cortex; they are important for the programming of saccades concerned with intentional exploration of the visual environment. The supplementary eye fields lie in the posteromedial portion of the superior frontal gyrus and are important in programming saccades concerned with complex motor behaviors. The

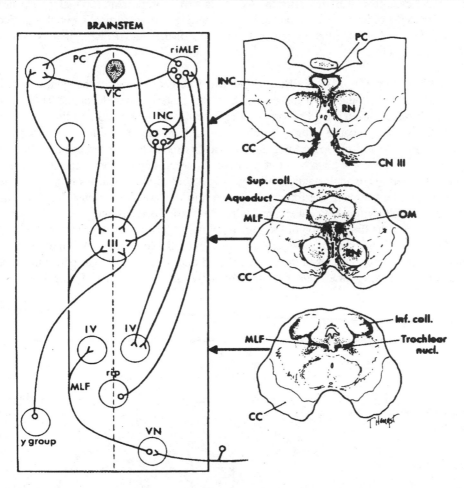

Figure 4-6 Anatomic pathways important in the synthesis of vertical and torsional eye movements. Vestibular inputs from the vertical semicircular canals synapse in the vestibular nuclei (VN) and ascend in the medial longitudinal fasciculus (MLF) and brachium conjunctivum (not shown) to contact neurons in the trochlear nucleus (IV), oculomotor nucleus (III), interstitial nucleus of Cajal (INC), and rostral interstitial nucleus of the medial longitudinal fasciculus (riMLF). The riMLF, which lies in the prerubral fields, also receives an input from omnipause neurons of the nucleus raphe interpositus (rip), which lies in the pons. The riMLF contains saccadic burst cells that project ipsilaterally to the motorneurons of III and IV and also send an axon collateral to the INC. Connections between the right and left riMLF may pass in or near the posterior commissure (PC) and ventral commissure (VC). Cells in the INC that may encode vertical eye position (contributing to the neural integrator) also project to III and IV; projections to the elevator subnuclei (innervating the superior rectus and inferior oblique muscles) pass above the aqueduct of Sylvius (A) in the posterior commissure; projections to the depressor subnuclei (innervating the inferior rectus and superior oblique) pass ventrally. Signals contributing to vertical smooth pursuit and eye-head tracking reach III from the y group via the brachium conjuntivum and a crossing ventral tegmental tract. The anatomic sections on the right correspond to the level of the arrowheads in the schematic on the left. CC = crus cerebri; CN III = oculomotor nerve; RN = red nucleus; Sup. coll. = superior colliculus; Inf. coll. = inferior colliculus; OM = oculomotor nucleus. (Adapted from Leigh and Zee, 1991.)

dorsolateral prefrontal cortex (Brodmann's area 46) is important for making accurate saccades to the remembered spatial locations of targets. These cortical eye fields projects in parallel to the brainstem reticular formation (riMLF and PPRF), mainly via the superior colliculus.

INNERVATION OF THE PUPIL   The central cells of origin for the sympathetic innervation of the iris dilator of the *pupil* are in the posterior hypothalamus. Their axons project diffusely through the brainstem, lying laterally in the medulla, to the spinal cord levels C7 to T1 to synapse in the ciliospinal center of Budge in the intermediolateral cell column (Fig. 4-8). From there, preganglionic axons pass close to the apex of the lung, through the stellate ganglion without synapse, to reach the superior cervical ganglion, where they terminate on postganglionic neurons. Axons of these neurons follow the internal carotid artery through the foramen lacerum into the cavernous sinus. For a few millimeters, pupillosympathetic fibers run with the sixth nerve as they leave the carotid artery to reach the first division of the trigeminal nerve. Then they enter the orbit with the ophthalmic division of cranial nerve V and travel with the long posterior ciliary nerves to innervate the dilator muscles of the iris and the lid muscle of Müller. The parasympathetic innervation of the intraocular muscles probably arises from the Edinger-Westphal

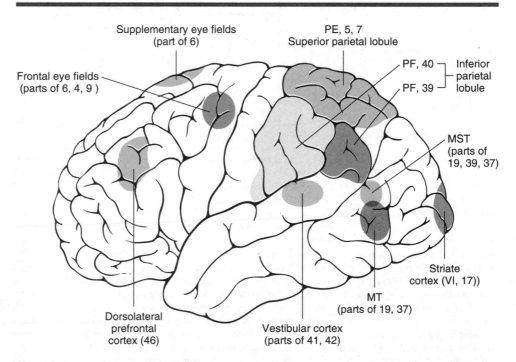

Figure 4-7   Probable location of cortical areas important for eye movements in the human brain. MT = middle temporal visual cortex homolog (V5); MST = medial superior temporal visual cortex homolog; both are important for "motion vision." (Adapted from Leigh and Zee, 1991.)

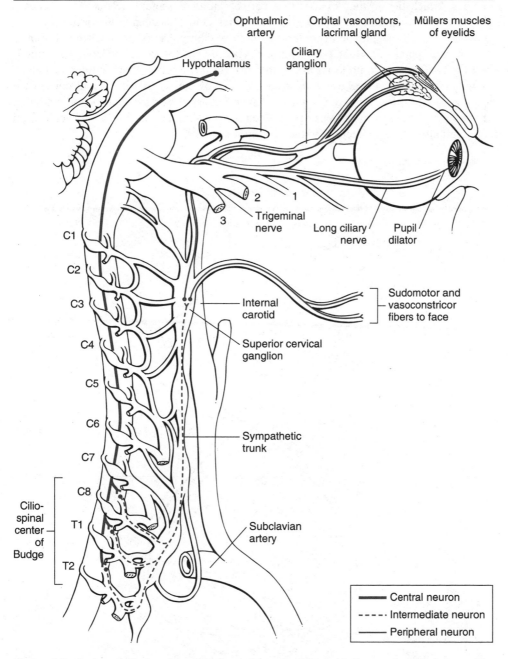

Figure 4-8 Oculosympathetic pathway. The first-order neuron is located in the posterior hypothalamus. The second-order neuron is in the intermediolateral column of the lower cervical and upper thoracic cord. The third-order neuron is in the superior cervical ganglion. (Adapted from Bonner and Jaeger Bonner, 1991.)

nucleus, which lies in the dorsal-rostral part of the oculomotor nucleus. The preganglionic fibers synapse in the ciliary ganglion, which is located deep in the orbit (Figs. 4-8 and 4-9). The postganglionic fibers follow the short ciliary nerves into the sclera to innervate the iris sphincter and the ciliary muscle. The afferent pathways subserving the pupillary light reflex pass to pretectal nuclei that project bilaterally to the oculomotor nuclei, so that stimulation of one eye causes constriction of both eyes (direct and consensual responses). The afferent pathways that mediate pupillary constriction and accommodation of the lens of the eye in response to viewing a near stimulus depend on cortical visual areas and also project bilaterally to the oculomotor nuclei.

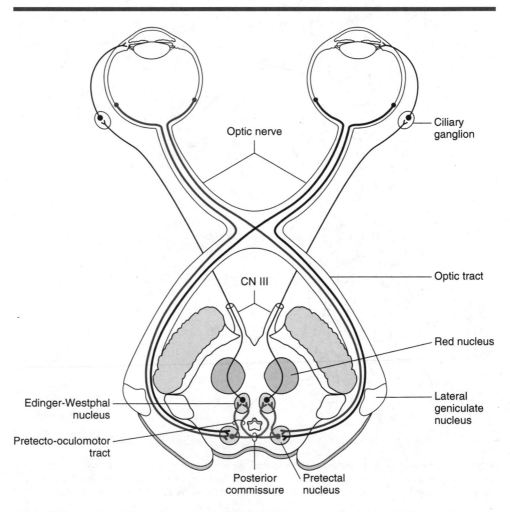

Figure 4-9 Pupillary light reflex pathway and parasympathetic innervation of the pupil. (Adapted from Bonner and Jaeger Bonner, 1991.)

INNERVATION OF THE EYELIDS Eyelid opening is achieved mainly by the levator palpebrae superioris muscle, which is innervated by the superior division of cranial nerve III. The muscle of Müller lies embedded in the levator and is sympathetically innervated; it adjusts the width of the palpebral fissure. During extreme efforts to open the lids (and in far upgaze), the frontalis muscle contracts; it is supplied by the facial nerve. Gentle lid closure is achieved by relaxation of the levator. Firm lid closure brings the orbicularis oculi muscle into action; it is supplied by the facial nerve. The eyelid follows vertical eye movements except during forceful lid closure, when the eyes deviate up—Bell's phenomenon.

Cranial nerve III neurons supplying the levator are located bilaterally in the central caudal subdivision of the oculomotor nucleus. A nearby "M" nucleus is important for coordinating vertical eye and lid movements, and the nuclei of the posterior commissure may send tonic inhibition to it (Schmidke and Büttner-Ennever, 1992). The extrapyramidal dopaminergic system influences the execution of blinks, and the cerebral cortex, especially the right parietal lobe, influences the tonic level of levator activity and voluntarily lid opening (Averbuch-Heller et al, 1996).

Clinical Examination

Before examining the range of eye movements, ask about the presence of diplopia. Diplopia that is still present with one eye covered (monocular diplopia) commonly is due to astigmatism or cataract. If diplopia is binocular, determine whether the images are separated horizontally, vertically, or diagonally and whether it is worse on gaze in one specific direction, worse when viewing near or distant objects, and worse at the beginning or the end of the day. Also inquire about a past history of strabismus or eye muscle surgery.

Next, examine movements of the eyes and then the pupils and eyelids. Clinical examination of eye movements has two main components. First, examine the static alignment and range of eye movements. This part of the examination of especially important in patients who complain of double vision (diplopia). Second, observe the dynamic properties of each functional class of eye movements. This part of the examination is likely to shed light on a wide range of diseases of the nervous system.

Test the range of eye movement with one eye viewing (ductions) and then with both eyes viewing (versions). Ask the patient to follow a small target through the full range of movement, including the position shown in Fig. 4-10, noting any limitation of movement or deviation (misalignment of the visual axes). Ask the patient to look at a penlight while you keep yourself aligned with the stationary penlight as the patient rotates his or her head to carry the eyes into the positions indicated in Fig. 4-10. If the images from the two corneas appear centered, the visual axes are usually correctly aligned. This technique is useful in patients with facial asymmetries, ptosis, or broad epicanthic folds (especially young children). Although the scheme shown in Fig. 4-10 is a simplification of the orbital positions at which the named muscles have their major horizontal or vertical effects, it often helps identify the weak muscle or muscles. In more complicated cases, a variety of other clinical tests are available (Leigh and Zee, 1999).

Next, test the different functional classes of eye movements (Table 4-1). First test the *visual fixation* of a stationary target, such as the tip of a pencil, with the eyes close to central position and then with them turned to the extremes of horizontal and vertical gaze.

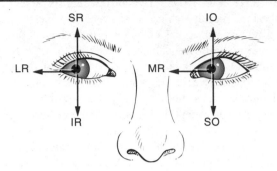

Figure 4-10 Simplified scheme for testing the major pulling actions of extraocular muscles. IO = inferior oblique; IR = inferior rectus; LR = lateral rectus; MR = medial rectus; SO = superior oblique; SR = superior rectus.

Look for any abnormal movements, such as nystagmus, that disrupt steady fixation. Nystagmus is an involuntary oscillation of the eyes that consists of a slow drift and usually a corrective eye movement (saccadic quick phases). If nystagmus is present with the eyes in eccentric gaze (e.g., directed to the far right), note whether it is sustained and in what direction the quick phases carry the eye (e.g., rightward or downward). Low-amplitude nystagmus and abnormal saccades that intrude on steady fixation (square-wave jerks) may be detected only by viewing the patient's retina with an ophthalmoscope (Zee, 1978); note, however, that the direction of horizontal or vertical nystagmus is inverted when viewed through the ophthalmoscope. Next, test the *vestibulo-ocular reflex*. Ask the patient to fix vision on a distant object; hold the patient's head firmly with your palms against the cheeks and effect a rapid, small head turn. If the reflex movement of the eyes is inappropriate (too small or too big), it will be followed by a corrective (saccadic) movement. The interpretation of this test is discussed further in the section on cranial nerve VIII. Test *saccades* by asking the patient to alternately look at a pencil tip and the tip of your nose. Change the position of the pencil to elicit horizontal or vertical saccades. Note the ease of initiation, the accuracy of the saccades (and whether any correction is necessary), and the speed of the movement. Test *smooth pursuit* by asking the patient to follow the pencil tip as you slowly move it first horizontally and then vertically across the field of gaze. Look for corrective saccades, which indicate that the pursuit is not holding the eye on the moving target. It is sometimes useful to ask the patient to follow the stripes on a small optokinetic drum or tape; this induces "optokinetic nystagmus," which consists of a series of smooth pursuit movements and resetting saccadic quick phases. Look for any asymmetry of the response when the stimulus is moved in opposite direction (right versus left, up versus down). Test *convergence* by asking the patient to follow a visual target (pencil tip or the patient's thumb) as it is brought from distance along the midsagittal plane toward the patient's nose.

Observe the resting size and shape of the *pupils* in ambient light. Ask the patient to fixate a distant target such as letter or another symbol to impose a fixed state of accommodation and measure pupillary size. Then test the pupillary responses to light. Swiftly move a penlight in from the temporal side to shine the beam into one eye and test the direct pupillary light reaction. Remove the beam and then repeat the procedure for the other eye.

Although the consensual response of the other pupil can be observed during such testing, it is more convenient to compare the direct and consensual responses. This is achieved by rapidly moving the penlight from one eye to the other and holding it at its new location for about 5s. If the pupil dilates when the flashlight is beamed into it, the prior consensual response was greater than the present direct response; this is "relative afferent pupillary defect" or "Marcus Gunn pupil" and indicates an abnormality of the anterior visual pathway of that eye. Test the pupillary component of the near triad response (convergence, accommodation of the pupil, and pupillary constriction) by asking the patient to change fixation from a distant to a near target and looking for miosis.

Observe the resting position of the *eyelids* with the eyes in midposition and in each direction of gaze, noting whether the lids follow vertical eye movements. When the eyes are in midposition, the upper lid normally just covers the upper cornea but the lower lid lies below the cornea. Compare the two palpebral fissures and measure any differences. Observe whether there is any contraction of the frontalis muscles, which may be seen when patients with partial ptosis attempt to open their eyes. In such cases, the patient may be unable to open the eyes if the frontalis muscle is fixed with a finger. Also note any proptosis.

Disorders of Eye Movements

NUCLEAR AND INFRANUCLEAR LESIONS OF CRANIAL NERVES III, IV, AND VI Misalignment of the visual axes during binocular viewing usually causes diplopia unless the patient can suppress the image from one eye. Such a deviation, or tropia, may be due to childhood strabismus or neurologic disease. In the case of childhood strabismus, diplopia is seldom a complaint and the deviation is similar in all gaze angles; that is, it is concomitant. In the case of acquired disease, diplopia is the rule and the deviation is greatest when the eye is directed into the field of action of the paretic muscle.

In the case of abducens palsy, the diplopia is horizontal and is worse when looking at objects located at a distance and on the side of the palsy; the affected eye fails to abduct fully. Leading causes of abducens palsy are nerve infarction in association with diabetes or hypertension, craniocerebral trauma, and intracranial tumor. The latter two causes often reflect traction on cranial nerve VI as it bends sharply over the petrous temporal bone (Fig. 4-5). A benign form that is more common in children occurs after viral infections and immunizations. A lesion of the abducens nucleus affects both motoneurons and the internuclear neurons that project to the contralateral medial rectus portion of the third cranial nerve; this causes an ipsilateral, conjugate gaze palsy. An ipsilateral peripheral facial palsy often coexists because of the genu of cranial nerve VII, which encircles the abducens nucleus.

With trochlear palsy, the diplopia is vertical and is worse when viewing objects in the inferior field; the adducted eye may not depress fully. A head tilt to the contralateral side of the lesion may be present. Chronic fourth nerve palsy may be difficult to diagnose accurately, but tilting the head (ear to shoulder) toward the affected, higher eye increases the vertical deviation (Fig. 4-11). An isolated vertical deviation that does *not* change with head tilt is likely to be a skew deviation, which is due to abnormality of prenuclear inputs from the otolithic organs of the ear. These projections synapse in the vestibular nucleus

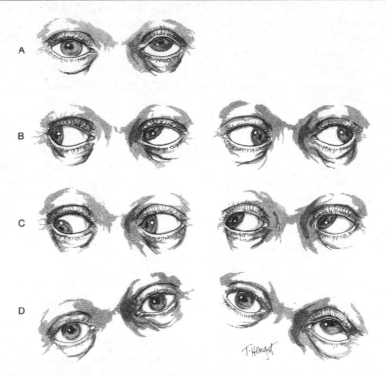

Figure 4-11   The diagnosis of vertical ocular deviation. The steps in the diagnosis of a left superior oblique palsy are shown. *A.* In the primary position there is a left hypertropia. This could be due to weakness of elevators of the right eye or depressors of the left eye. *B.* The deviation becomes worse on gaze to the right. This implies weakness of the right superior rectus or the left superior oblique. *C.* With the eyes in right gaze, the deviation is more marked on looking down. This implies weakness of the left superior oblique muscle. *D.* The Bielschowsky head-tilt test. With a rightward head tilt, there is no detectable vertical deviation of the eyes (this would be the patient's preferred head position). With the head tilted to the left, there is an exaggeration of the left hypertropia. (Adapted from Leigh and Zee, 1991.)

and ascend in the contralateral MLF to the interstitial nucleus of Cajal. Fourth nerve palsy most commonly follows head trauma; when it is bilateral, this is probably due to forces transmitted by the tentorial edge to the nerves as they emerge from the dorsal surface of the brainstem (Fig. 4-5).

Fully developed third cranial nerve palsy is characterized by complete ptosis, a fixed middilated pupil, and a resting eye position that is "down and out." An isolated paresis of adduction of the eye is unlikely to be due to cranial nerve III palsy; this finding usually is due to internuclear ophthalmoplegia (Fig. 4-4). The most common causes of cranial nerve III palsy are nerve infarction in association with diabetes or hypertension and aneurysms of the carotid artery. Sparing of the pupil cannot be relied on to distinguish these etiologies. Lesions of the nucleus of cranial nerve III are rare and may be characterized by bilateral ptosis and superior rectus weakness (reflecting the innervation of these muscles; see above).

Combined lesions of cranial nerves III, IV, and VI may occur with lesions in the region of the cavernous sinus, generalized neuropathies such as Guillain-Barré and Miller Fisher syndromes, and trauma. When the examination suggests involvement of one or more motor cranial nerves, disease at the neuromuscular junction—especially myasthenia gravis—should be considered.

PRENUCLEAR AND SUPRANUCLEAR LESIONS

Pons and Medulla.   Lesions of the medial longitudinal fasciculus (Fig. 4-4) produce internuclear ophthalmoplegia (INO), which is characterized by paresis of adduction for conjugate movements on the side of the lesion and "dissociated nystagmus" characterized by abduction overshoot of the eye contralateral to the lesion. A combined lesion of one

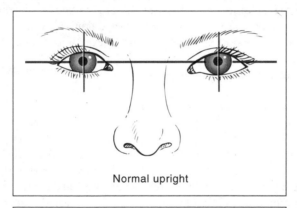

Normal upright

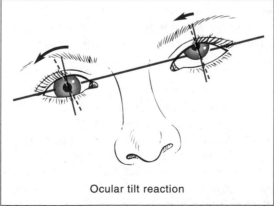

Ocular tilt reaction

Figure 4-12   The ocular tilt reaction represented as a "motor compensation" of a lesion-induced apparent eye-head tilt (dashed line), which would be opposite in direction to the apparent tilt. Eyes and head are continuously adjusted to what the lesioned brain computes as being vertical. (Adapted from Brandt and Dieterich, 1987.)

MLF and the adjacent abducens nucleus (Fig. 4-4) produces paralysis of all conjugate movements except for abductio.. of the eye contralateral to the side of the lesion, the "one-and-a-half" syndrome. Discrete lesions of the PPRF, which contains saccadic burst neurons, cause loss of saccades and quick phases of nystagmus to the side of the lesion. Smooth pursuit, the vestibulo-ocular reflex, and gaze-holding ability may be spared, but the lesion often involves the adjacent fibers serving these functions. The best known example of the effects of disease that affects the vestibular nuclei is *Wallenberg syndrome* (lateral medullary infarction). This syndrome consists of ipsilateral impairment of pain and temperature sensation over the face, Horner syndrome, limb ataxia, dysarthria, and dysphagia, as well as, contralaterally, impairment of pain and temperature sensation over the trunk and limbs. The disorder most commonly is due to occlusion of the ipsilateral vertebral artery. The characteristic disorder of eye movements is lateropulsion: The eyes deviate conjugately toward the side of the lesion if the eyes are closed or with saccades. Spontaneous nystagmus in Wallenberg syndrome is usually horizontal or mixed horizontal-torsional with the slow phases directed toward the side of the lesion, although it may reverse direction in eccentric positions, suggesting coexistent involvement of the gaze-holding mechanism. In addition, an ipsilateral *ocular tilt reaction* may be present: a skew or deviation (ocular deviation with the ipsilateral eye down), extorsion of the ipsilateral eye (upper pole out), intorsion of the contralateral eye (upper pole in), and ipsilateral head tilt (Fig. 4-12). The ocular tilt reaction reflects an imbalance of otolithic inputs (Brandt and Dieterich, 1994).

Midbrain.   Bilateral infarction in the region of the riMLF (Fig. 4-6) causes deficits of either downward of both upward and downward saccades. Lesions of the interstitial nucleus of Cajal (INC) may impair gaze-holding function in the vertical plane and produce a contralateral ocular tilt reaction. Bilateral lesions of the medial longitudinal fasciculus (bilateral INO) impair vertical vestibular and pursuit movements and cause vertical gaze-evoked nystagmus but spare vertical saccades, which are generated in the riMLF. Lesions of the posterior commissure cause a loss of upward gaze; usually all types of eye movement are affected, although the vestibulo-ocular reflex and Bell's phenomenon sometimes may be spared. Other findings with dorsal midbrain lesions include slowing of vertical saccades below the horizontal meridian, disorders of convergence and "convergence-retraction nystagmus," light-near dissociation of the pupils, and eyelid retraction.

Cerebellum.   Disease affecting the flocculus and paraflocculus of the cerebellum (classically with Chiari malformations) causes downbeat nystagmus, deficient smooth pursuit, gaze-evoked nystagmus, and rebound nystagmus. Rebound nystagmus occurs after one attempts to hold the eye in far eccentric gaze. For example, after the eyes have been held in far right gaze and are returned to midposition, rebound nystagmus beating to the right may occur. When disease affects the midline cerebellar nodulus, patients may show periodic alternating nystagmus, in which the horizontal direction of the quick phases changes about every 2 min. Lesions affecting the dorsal vermis produce dysmetria or inaccuracy of saccades, typically with overshoots. When the fastigial nucleus is also involved, a severe form of saccadic dysmetria may occur in which the eyes repetitively overshoot a stationary target, so-called macrosaccadic oscillations. Smooth pursuit also may be impaired.

Cerebral Hemispheres, Basal Ganglia, and Superior Colliculus. An acute lesion of one cerebral hemisphere—especially if it is large, right-sided, or posterior—causes conjugate deviation of the eyes toward the side of the lesion. Unilateral lesions of the temporoparietal region produce impairment of smooth pursuit that is more marked when the stimulus moves toward the side of the lesion. With a hand-held "optokinetic" tape or drum, less nystagmus is generated as the stimulus moves toward the side of the lesion. Bilateral parietofrontal lesions may cause acquired oculomotor apraxia, in which there is loss of voluntary control of eye movements (in response, for example, to "look right") but preservation of vestibular slow and quick phases of nystagmus with rotation in an office chair. Oculomotor apraxia and peripheral visual inattention and optic ataxia (inaccurate reaching of the limbs to visual targets) are components of Balint syndrome.

Nystagmus is a repetitive to-and-fro movement of the eyes that includes smooth sinusoidal oscillations and alternation of slow drift and the corrective quick phase. Normal subjects show nystagmus during self-rotation in response to vestibular and optokinetic stimulation; this nystagmus preserves clear vision. Pathologic nystagmus reflects failure of the normal mechanisms that hold gaze steady: visual fixation, the vestibulo-ocular reflex, and the mechanism for holding the eyes at an eccentric position in the orbit. Pathologic nystagmus impairs clear vision and can cause oscillopsia—illusory motion of the environment. Impairment of vision (e.g., as a result of a tumor of the optic nerve) may lead to nystagmus (which may be monocular). Disease of the vestibular labyrinth is discussed in the section on cranial nerve VIII. Nystagmus induced by assuming an eccentric position in the orbit it called gaze-evoked nystagmus; it reflects inadequacy of the tonic signal required to hold the eyes away from the midposition and occurs with cerebellar and medullary lesions. Seesaw nystagmus is characterized by oscillations in which one half cycle consists of elevation and intorsion of one eye and synchronous depression and extortion of the other eye; during the next half cycle, the vertical and torsional movements reverse. Seesaw nystagmus occurs with lesions that affect the INO and with large parasellar lesions, such as pituitary tumors, that compress the upper brainstem. It is important to differentiate these acquired disorders from congenital nystagmus, which requires no neurologic investigation. Congenital nystagmus is characterized by horizontal, conjugate oscillations that often suppress on convergence and by waveforms that show "foveation periods" when the eyes are momentarily still. Long-standing head turns are common. "Latent nystagmus" occurs or increases when one eye is covered; it occurs in patients who lack binocular vision and often have strabismus.

Saccadic intrusions differ from nystagmus in that the abnormal movement that takes the eye off the target is an inappropriate saccade rather than the slow drift of nystagmus. The most common are square-wave jerks, which are small saccades that take the eye away from the fixation position and return it after a period of about 200 ms. They occur in normal subjects but are more common in cerebellar disorders, progressive supranuclear palsy, and cerebral hemispheric disease. Macro square-wave jerks (square-wave pulses) are large oscillations that occurs at a frequency of about 2 to 3 Hz and after taking the eye off the target, return it with a latency of about 80 ms. They are encountered in disease states that disrupt cerebellar outflow, such as multiple sclerosis. Macrosaccadic oscillations usually consist of horizontal saccades that occurs in bursts, building up and then decreasing in amplitude, with intersaccadic intervals of about 200 ms. The occur in disease affecting the cerebellum, especially the fastigial nucleus. Saccadic oscillations without an intersaccadic interval may occur in one direction, usually the horizontal plane (ocular flutter), or may be multivectorial (opsoclonus or saccadomania). The frequency of oscillations is high, typically 10 to 15 cycles per second, and is higher with smaller-size movements. Ataxia and encephalopathy also may accompany opsoclonus. Opsoclonus may be postviral, caused by drug intoxication, or a manifestation of a remote tumor (especially neuroblastoma in children and ovarian cancer in adults).

Disorders of Pupillary Function

The most common diagnostic problem is pupillary inequality (anisocoria). Healthy individuals may show anisocoria of 0.5 mm or more; however, their pupils respond normally to light. Ocular disease or prior trauma may cause anisocoria. The three most important neurologic causes of anisocoria are Horner syndrome, Adie syndrome, and cranial nerve III palsy. These disease entities should be differentiated from anisocoria resulting from drugs. An algorithm for diagnosing anisocoria is useful (Fig. 4-13).

Horner syndrome consists of miosis, ptosis, and anhydrosis and results from a lesion of the sympathetic pathways at some site from the hypothalamus to the orbit. In practice, diagnosing Horner syndrome rests on testing the pupils because lid asymmetries are common (see below) and anhydrosis is difficult to demonstrate at the beside. The anisocoria becomes more evident in dim illumination, and there is a "dilatation lag" of the affected pupil when the lights are turned down. The diagnosis is confirmed by applying 2 drops of 10% cocaine to both eyes and measuring pupil size after 45 min. If the miotic pupil fails to dilate (compared with the other eye), Horner syndrome is confirmed. To determine if the Horner syndrome is due to a pre- or postganglionic lesion of the sympathetic pathway, apply 2 drops of 1% hydroxyamphetamine (Paredrine) to each eye. If the miotic pupil dilates less than does the other pupil, the lesion is most likely postganglionic. The interval between the cocaine and hydroxyamphetamine tests must be at least 72 h. Postganglionic Horner syndrome may be due to carotid or cavernous sinus disease. Preganglionic Horner syndrome raises the possibility of apical lung tumor and a spinal or brainstem process (e.g., lateral medullary syndrome).

Anisocoria may be due to *Adie's tonic pupil*, which is caused by degeneration of postganglionic neurons in the ciliary ganglion and is usually unilateral. The affected pupil is usually mydriatic and responds poorly to light. With a near stimulus, the pupil constricts in a brisk and sustained (tonic) manner and redilatation is slow. An associated finding is reduced deep tendon reflexes; however, affected individuals may be otherwise healthy. Diagnosis rests on demonstrating denervation hypersensitivity with 0.125% pilocarpine. Forty-five min after the application of 2 drops to each eye, only the tonic pupil will have constricted.

A more serious cause of anisocoria resulting from unilateral mydriasis is *cranial nerve III palsy*. Pupillary dilatation may be the first sign of compression of the oculomotor nerve by aneurysm or during uncal herniation because the parasympathetic fibers lie peripherally in nerve. Often, however, anisocoria results from the effects of mydriatic drugs such as atropine. To determine whether a fixed, dilated pupil is due to cranial nerve III palsy or mydriatic agents, apply pilocarpine 1% eyedrops (Fig. 4-13); they will cause the former but not the latter to constrict. Argyll Robertson pupils resulting from neurosyphilis

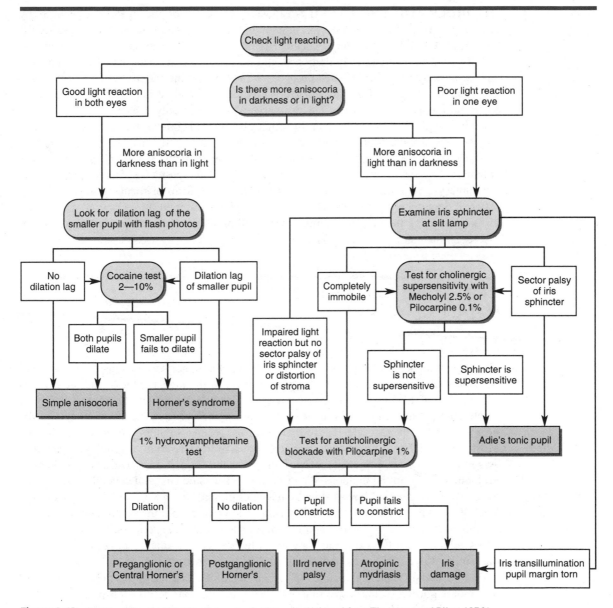

Figure 4-13 An algorithm to aid in the diagnosis of anisocoria. (Adapted from Thompson and Piley, 1976.)

are now rare; however, small, irregular pupils that constrict with a near stimulus but not with light are encountered in other disorders, such as diabetes.

Lesions of the optic pathway such as optic neuritis do not cause anisocoria because of the consensual light reflex. However, by using the swinging flashlight test, a relatively afferent pupillary defect can be demonstrated: The pupil of the affected eye dilates as the flashlight is moved over to stimulate it.

DISORDERS OF THE EYELIDS Ptosis—drooping of the eyelid—is caused by several processes. Lid dehiscence is common in the elderly and is of no neurologic significance. Diseases affecting the extraocular muscles and lids, such as ocular myopathies, usually produce symmetric limitation of the lids and vertical gaze. Neuromuscular disease, especially myasthenia, often produces variable, asymmetric ptosis that worsens during sustained upgaze. The ptosis of Horner syndrome is slight but often also affects the lower lid ("upside-down ptosis"). Third nerve palsy commonly causes monocular ptosis except when the location is nuclear, in which case ptosis is bilateral. Supranuclear lesions cause bilateral ptosis; most frequently this occurs with right hemispheric lesions (Averbuch-Heller, 1996). Eyelid opening apraxia describes patients who can open their eyes spontaneously but cannot do so on command. Blepharospasm consists of paroxysmal, involuntary contractions of the orbicularis oculi; it is a form of focal dystonia and may reflect a dopaminergic disorder in the basal ganglia. Sustained lid retraction occurs with lesions affecting the posterior commissure (Collier's sign) but is also a feature of orbital disorders, including Graves disease.

THE TRIGEMINAL NERVE (CRANIAL NERVE V)

Anatomy and Physiology

The trigeminal nerve contains somatic motor fibers that innervate the muscles of mastication and somatic sensory fibers that supply the skin of the face, the teeth, and the mucous membranes of the mouth and nasal cavities. The cell bodies of the motor fibers are located in the trigeminal motor nucleus in the pons, which lies in the lateral margin of the floor of the fourth ventricle. These motorneurons receive bilateral corticobulbar inputs. Most somatic afferent fibers have their cell bodies in the gasserian or semilunar ganglion. Trigeminal afferents project to one of three nuclei (Fig. 4-14): rostrally, the mesencephalic nucleus; in the midpons, the principal sensory nucleus; and caudally, the nucleus of the spinal trigeminal tract ("spinal nucleus of cranial nerve V"), which extends to the level of C4. The motor and sensory roots emerge together from the ventrolateral aspect of the midpons. The nerve passes ventrally through the pontine cistern, and the sensory portion swells to form the gasserian ganglion, which rests in a small groove on the apex of the temporal pyramid bone, empouched in dura. After piercing the dura, the nerve splits into three division: the ophthalmic (V1), the maxillary (V2), and the mandibular (V3). The motor portion of the nerve runs with V3. The ophthalmic division passes ventrally and rostrally through the lateral wall of the cavernous sinus, below the trochlear nerve, to reach to the superior orbital fissure. There it gives branches that supply the dura mater. After passing through the superior orbital fissure, it supplies the lacrimal gland, skin of the forehead to the vertex, cornea, conjunctiva, sphenoid sinus, and mucous membrane of the anterior part of the nose. The maxillary division lies below the cavernous sinus, where it gives small meningeal fibers before passing through the foramen rotundum. It emerges through the infraorbital foramen to innervate the skin of the maxilla, the anterior part of the temple and teeth of the upper jaw, and the mucous membrane of the posterior nasal cavity and hard palate. The mandibular division leaves the skull through the foramen

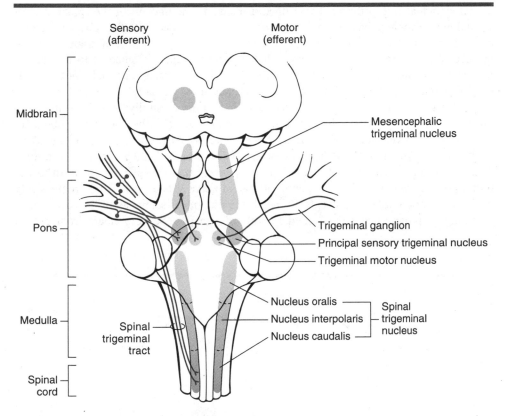

Figure 4-14 Location of sensory *(left)* and motor *(right)* components of the trigeminal system. (Adapted from Kandel, Schwartz, and Jessell, 1991.)

ovale, where it splits into auriculotemporal, lingual, long buccal, inferior dental, and masticatory branches. The last of these branches supplies the muscles of mastication—temporalis, masseter, and external and internal pterygoids—as well as the tensor veli palatini and tensor tympani muscles. The distribution of the cutaneous branches is summarized in Fig. 4-15.

In interpreting findings from an examination of the trigeminal nerve, it is helpful to understand the somatotopic organization of afferent projections to the trigeminal nuclei (Fig. 4-14). The afferent fibers that project to the mesencephalic nucleus are anatomically peculiar, since their cell bodies are located centrally in this nucleus rather than in the gasserian ganglion. They are thought to convey proprioceptive inputs concerned with jaw movements but not eye movements (Porter et al, 1983). The principal sensory nucleus lies lateral to the trigeminal motor nucleus and receives thick fibers that probably are concerned with the perception of touch. On the other hand, the fibers that project to the spinal nucleus of cranial nerve V are predominantly thin and are concerned mainly with pain perception. After entering the pons, most trigeminal afferent fibers run caudally in the spinal tract of cranial nerve V, which lies just under the lateral surface of the medulla and extends as low as the fourth cervical segment, where it becomes continuous with the lateral spinothalamic pathway. These fibers synapse in the nucleus of the spinal tract of cranial nerve V, which lies medial to the tract and is continuous with the substantia gelatinosa of the spinal cord. The neurons of the nucleus of the spinal tract of cranial nerve V project across the midline to the quintothalamic tract, which is adjacent to the medial lemniscus, and ascend to the ventral posterior medial and intralaminar nuclei of the thalamus. Fibers from the ophthalmic division terminate most caudally in the nucleus of the spinal tract of cranial nerve V, the maxillary fibers more rostrally, and the mandibular fibers most rostrally. Within the spinal tract of cranial nerve V, the ophthalmic fibers are distributed most ventrally, the maxillary fibers more dorsally, and the mandibular fibers most dorsally. An alternative scheme proposed by Dejerine is that there is an "onion skin" distribution (Fig. 4-15), with afferents from the perioral skin synapsing in the most rostral portion of the nucleus of the spinal tract of cranial nerve V and fibers from progressively more concentric circles that eventually reach the outermost segments of the face, corresponding to progressively more caudal levels of synapse. Sensory fibers from cranial

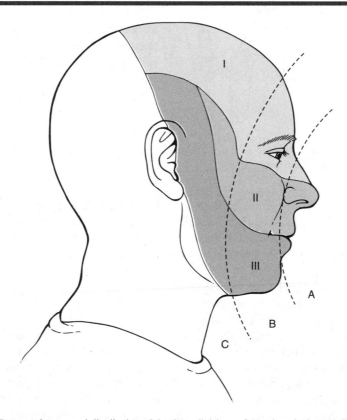

Figure 4-15 Pattern of segmental distribution of the three divisions of the trigeminal nerve. The dashed concentric lines represent the alternative onion skin distribution of afferents in the nucleus of the spinal tract. The perioral region *(A)* is represented in the most rostral portion of the nucleus, and *B* and *C* are represented progressively more caudally. (Adapted from Kandel, Schwartz, and Jessell, 1991.)

nerves VII, IX, and X also enter the descending tract of the fifth cranial nerve, carrying inputs from the external ear and the mucous membrane of the larynx and pharynx.

Clinical Examination

In examining the sensory functions of the trigeminal nerve, the most important modality to be tested is pain. Use a sterile pin and ask the patient to compare the sharpness of the stimulus when it is applied to the right side and then the left side of each of the three divisional dermatomes (Fig. 4-15). If sensory loss is present, determine whether it is worse in a divisional or a segmental pattern (Fig. 4-15). Touch and temperature and be tested in a similar manner. Sometimes it is useful to test sensation over the nasal mucosa by tickling with a cotton swab. Test the corneal reflex by touching the cornea (not the sclera) with cotton while the patient looks up. Observe both the direct and the consensual responses and ask the patient whether the sensation is the same on both sides.

Examine motor function of the trigeminal nerve by palpating the masseter and temporalis muscles as the patient clenches the teeth. Ask the patient to open the mouth and look for a deviation; the jaw will deviate laterally to the side of the weak pterygoid muscle. If there is jaw deviation, compare the power of the pterygoid muscles as the patient attempts to laterally deviate the open jaw laterally. Test the jaw jerk by striking your finger placed on the patient's chin with the patient's mouth slightly opened. Many normal individuals lack a jaw jerk; when it is increased, it may help determine whether a corticospinal lesion lies above the level of the pons. Since the jaw jerk is the only muscle stretch reflex that can be tested easily in the cranial nerves, it can be used to detect a corticospinal tract lesion above the level of the cervical cord.

Disorders of Function

Among the more common disorders that affect the trigeminal nerve are local processes within the face and paranasal sinuses; in such cases, involvement may be restricted to individual divisions of cranial nerve V, including the motor division. When the trigeminal nerve is involved by disease within the cavernous sinus, such as a tumor, aneurysm, or inflammation, the nerves supplying the extraocular movements often are also involved, producing the picture of "painful ophthalmoplegia." Involvement of the gasserian ganglion by herpes zoster most often causes pain and skin rash in the ophthalmic division. The ganglion also may be involved by an inflammatory process affecting the underlying temporal bone, and in this case, pain is usually in V1 and may be accompanied by ipsilateral sixth nerve palsy (Gradenigo syndrome). This entity also can be produced by tumors, such as nasopharyngeal carcinoma growing up through the foramen lacerum. A common disorder involving cranial nerve V is trigeminal neuralgia. Lancinating pain may affect one or more divisions and be triggered by cold or other tactile stimuli. In this condition, also known as tic douloureux, the trigeminal nerve examination is normal. The trigeminal nerve also is often affected by brainstem disorders because of the long rostrocaudal extent of its nuclei. Thus, pain sensation in the face may be impaired in syringobulbia, which affects crossing fibers, and in Wallenberg syndrome, in which lateral medullary infarction involves the spinal tract of cranial nerve V and its nucleus. Cerebral hemispheric disease seldom produces either sensory or motor findings confined to the face. Finally, facial sensory symptoms—pain and numbness—are common in psychologic disorders; in these cases, careful attention to whether the symptoms conform to the dermatomes of the trigeminal nerve is crucial.

THE FACIAL NERVE (CRANIAL NERVE VII) AND THE INTERMEDIATE NERVE

Anatomy and Physiology

The facial nerve contains somatic motor fibers that supply the muscles of facial expression. The intermediate nerve, which runs with it, carries visceral efferent and afferent fibers. The visceral afferents, which convey taste, have their cell bodies in the geniculate ganglion and synapse in the nucleus of the solitary tract (Fig. 4-16). The somatic motor fibers originate in the facial nucleus, which lies deep in the reticular formation of the caudal pons, ventromedial to the nucleus of the spinal tract of cranial nerve V. Visceral efferent neurons lie in the superior salivary nucleus, which is located dorsolateral to the caudal end of the somatic motor nucleus. From this double origin, axons pass dorsomedially, hooking over the abducens nucleus, just beneath the fourth ventricle, and then run ventrolaterally to leave the brainstem between the olive and the inferior cerebellar peduncle, in the cerebellopontine angle.

The facial nerve, the intermediate nerve, and cranial nerve VIII enter the internal auditory meatus surrounded by a common dural sheath. Thereafter, the facial and intermediate nerves enter the facial canal of the temporal bone and after a short distance make a sharp bend posteriorly; at this point, the intermediate nerve swells to form the geniculate ganglia and gives off the greater superficial petrosal nerve. This nerve reenters the skull to leave again via the foramen lacerum, passes through the pterygoid canal, and synapses in the sphenopalatine ganglion to innervate the lacrimal gland. As it continues its course in the facial canal, cranial nerve VII runs close to the wall of the tympanic cavity, where it gives off somatic efferent fibers to the stapedius muscle. Subsequently, the intermediate nerve gives off the chorda tympani branch, which runs submucously in the tympanic cavity and then leaves to join the lingual nerve, a branch of cranial nerve V. In this way, visceral efferent fibers innervate the submandibular and sublingual salivary glands and visceral afferents, conveying taste from the anterior two-thirds of the tongue, project to the brainstem nucleus of the solitary tract. The facial nerve then bends for a second time and runs downward to the stylomastoid foramen, where it exits the skull. In its extracranial course, it penetrates the parotid gland, where it forms a plexus and splits into branches to innervate the facial muscles, the stylohyoid, the posterior belly of the digastric, and the platysma. The facial nerve also carries a small and variable somatic afferent component that supplies the skin in the external auditory meatus and the concha of the ear.

Corticobulbar fibers that mediate voluntary movements of the face project to the pons. Although the cortical innervation of the facial muscles is incompletely understood (Jenny

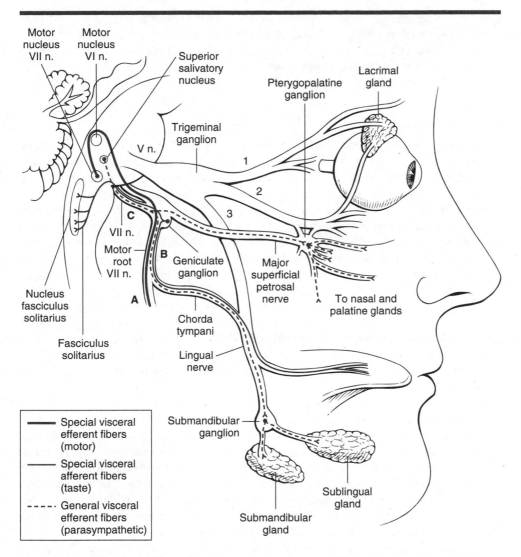

Figure 4-16 Schematic representation of the anatomic pathways of the facial nerve. *A*, *B*, and *C* denote lesions of the facial nerve at the stylomastoid foramen, distal and proximal to the geniculate ganglion, respectively. Dashed lines indicate the parasympathetic fibers, full lines indicate motor fibers, and dash and dot lines indicate visceral afferent fibers (taste). (Adapted from Carpenter, 1978.)

and Saper, 1987; Meyer et al, 1994), muscles above the palpebral fissure appear to receive bilateral projections, whereas muscles below the palpebral fissure receive crossed projections. Other projections to the facial nucleus, perhaps from limbic structures and the basal ganglion, which mediate emotional facial movements, may be bilateral. The facial muscles are involved in several reflexes, notably blinking in response to corneal stimulation (corneal reflex) or bright illumination, and contraction of the stapedius muscle (which controls the compliance of the auditory ossicular chain) in response to loud sounds. Taste inputs from chorda tympani synapse in the nucleus of the solitary tract and are relayed to a pontine "taste center" that lies adjacent to the parabrachial nucleus, next to the thalamus, and finally to the insular cortex, where there is convergence with olfaction (Zatorre and Jones-Gotman, 1992).

Clinical Examination

In evaluating the facial nerve, usually two main judgments must be made: (1) Is there any facial weakness and (2) if there is facial weakness, is it due to an *upper motor lesion* (e.g., after a hemispheric stroke causing hemiplegia) or a *lower motor lesion* (peripheral facial palsy)? The first question can be addressed by looking for asymmetry of the patient's nasolabial folds (from the edge of each nostril to the corner of the mouth) both at rest and during movement when the patient is asked to "show me your teeth." Asymmetry, especially of the movement, indicates facial weakness. The second question can be answered best by noting the symmetry of eyebrow raising; weakness of the frontalis muscle indicates a lower motor neuron lesion. In addition, eye closure (orbicularis oculi), blowing out the cheeks (buccinator), pursing the lips (orbicularis oris), and movements of the skin of the neck (platysma can be tested). Ask the patient to blink repetitively and note whether synkinetic movements of other facial muscles occur, such as "jaw winking." This Marcus Gunn sign results from aberrant regeneration of the facial nerve after a prior palsy. Note whether tearing is present; not only is this helpful in localization, it is important for managing eye care if the patient cannot close the lid adequately.

The complaint of loss of taste often results from olfactory loss; most of our ability to detect the flavor of foods depends on smell. True taste is the sensory information obtained from the gustatory system and includes sweet, salty, sour, bitter, and possibly a metallic sensation; it appears to be more resistant to the effects of aging and disease than is olfaction. In patients with facial nerve palsy, test taste by holding the protruded tongue, using cotton gauze and placing test solutions on one or the other side of the anterior two-thirds of the tongue with cotton-tip applicators. Make up separate solutions with salt, sugar, sour (lemon), and bitter (quinine or crushed acetaminophen tablets). Instruct the patient to indicate the taste of the stimulus by pointing to written labels.

Several facial reflexes can be tested (apart from the corneal reflex described in the section on cranial nerve V). The glabellar reflex is elicited by tapping the forehead between the eyes; the orbicularis oculi muscles reflexly contract. In normal subjects, this response habituates with repeated stimuli, but it persists in some patients with parkinsonian syndromes. Light percussion over the lips may induce contraction of the levator anguli oris muscles (the "snout" or "pout" reflex). This and the suck reflex (elicited by stroking the lips with a tongue depressor) normally are present only during the first year of life but return in patients with a variety of bihemispheric or degenerative disorders.

Disorders of Function

Facial palsy is the most common cranial nerve disorder. Injuries to the face or the parotid gland may cause partial facial weakness. Idiopathic Bell's palsy, which often occurs in the setting of an upper respiratory tract illness, probably affects the nerve in the facial canal after the greater superficial petrosal nerve comes off, since tearing usually is preserved. Infections involving the middle ear and the temporal bone may cause facial palsy, as may temporal bone fractures. Such lesions also may affect the chorda tympani. The best documented disorder affecting the geniculate ganglion is herpes zoster, which causes pain in the ear, vesicles in the external auditory canal, facial palsy, and often vertigo or hearing loss from involvement of the adjacent cranial nerve VIII. Lesions in the cerebellopontine angle—classically schwannomas of cranial nerve VIII—also may lead to deafness, vertigo, and facial palsy. Such lesions, which are central to the point where the greater superficial petrosal nerve comes off, also cause loss of tearing. Disease prior to the departure of the chorda tympani causes loss of taste in the anterior two-thirds of the homolateral half of the tongue. Lesions central to the point where the tensor tympani is given off, corresponding to the pyramidal eminence in the tympanic cavity, cause hyperacusia—sounds seeming too loud. Bilateral peripheral facial palsy usually indicates an infectious or carcinomatous meningitic process, sarcoid, Lyme disease, or the Guillain-Barré syndrome. Within the brainstem, lesions in the pontine tegmentum also affect the fascicles of cranial nerves VII as they hook over the abducens nucleus; the result is a horizontal gaze palsy and ipsilateral facial palsy. After recovery from facial palsy, synkinetic movements such as eyelid closure with forced mouth closure reflect aberrant regeneration. The most common is "jaw winking" (see above).

Unilateral facial weakness is a common feature of disease affecting the pyramidal tracts as they descend from cortex to brainstem. Such patients with "central facial weakness" show sparing of the frontalis muscles and relative sparing of the orbicularis oculi, but the muscles of the lower face are weak. Other descending pathways project bilaterally to all the facial muscles so that a dissociation between the voluntary and emotional facial movements may be observed. Thus, certain patients with central facial weakness may be able to smile symmetrically in response to a joke but not when they mimic the examiner's smile.

As noted above under "Disorders of the Eyelids," voluntary blinking is under corticobulbar control, but spontaneous blinking and emotional blinking are influenced by the basal ganglia and substantia nigra. Thus, blink rate is decreased in some parkinsonian syndromes and increased in drug-induced dyskinesias and in Tourette syndrome. Blepharospasm may be associated with oromandibular dystonia, in which case it is called Meige syndrome. Intermittent, involuntary contractions of the facial muscles on one side—hemifacial spasm—may reflect compression of the facial nerve by blood vessels or tumors in the cerebellopontine angle.

THE VESTIBULOCOCHLEAR NERVE (CRANIAL NERVE VIII)

The vestibulocochlear nerve subserves two different senses—balance and hearing—both of which depend on a similar mechanical-neural transduction process that is achieved by "hair cells" of the vestibular labyrinth and the organ of Corti.

THE VESTIBULAR NERVE

Anatomy and Physiology

The vestibular nerve carries impulses from the cristae of the semicircular canals, which sense head rotation, and the maculae of the utricle and saccule, which sense linear motion and static tilt of the head. Both the cristae and the maculae contain hair cells which possess cilia that transduce mechanical shearing forces into neural impulses. In the semicircular canals, the hair cell cilia project into a gelatinous saillike structure called the cupula. Angular acceleration of the head displaces the endolymph of the semicircular canals, and this bends the cupula and the cilia of the hair cells. The cilia of hair cells in the maculae of the utricle and saccule project into a gelatinous membrane in which are embedded crystals of calcium carbonate — the ear stones, or otoconia. Movement of the otoconia in response to linear acceleration and gravity stimulates cilia of these hair cells. Certain physiologic properties of the vestibular organs have a direct bearing on clinical disturbances. First, even with the head stationary, there is a resting discharge in the primary vestibular afferents. Second, with head movements the discharge from afferents from one ear increase whereas the inputs from the other decrease. Third, the central vestibular system is constantly "recalibrating" so that it can accurately interpret differences between the discharges of the vestibular afferents as head movements.

A superior branch of the vestibular nerve carries information from the anterior and lateral semicircular canals and utricle and an inferior branch from the posterior semicircular canals and saccule. The superior branch runs with the facial nerve, and the inferior branch runs with the cochlear nerve. The vestibular nerve has its bipolar cell bodies in the vestibular ganglion of Scarpa, which lies at the bottom of the internal auditory meatus. The vestibular nerve passes through the cerebellopontine angle to enter the medulla between the inferior cerebellar peduncle dorsally and the spinal tract of cranial nerve V ventrally. The vestibular nuclear complex lies in the floor of the fourth ventricle, mainly in its lateral recess. The medial and superior vestibular nuclei are concerned primarily with vestibulo-ocular reflexes, whereas the lateral and descending nuclei are more concerned with vestibulospinal reactions. The vestibular nuclei have a commissural connection and project extensively to other brainstem structures and the cerebellum and, via the ventroposterior lateral thalamic nucleus, to cortical areas, especially the insular cortex of the temporoparietal junction.

Clinical Examination

In a patient who complains of "dizziness," before preceding with the examination, it is useful to determine whether the symptom is a form of vertigo (the illusion of movement) or is due to another process, such as presyncope, postural unsteadiness, or psychologic feelings such as panic. In patients who complain of vertigo at the time they are evaluated, look for nystagmus and note its characteristics. Determine whether the nystagmus increases when visual fixation is prevented, using Frenzel goggles (plus 20-diopter lenses, with a flashlight to view the eyes will suffice) or by transiently covering the viewing eye during ophthalmoscopy in an otherwise dark room.

Evaluate the *vestibulo-ocular reflex*, which generates eye movements to compensate for head movements so that the line of sight remains steady (Fig. 4-17). Vestibularly evoked eye movements are generated much more promptly (latency to onset less than 16 ms) than are visually mediated eye movements (latency to onset greater than 100 ms), and this difference can be applied to beside testing. The vestibulo-ocular reflex also can be tested by ophthalmoscopy, observing (through glasses, if worn) the optic nerve and retinal vessels as the patient shakes the head from side to side in small movements at about 2 cycles per second and fixates on a distant, stationary target. If the reflex is appropriate, eye and head movements cancel out and the retinal vessels and optic disc appear stationary.

The contribution of each ear to the vestibulo-ocular reflex is best tested by *caloric stimulation*, and when indicated, this can be performed at the beside. After verifying that the tympanic membrane is intact and that wax is absent, elevate the patient's head 30° on a pillow to place the lateral semicircular canal in a vertical position. Ideally, eye move-

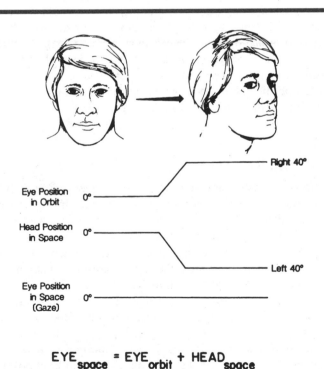

$$EYE_{space} = EYE_{orbit} + HEAD_{space}$$

Figure 4-17 The function of the vestibulo-ocular reflex. As the head is rapidly turned to the left, the eyes move by a corresponding amount in the orbit to the right. Below, head position in space and eye position in the orbit are plotted against time. Because the movements of head and eye in orbit are equal and opposite, the sum, eye position in space (the angle of gaze or gaze), remains zero (bottom equation). If gaze is held steady, images do not slip on the retina and vision remains clear. (Adapted from Leigh and Zee, 1991.)

ments should be observed behind Frenzel goggles or recorded in darkness to avoid the effects of visual fixation. A normal response can be elicited with as little as 0.2 mL of ice-cold water. The strategy of this "minimal ice-water caloric" test is to compare the thresholds for inducing nystagmus from the two ears.

In patients who report vertigo when they change head position (see below), carry out *positional testing*. Start with the patient seated on the examination table. Explain the nature of the testing and the importance of keeping the eyes open and reporting symptoms as they occur. Then, after turning the patient's head to one shoulder, swiftly move the patient's head and neck "en bloc" into a head-hanging (down 30 to 45 degrees) position. Note the presence of any latency period and the nature of any nystagmus that follows. After about 30 to 60 s (or resolution of symptoms and signs), return the patient to the sitting position and again note the characteristics of any vertigo and nystagmus so induced.

The *vestibulospinal reflexes* can best be evaluated by asking the patient to stand with the feet together and the arms flexed at the elbows and pulled taught against the fingers of each hand, which are hooked under each other against the chest (Jendrassik's maneuver). In this situation, three factors contribute to balance: vision, proprioception (largely at the ankle), and the vestibulospinal reactions. The effects of vision can be excluded by asking the patient to close the eyes. The effects of proprioception can be largely negated by asking the patient to stand on a soft pillow. In this way, the vestibulospinal contributions to steady posture can be "isolated." Ask the patient to walk in place with the eye closed and note tendency to turn in one direction (the Fukuda stepping test). Patients with postural instability can be tested for stability during sitting with the eyes closed (truncal stability). Test for past pointing of the limbs by asking the patient to bring the outstretched upper limb from an initial position above the head downward so that the index finger meets the examiner's index finger. After a trial run with the eyes open, the test is performed with the eyes closed.

Disorders of Function

When disease affects the vestibular organ, the first consequence is an imbalance of inputs from the two ears. As was indicated above, in health, such an unequal discharge rate from the right and left vestibular afferents indicates head movement. In the case of disease, however, the head is stationary and an illusion of movement occurs—vertigo. Vestibular imbalance also causes nystagmus, which is usually mixed horizontal and torsional and is suppressed by visual fixation. In general, the slow phase of nystagmus, the direction of past pointing, and the tendency to fall are all to the side of the lesion. Such a constellation of findings commonly results from viral or other infections that affect the vestibular labyrinth or its nerve. Because of central "recalibration" processes, recovery usually occurs within days.

The most common vestibular disorder is *benign positional vertigo*. Affected patients report brief episodes of vertigo induced by specific changes in head position. During positional testing, after a latency of a few seconds, the patient reports vertigo and develops a mixed torsional-upbeat nystagmus which lasts up to 30 s. When the patient is brought back up to the sitting position, vertigo may be experienced again, this time with down-beating-torsional nystagmus. Benign positional vertigo is thought to be due to detached otoconia that have migrated into one (usually the posterior) semicircular canal. During positional testing, the otoconial debris impedes the normal movement of the cupula and leads to vertigo and nystagmus. Treatment consists of maneuvers and exercises that extricate the otoconial debris from the canal (Brandt et al, 1994). The combination of recurrent vertigo and progressive deafness may be due to ear disease (e.g., Ménière disease), but the possibility of a cranial nerve VIII schwannoma should be considered.

The *central vestibular structures,* such as the nuclei, frequently are involved in a number of disorders of the central nervous system, such as stroke and multiple sclerosis. In such disorders, nystagmus is more commonly in one plane (e.g., downbeat, upbeat, torsional) and is not suppressed by visual fixation. Signs of involvement of adjacent structures, such as the long tracts, often coexist.

THE COCHLEAR NERVE

Anatomy and Physiology

The organ of Corti consists of a spiral array of hair cells and support cells that lie on a basilar membrane covered by a tectorial membrane. Mechanical vibrations of the basilar membrane generate neural impulses. The cell bodies of bipolar neurons that innervate the hair cells are located in the spiral ganglion, which sits in a bony channel that travels in a spiral direction from the base to the apex of the cochlea. The central processes of these neurons run toward the base of the cochlea, enter the internal auditory meatus, and fuse to form the cochlear nerve. The cochlear nerve runs with the vestibular and facial nerves through the cerebellopontine angle to enter the brainstem at the lower border of the pons, dorsolateral to the inferior cerebellar peduncle, and reach the dorsal and ventral cochlear nuclei (Fig. 4-18). The dorsal cochlear nucleus lies lateral to the vestibular complex, producing an "acoustic tubercle" on the dorsal aspect of the inferior cerebellar peduncle. The ventral cochlear nucleus lies lateral to the inferior cerebellar peduncle. Many primary auditory fibers bifurcate and project to both nuclei. Secondary auditory neurons mainly project through the contralateral lateral lemniscus to the inferior colliculus, with some synapsing first in the superior olivary nucleus. From the inferior colliculus, fibers continue via the medial geniculate nucleus of the thalamus and the posterior limb of the internal capsule to terminate in the upper bank of the temporal lobe (Brodmann's areas 41 and 42).

Clinical Examination

Before testing hearing, ensure that the external auditory meatus is clear and the tympanic membrane is intact. In a patient with hearing complaints, screen hearing by detection of finger rub or test by using a 256-Hz tuning fork, comparing the patient's threshold with yours. A sensitive bedside test makes use of the stethoscope (Arbit, 1977). Apply the lightly vibrating tuning fork to the diaphragm of the stethoscope while the patient listens. By alternately clamping the tubing going to one or the other ear piece, compare hearing in the two ears.

Next compare air with bone conduction by alternately placing the vibrating tuning fork on the mastoid process (bone conduction) and holding it in front of the external auditory meatus (air condition); this is Rinne's test. In a normal individual, the tuning fork is heard

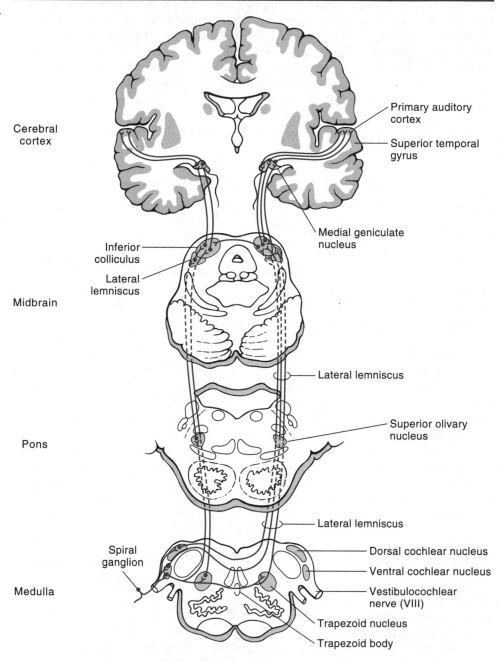

Figure 4-18   Summary of the central auditory pathway. (Adapted from Kandel, Schwartz, and Jessell, 1991.)

louder and longer by air than by bone conduction. In conduction deafness (e.g., that caused by middle ear disease), bone conduction is superior. In sensorineural deafness, both air and bone conduction are reduced but air conduction remains better. Finally, place the vibrating tuning fork over the middle of the forehead and inquire whether the vibration is heard more in one ear; this is Weber's test. Normal subjects cannot lateralize the vibration to either ear. In conductive deafness, the stimulus it is heard better in the affected ear. In sensorineural deafness, the stimulus is heard better in the normal ear.

Disorders of Function

Decreased hearing may be due to wax in the external ear, abnormalities of the tympanic membrane such as perforation, and middle ear disease such as effusion or disorders of the ossicular chain (e.g., otosclerosis). These are all forms of *conductive hearing loss*. Patients with a facial palsy may report hyperacusia if the nerve to the stapedius is involved, since this muscle usually adjusts transmission in the ossicular chain to reduce loud sounds.

Sensorineural hearing loss may be due to disease of the cochlea or the cochlear nerve and its central connection ("retrocochlear"). Disorders of the cochlea such as Ménière disease produce deafness that is greatest for lower frequencies, tinnitus, and the phenomenon of recruitment, in which loud sounds are perceived as too loud, distorted, and discomforting. With cochlear disease, loss of acuity for pure tones and speech discrimination tends to be similar.

Dysfunction of the cochlear nerve and its central projections causes tinnitus and hearing loss that is more pronounced for higher tones. Loss of speech discrimination is greater than that of pure tones. Recruitment is not a feature of retrocochlear disease. The cochlear nerve may be damaged with fractures of the temporal bone. Progressive, insidious sensorineural hearing loss is a classic presentation of a schwannoma of cranial nerve VIII.

THE GLOSSOPHARYNGEAL NERVE (CRANIAL NERVE IX)

Anatomy and Physiology

The glossopharyngeal nerve supplies the tongue and pharynx. It is closely related to the vagus nerve and contains somatic motor, visceral efferent, visceral sensory, and somatic sensory fibers. The glossopharyngeal somatic motor fibers arise from the rostral part of the nucleus ambiguus, which is situated in the medulla, medial to the spinal tract and nucleus of cranial nerve V (Fig. 4-19). Its visceral efferent fibers arise from the inferior salivatory nucleus, which is immediately rostral to the dorsal motor nucleus of the vagus. The visceral afferents have their cell bodies in the petrosal ganglion and synapse in the nucleus of the solitary tract. The somatic sensory fibers have their cell bodies in the superior ganglion and synapse in the spinal trigeminal nucleus. The rootlets of the glossopharyngeal nerve exit the medulla just dorsal to the inferior olive.

The glossopharyngeal nerve exits the skull through the jugular foramen and then

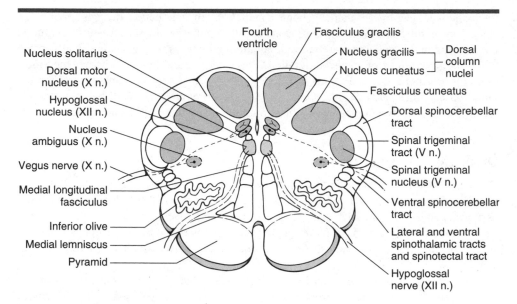

Figure 4-19   The locations of cell groups and fibers of cranial nerves IX through XII in a brain section cut through the medulla. (Adapted from Brodal, 1981.)

arches down and forward, on the lateral wall of the pharynx, turning medially to reach the base of the tongue, where it splits into its terminal branches. The superior ganglion is located within the jugular foramen, and the petrosal ganglion is located just outside the jugular foramen, in the petrosal fossa. The somatic motor fibers supply the stylopharyngeus muscle, which helps elevate the larynx during swallowing. The visceral efferent fibers pass via the lesser superficial petrosal nerve to synapse in the otic ganglion, which is located below the foramen ovale; postganglionic fibers innervate the parotid gland and salivary glands in the posterior tongue. The visceral afferents mediate taste from the posterior third of the tongue. A carotid branch leaves cranial nerve IX just below the skull and descends to the carotid bifurcation, where it innervates the carotid sinus and body. The somatic afferent fibers supply sensation over the posterior tongue, palate, and pharynx, where they anastomose with vagal fibers to form the pharyngeal plexus. A small auricular branch innervates skin over the concha.

Clinical Examination

The most reliable test of glossopharyngeal nerve function is taste over the posterior third of the tongue. (Testing of taste is described above, in the section on the facial nerve.) The innervation of the parotid gland by cranial nerve IX can be tested by reflexly inducing secretion of saliva (by placing seasoned food over the tongue) and observing saliva flowing from Stensen's duct. Sensation in the posterior pharyngeal wall also should be tested, although this and the gag reflex probably depend mostly on the vagal contribution to the pharyngeal plexus.

Disorders of Function

Isolated lesions of the glossopharyngeal nerve are unusual; more commonly, the vagus nerve also is involved. Glossopharyngeal nerve palsy would be expected to produce only slight dryness of the mouth, changes in taste, and minor difficulties in swallowing. Glossopharyngeal neuralgia causes lancinating pain typical of tic douloureux but located in the throat or tonsillar region, with radiation into the ear. Sometimes syncope or cardiac arrest is associated. Patients with metastases to the region of the jugular foramen may suffer attacks of severe pain lasting up to 30 min, located in the neck, ear, or side of the head and accompanied by syncope (Posner, 1995).

THE VAGUS NERVE
(CRANIAL NERVE X)

Anatomy and Physiology

The vagus nerve contains somatic motor, visceral efferent, visceral sensory, and somatic sensory fibers. The motor fibers originate in the nucleus ambiguus in the medulla (Fig. 4-19); this structure receives corticobulbar innervation that is bilateral but predominantly crossed. The visceral efferent fibers originate in the dorsal nucleus of the vagus, which is located lateral to the hypoglossal nucleus under the fourth ventricle. The visceral sensory fibers have their cell bodies in the nodose ganglion and terminate in the nucleus of the solitary tract. The somatic sensory fibers have their cell bodies in the jugular ganglion and terminate in the spinal trigeminal nucleus. The fiber bundles of the vagus emerge from the medulla just dorsal to the inferior olive.

After leaving the medulla, the vagus exits the skull—along with cranial nerve IX, cranial nerve XI, and the jugular vein—through the jugular foramen. At this site, the vagus show a small swelling, the jugular ganglion, which receives somatic sensation from an auricular branch that supplies the dorsal wall of the auditory meatus and fundus of the auricle, and a meningeal branch that supplies the dura of the posterior fossa. Soon afterward, the vagus shows a second, larger swelling, the nodose ganglion. At this level a pharyngeal branch comes off to supply the pharyngeal constrictors and muscles of the palate and carries visceral afferent fibers that mediate taste on the posterior third of the tongue. The superior laryngeal nerve is also given off at the level of the nodose ganglion and innervates the cricothyroid muscle and the mucous membranes of the larynx. The vagus descends in the neck in the carotid sheath, lying medial to the jugular vein. When the right vagus reaches the thoracic aperture, it descends anterior to the subclavian artery and passes to the posterior aspect of the right main bronchus. The right recurrent laryngeal nerve comes off at the anterior aspect of the subclavian artery, and after hooking under this vessel, it ascends close to the thyroid gland to innervate all laryngeal muscles except the cricothyroid. The left vagus descends through the thoracic aperture anterior to the subclavian artery and aortic arch to reach the left mainstem bronchus. The left recurrent laryngeal nerve arises from the left vagus at the level of the aortic arch and, after hooking under this vessel, ascends to the larynx. In the thorax, the vagus innervates the heart, lungs, and esophagus; terminal branches pierce the diaphragm to innervate the stomach, intestines, kidneys, pancreas, spleen, and liver.

Clinical Examination

Although the vagus nerve has many function, clinical evaluation largely depends on testing the somatic motor functions it subserves. Observe the *soft palate* and *uvula* in the resting position. Deviation of the uvula may be due to old tonsilar scarring; however, pay attention to whether the palate elevates symmetrically when the patient says "aah" (the palatal reflex). The palate will elevate less on the side of weakness, and the uvula will deviate toward the intact side. Bilateral palatal weakness causes difficulty in closing the posterior pharynx, which gives a nasal quality to speech so that, for example, "k" becomes "ng."

Test *pharyngeal sensation* over the posterior wall of the pharynx by touching each side with a cotton-tip applicator; ask the subject whether the stimulus is perceived on each side. Note, however, that the glossopharyngeal nerve also contributes to pharyngeal sensation. The pharyngeal ("gag") reflex may be induced by stimulating the posterior pharyngeal wall; its threshold varies idiosyncratically, but asymmetries of response are more reliable. It is often useful to watch the patient swallow liquids.

Test *laryngeal function* by asking the patient to speak (listening for hoarseness), cough, and imitate a high-pitched "ee" sound, which requires apposition of the vocal cords. Abnormalities can be further clarified by laryngoscopy, which allows inspection of the vocal cords during phonation.

Bedside testing of *autonomic functions* supplied by the vagus nerve is limited. However, a change in pulse rate during a Valsalva maneuver, especially the slowing that subsequently occurs, implies intact vagal cardiac innervation. Massage of the carotid sinus to induce bradycardia carries risk and should not be used as a bedside test (see Chap. 8 on autonomic testing).

Although the vagus nerve supplies the tympanic membrane and skin over the external acoustic meatus, several other nerves also contribute, and thus examination of somatic sensory function at this site is seldom helpful.

Disorders of Function

Because of its long course, the branches of the vagus nerve are susceptible to diverse disease processes. In the neck, common causes of dysfunction are trauma, tumor, and thyroid gland surgery; in the thorax, tumor, infections, and aneurysm are common causes. In the brainstem, involvement of the nucleus ambiguus may disrupt the pharyngeal and laryngeal functions necessary for respiration. Previously, the nucleus ambiguus dysfunction commonly was due to poliomyelitis, but it is now encountered after brainstem stroke and in the progressive bulbar palsy variant of motorneuron disease.

A unilateral vagal palsy causes paresis of the soft palate, pharynx, and larynx on the affected side. The most useful sign is asymmetry of the palatal reflex, with deviation of the uvula away from the abnormal side. Pharyngeal sensation and the gag reflex may be reduced on the affected side. Acutely, there may be some difficulty swallowing both solid and liquids, and the voice may be hoarse or nasal in quality. Bilateral vagal palsy is life-threatening because it leads to paralysis of the palate, pharynx, and larynx. In addition, cardiac dysryhthmia and disturbance of respiration may occur. In any patient with such disturbances, emergency measures such as tracheostomy are required. Consideration should be given to neuromuscular disorders that imitate bilateral vagal dysfunction: myasthenia gravis, botulism, and organophosphate poisoning.

THE ACCESSORY NERVE (CRANIAL NERVE XI)

Anatomy and Physiology

The accessory nerve arises from both cranial and spinal roots. The cranial root originates in the nucleus ambiguus (Fig. 4-19); after joining the spinal root, it soon leaves and joins the vagus nerve above the nodose ganglia. Thus, the cranial root can be viewed as an aberrant portion of the vagus nerve. The accessory nerve proper depends on the spinal root, which emerges from the lateral funiculus of the spinal cord from the second to sixth cervical segments; these are purely somatic efferent fibers. The spinal roots ascend through the vertebral canal to enter the cranial cavity through the foramen magnum and join the cranial root. The fused cranial and spinal roots leave the skull through the jugular foramen, after which the cranial fibers leave to join the vagus nerve. The spinal accessory nerve descends close to and usually behind the internal jugular vein. It passes anterior to the transverse process of the atlas vertebra and enters the sternocleidomastoid on its medial surface to innervate that muscle. Branches of the accessory nerve leave from the middle posterior aspect of the sternocleidomastoid muscle and pass inferiorly and posteriorly through a region occupied by lymph nodes, to terminate in the upper part of the trapezius muscles. In the neck, the accessory nerve anastomoses with fibers from the cervical plexus (from the third and fourth cervical segments), and these fibers may supply the lower part of the trapezius muscle.

Clinical Examination

Observe the size and symmetry of the sternocleidomastoid and trapezius muscles and look for any abnormal neck postures such as torticollis. Test the right sternocleidomastoid muscle by asking the patient to turn the chin forcefully to the left (horizontal head rotation) against the examiner's hand; observe and feel contraction of the muscle belly. Test the left sternocleidomastoid during a rightward head turn. The sternocleidomastoid is one of several cervical muscles (such as the splenius capitis) that contribute to head turning, and so paralysis of the sternocleidomastoid alone may not cause detectable weakness; thus, it is important to observe and palpate the muscle belly during testing. Depending on body habitus, it may be possible to compare the sternocleidomastoid muscles as the patient attempts to flex the neck while the examiner opposes by pressing on the patient's forehead. With severe bilateral involvement, the patient may have difficulty lifting the head off the pillow.

Look for any asymmetry of the trapezius muscles and shoulder droop. Test the trapezius by asking the patient to shrug and retract the shoulders against resistance. The two trapezius muscles also can be tested by asking the patient to extend the neck against resistance. With severe, bilateral trapezius weakness, the patient's head tends to fall forward. In addition, the patient will show weakness of elevation of the arm, because the trapezius assists the serratus anterior in rotating the scapula about its dorsoventral axis. Winging of the scapula may occur.

Disorders of Function

Isolated lesions of the *spinal accessory nerve* are rare, occurring when a tumor or infection involves the cervical lymph nodes in the posterior triangle of the neck. More commonly, cranial nerve XI is involved along with the vagus and glossopharyngeal nerves as they pass through the jugular foramen as a result of skull base disease such as tumor or trauma. Bilateral weakness of the sternocleidomastoid and trapezius muscles usually results from muscle disease, such as myotonic dystrophy (in which there is atrophy of the sternocleidomastoid), polymyositis, and myasthenia gravis.

Patients who have suffered a unilateral cerebral lesion often show some weakness of the sternocleidomastoid ipsilateral to the side of the cerebral lesion (recall that the sternocleidomastoid turns the head to the contralateral side). Thus, a right hemispheric lesion may produce a head rotation to the right and weakness of the right sternocleidomastoid but a left hemiplegia, with involvement of the left trapezius muscle. This phenomenon suggests that the descending pathways to the sternocleidomastoid undergo a double decussation (Geschwind, 1981). Thus, brainstem lesions may cause sternocleidomastoid weakness and hemiparesis on the same side (Mastaglia et al, 1986), presumably because the lesions are below the first decussation for the sternocleidomastoid but above the second. The site of the second decussation may be in the high spinal cord since hemicord section at C1 on the right has been reported to cause right hemiparesis with sparing of the right sternocleidomastoid but weakness of the left sternocleidomastoid (Iannone and Gerber, 1982). Furthermore, lesions at C4 have beeen reported to cause paralysis of the trapezius and quadriparesis but spare the sternocleidomastoid (Manon-Espaillat and Ruff, 1988; Modi et al, 1989).

Another disorder affecting the sternocleidomastoid is *torticollis* or *wryneck,* in which the head and occiput are pulled to the side of the affected muscle and the face is turned in the opposite direction. When persistent, these spasmodic movements may be accompanied by dystonic movements of the limbs. The site in the nervous system responsible for the disorder is presumed to be the basal ganglia. Sustained anterocollis and retrocollis occur in parkinsonian syndromes, especially progressive supranuclear palsy.

(THE HYPOGLOSSAL NERVE (CRANIAL NERVE XII)

Anatomy and Physiology

The hypoglossal nerve is the motor nerve of the tongue. Its nucleus consists of a longitudinal column of nerve cells approximately 2 cm long located in the medulla, just lateral to the midline and underlying the floor of the fourth ventricle (Fig. 4-19). The hypoglossal nerve innervates the ipsilateral side of the tongue. Most pyramidal tract fibers project to the hypoglossal nucleus after crossing the midline. The nucleus probably also receives projections from the sensory trigeminal nucleus and the nucleus of the solitary tract, which are involved in the reflex behaviors of sucking, swallowing, and chewing.

The hypoglossal fibers emerge on the ventral surface of the medulla between the pyramid and the inferior olive (Fig. 4-19). They leave the skull through the anterior condyloid foramen (the hypoglossal canal) in the occipital bone. The nerve courses between the vagus and the internal carotid artery toward the root of the tongue to innervate the genioglossus (intrinsic tongue muscle) and the hyoglossus, styloglossus, and geniohyoid muscles. The hypoglossal nerve is joined by fibers from the first and second cervical roots until the place where cranial nerve XII crosses the carotid artery; thereafter, they separate and become the descending hypoglossal ramus, which anastomoses with other cervical branches to form the *ansa hypoglossi*. The ansa hypoglossi innervates the infrahyoid muscles: sternohyoid, omohyoid, and sternothyroid.

Clinical Examination

Observe the tongue as it rests on the floor of the mouth. Look for atrophy and fasciculations. A reduced volume and a wrinkled appearance of the mucosa indicate atrophy. Fasciculations are fine involuntary movements that usually are detected at the sides of the tongue, posteriorly. In judging whether any involuntary movements are present, bear in mind that normal subjects cannot hold the tongue perfectly still but are able to prevent protrusion from the mouth and sustain protrusion. Ask the patient to protrude the tongue and look for any lateral deviation. In patients with unilateral facial weakness, it is important to use a reliable fiduciary of the midline or the tongue will be misinterpreted as deviating laterally. In such patients, gently lift the weak side of the face with one hand and place the index finger of the other hand at the middle of the lower lip; then ask the patient to protrude the tongue. Test the mobility of the tongue by asking the patient to make rapid side-to-side movements of the tongue, illustrating with your own example. Test the strength of the tongue by asking the patient to push the tongue into each cheek in turn, feeling the force generated with your fingers. The contribution of the tongue to speech can be evaluated by asking the patient to say "la-la-la-la" repetitively and count quickly from 1 to 20. Test the infrahyoid muscles by asking the patient to press down the lower jaw against resistance; these muscles (especially the omohyoid) can be felt to contract.

Disorders of Function

With a unilateral lesion of the *hypoglossal nucleus or nerve*, the tongue shows hemiatrophy and, on attempted protrusion, deviates toward the affected side (because the intact genioglossus muscle pulls its half of the tongue forward). Unilateral paralysis of the tongue usually does not interfere with swallowing, but bilateral paralysis does. Fasciculations of the tongue suggest a nuclear process, usually a motor neuron disease. Cranial nerve XII may be involved in its intramedullary course, and classically this causes ipsilateral tongue weakness and contralateral hemiplegia. With such brainstem lesions, the infrahyoid muscles are spared; they may be involved if the hypoglossal nerve is affected by disease in the neck.

When impaired tongue movements are due to *supranuclear disease*, there is no atrophy and the weakness is usually bilateral. However, when bilateral pyramidal tract disease causes pseudobulbar palsy, the tongue appears small and patients cannot make rapid side-to-side movements. Tremors of the tongue occur in parkinsonian disorders. In chorea and oral-facial dyskinesia (e.g., after neuroleptic drug administration or during the administration of dopaminergic agents), the patient often cannot hold the tongue in the mouth or sustain protrusion because of involuntary movements.

Disturbance of *speech* as a result of a peripheral cranial nerve XII lesion usually is identified by a selective difficulty in enunciating lingual sounds and the abnormal signs described in the paragraph above. Disease of the cerebral hemispheres that causes language disturbance (aphasia) may lead to apraxia of tongue movements and inability to protrude the tongue to command, but without wasting or weakness. In pseudobulbar palsy, speech is slow, difficult, and "explosive" in nature; these patients are unable to sustain the effort required to talk and often cry or laugh without clear provocation.

SUGGESTED READINGS

Arbit E: A sensitive bedside hearing test. *Ann Neurol* 2:250, 1977.

Averbuch-Heller L, Stahl JS, Remler BF, Leigh RJ: Bilateral ptosis and upgaze palsy with right hemispheric lesions. *Ann Neurol* 40:465, 1996.

Bonner JS, Jaeger Bonner J: *The Little Black Book of Neurology*. St. Louis, Mosby Year Book, 1991.

Brandt T, Dieterich M: Pathological eye-head coordination in roll: Tonic ocular tilt reaction in mesencephalic and medullary lesions. *Brain* 110:649, 1987.

Brandt T, Dieterich M: Vestibular syndromes in the roll plane: Topographic diagnosis from brain stem to cortex. *Ann Neurol* 36:337, 1994.

Brandt T, Steddin S, Daroff RB: Therapy for benign paroxysmal positioning vertigo, revisited, *Neurology* 44:796, 1994.

Brazis PW, Masdeu JC, Biller J: *Localization in Clinical Neurology*, 3d ed. Boston, Little, Brown, 1996.

Brodal A: *Neurological Anatomy in Relation to Clinical Medicine*, 3d ed. New York, Oxford University Press, 1981.

Büttner-Ennever J, Horn AKE: Upper eyelid premotor neurons in the rostral mesencephalon of the primate. *Soc Neurosci Abstr* 22:2035, 1996.

Büttner-Ennever JA, Akert, K: Medial rectus subgroups of the oculomotor nucleus and their abducens internuclear input in monkey. *J Comp Neurol* 197:17, 1981.

Carpenter MB: *Core Text of Neuroanatomy*, 2d ed. Baltimore, Williams & Wilkins, 1978.

Castro O, Johnson LN, Mamourian AC: Isolated inferior oblique paresis from brain-stem infarction: Perspective on oculomotor fascicular organization in the ventral midbrain tegmentum. *Arch Neurol* 47:235, 1990.

Dodd J, Castellucci VF: Smell and taste: The chemical senses, in Kandel ER, Scwartz JH, Jessell TM (eds.): *Principles of Neural Science*, 3d ed. Norwalk, CT, Appleton and Lange, 1991, p 512.

Geschwind N: Nature of the decussated innervation of the sternomastoid muscle. *Ann Neurol* 10:495, 1981.

Glaser JS: *Neuro-ophthalmology*, 2d ed. Philadelphia, Lippincott, 1990, p 1.

Horton JC, Hoyt WF: The representation of the visual field in human striate cortex: A revision of the classic Holmes map. *Arch Neurol* 109: 816, 1991.

Iannone AM, Gerber AM: Brown-Sequard syndrome with paralysis of head turning. *Ann Neurol* 12:116, 1982.

Jenny AM, Saper CB: Organization of the facial nucleus and cortico-facial projections in the monkey: A reconsideration of the upper motor neuron facial palsy. *Neurology* 37:930, 1987.

Keltner JL, Johnson CA, Spurr JO, et al: Baseline visual field profile of optic neuritis: The experience of the optic neuritis treatment trial: Optic Neuritis Study Group. *Arch Ophthalmol* 111:231, 1993.

Leigh RJ, Zee DS: *The Neurology of Eye Movements,* 3d ed. New York, Oxford University Press, 1999.

Manon-Espaillat R, Ruff RL: Dissociated weakness of sternocleidomastoid and trapezius muscles with lesions in the CNS. *Neurology* 38:796, 1988.

Mastaglia FL, Knezevic W, Thompson PD: Weakness of head turning in hemiplegia: A quantitative study. *J Neurol Neurosurg Psychiatry* 49:195, 1986.

Meyer BU, Werhahn K, Rothwell JC, et al: Functional organization of corticonuclear pathways to motoneurons of lower facial nucleus in man. *Exp Brain Res* 101:465, 1994.

Miller NR: *Walsh and Hoyt's Clinical Neuro-ophthalmology*, 4th ed. Baltimore, Williams & Wilkins, 1982, vol 1, p 108.

Modi G, Bill PLA, Hoffman MW: Sternocleidomastoid trapezius dissociation. *Neurology* 39:454, 1989.

Moschovakis AK, Scudder CA, Highstein SM: A structural basis for Hering's law: Projections to extraocular motoneurons. *Science* 248:1118, 1990.

Mott AE, Leopold DA: Disorders of taste and smell. *Med Clin North Am* 75:1321, 1991.

Porter JD, Guthrie BL, Sparks DL: Innervation of monkey extraocular muscles: Localization of sensory and motor neurons by retrograde transport of horseradish peroxidase. *J Comp Neurol* 218: 208, 1983.

Posner JB: *Neurologic Complications of Cancer*. Philadelphia, Davis, 1995.

Schmidtke K, Büttner-Ennever JA: Nervous control of eyelid function: A review of clinical, experimental and pathological data. *Brain* 115:227, 1992.

Thompson HS, Piley SJ: Unequal pupils: A flow chart for sorting out the anisocorias. *Surv Ophthalmol* 21:45, 1976.

Warwick R: Representation of the extra-ocular muscles in the oculomotor nuclei of the monkey. *J Comp Neurol* 98: 449, 1953.

Zatorre RJ, Jones-Gotman M: Human olfactory discrimination after unilateral frontal or temporal lobectomy. *Brain* 114:71, 1991.

Zee DS: Ophthalmoscopy in examination of patients with vestibular disorders. *Ann Neurol* 3:373, 1978.

Zeki S: *Vision of the Brain*. London, Blackwell Scientific, 1993.

ROGER L. ALBIN / JOHN J. WALD

CHAPTER 5

THE MOTOR SYSTEM

The motor system consists of a group of interrelated nuclei and pathways that are involved in the control of posture and movement. The definition of these nuclei and pathways as the motor system is arbitrary because normal motor performance requires the integrated activity of many neural systems, including those primarily involved in sensation, vestibular function, and the various aspects of cognition. Nonetheless, it is conceptually and practically advantageous to define some nuclei and pathways as components of the motor system. Conceptually, accumulated clinical and physiologic evidence suggests that these nuclei and pathways are involved primarily in the execution of movement. Practically, injury to these nuclei and pathways gives rise to characteristic disturbances of motor performance that have great value in the clinical localization and characterization of disease processes.

The motor system spans the entire neuraxis from the neocortex to muscle. The central components consist of the brain elements that develop the instructions for motor acts, the central pathways that transmit this information between different brain motor nuclei, and the pathways that funnel motor instructions to the spinal cord and brainstem motor nuclei. Spinal and brainstem motor neurons serve as an interface between the higher central nervous system elements and the peripheral nervous system and integrate descending, local, and segmental information. Spinal and brainstem motor neurons convey information via the nerve roots, plexuses, individual nerves, and neuromuscular junctions to the actors of movement: the muscles. Dysfunction of each of these motor system elements produces a unique pattern of clinical symptoms and findings that allow the clinical examiner to localize the site of pathology.

THE COMPONENTS OF THE MOTOR SYSTEM

Although the motor system operates as an integrated whole, it can be divided into a series of distinct subsystems which, when injured, give rise to various sets of clinical findings (Fig. 5-1). The motor system can be conceptualized as hierarchically organized with movement plans initiated in the *neocortex* and executed by individual *muscles*. Between these two poles of the motor system are several intermediate levels. In each of these levels, information is not transmitted slavishly from the upper element to the lower element; instead, considerable modification of instructions takes place.

In the brain, the neocortex originates an important avenue of transmitting motor information from the highest level of the motor system directly to the motor neurons of the spinal cord and brainstem: the *corticobulbar* and *corticospinal tracts.* Neocortical neurons in several regions give rise to axons that synapse on spinal cord and brainstem motor neurons. Additional pathways convey information from higher to lower levels of the motor system. The *rubrospinal, reticulospinal, tectospinal,* and *vestibulospinal* pathways are all important in the regulation of posture and motor performance; however, it is difficult to attribute specific clinical deficits to lesions of these pathways, while injury to the corticospinal system (including both corticobulbar and corticospinal fibers) produces distinct and clinically useful patterns of dysfunction.

Modulation of corticospinal tract function occurs at two important levels. The first level is in the neocortex, where input from two other important brain components of the motor system—the *cerebellar system* and the *basal ganglia*—modulates the activity of neurons that give rise to corticospinal axons. Both of these brain systems provide important inputs to neocortical regions that contain corticospinal neurons or to other neocortical regions that project to corticospinal neuron–containing regions. Consequently, outputs of the cerebellar system and the basal ganglia should be considered corticospinal system modulators. The *spinal cord* is the second level at which corticospinal function is modulated. Spinal neurons receive not only descending input from the corticospinal tract and other brain systems but also a steady flow of activity from sensory neurons conveying somatosensory and proprioceptive information. Cerebellar system outputs also influence other descending pathways that affect spinal neuron behavior, including the rubrospinal, reticulospinal, and vestibulospinal projections. The spinal cord contains heterogeneous populations of neurons that interact to modify the effects of descending inputs. The *anterior horn cells* of the spinal cord and the *primary motor neurons* of the brainstem, which give rise to the axons innervating muscles, are the final common pathway of central motor system function. After leaving the spinal cord in anterior root filaments, motor axons are bundled together with afferent sensory axons in the mixed spinal *nerve roots*, exit the spinal column, and combine with other spinal nerve roots to form the various *plexuses,* which give rise to individual *nerves.* The individual nerves terminate within the body of muscles in specialized zones referred to as *neuromuscular junctions.* All the complex acts of the motor system from the level of the neocortex to the neuromuscular junction are designed to lead to the patterns of muscle activation needed to perform motor acts efficiently.

EXAMINING THE MOTOR SYSTEM

The anatomy of the motor system lends itself to clinical evaluation of its individual components to localize the anatomic sites of motor dysfunction. The history should be considered an integral element of clinical evaluation. An experienced inteviewer often can garner information that provides clues regarding the site of pathology and guides the examination appropriately. No single clinical test or maneuver identifies pathology in a single component of the motor system. Because the motor system has several interconnected components, pathology within a single component may ramify throughout the

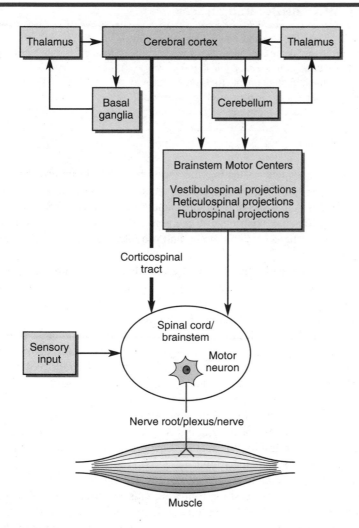

Figure 5-1 Schematic of the motor system.

motor system. It is the constellation of abnormal findings that permits anatomic localization of pathology. A thorough examination evaluating multiple aspects of motor function is necessary for accurate localization of pathology and will be described below.

Power

In conducting the motor examination, assess the strength or power of individual muscles or muscle groups. In many cases, individual muscles cannot be examined, but the power of muscle groups that act physiologically in concert can be evaluated. Since these muscle groups form functional units and the individual muscles usually are affected similarly by pathology at various levels of the motor system, information about the power of muscle

TABLE 5-1.   MRC Muscle Strength Scale

5	"Normal" power for given muscle in a given individual
4	Active movement; decreased power, moves joint against load greater than gravity alone
3	Active movement; moves joint against gravity *only*
2	Active movement, though unable to overcome gravity
1	Flicker of movement or visible muscle contraction
0	Absence of any muscle movement or contraction

groups usually is equivalent to testing the individual muscle components. A standard grading system developed under the auspices of the British Medical Research Council (MRC) during World War II has become the standard clinical descriptor of muscle power (Table 5-1). You need some experience to recognize the normal power of a given muscle group, but the MRC scale is easy to employ and provides a high degree of reproducibility across examiners.

The MRC grading describes the ability of a muscle group to move the joint it acts on. The MRC scale is nonlinear, with the 4 grade encompassing a very large range of power (from subtle weakness to overcoming gravity plus only a minimal additional load) (see Table 5-1). To compensate for the unequal weighting of grades, you can refine the scale with pluses and minuses, though this may limit reproducibility and understanding. Practically, you should use 5− MRC grading when you cannot be certain that power is normal, and you can use the plus and minus qualifiers to expand the 4 grade to 4+ (subtle weakness), 4 (moderate weakness), and 4− (just greater than antigravity). The plus and minus qualifiers are less useful with the lower strength grades. To evaluate a very weak muscle properly, position the limb to allow testing of the muscle or joint unit against gravity. If the muscle or joint unit does not have antigravity function, reposition the limb to allow testing with the effect of gravity eliminated. Encourage the patients to make a maximal effort; peak power is the parameter of interest.

Certain circumstances dictate extensive muscle testing, but in a general neurologic examination you should test at least the following muscle actions: neck flexion and extension, arm abduction (Fig. 5-2A and B), elbow flexion and extension (Fig. 5-2C and D), wrist flexion and extension (Fig. 5-3A), finger and thumb abduction (Fig. 5-3E and F), hip flexion and extension (Fig. 5-4A), knee flexion and extension (Fig. 5-4C), ankle dorsiflexion and plantar flexion (Fig. 5-5A), and great toe extension (Fig. 5-5C).

A guide for more extensive assessment of muscle and muscle group power is *Aids to the Examination of the Peripheral Nervous System* (Philadelphia, Bailliere Tindall, 1986). This concise book provides standard methods for evaluating virtually all clinically relevant muscles and muscle groups.

Muscle Bulk

A useful complement to examination of power is assessment of muscle bulk. Assess muscle bulk visually by observing muscle volume during contraction or by palpating the muscle group of interest during contraction. With experience, you can learn to distinguish reduced, normal, and increased muscle bulk.

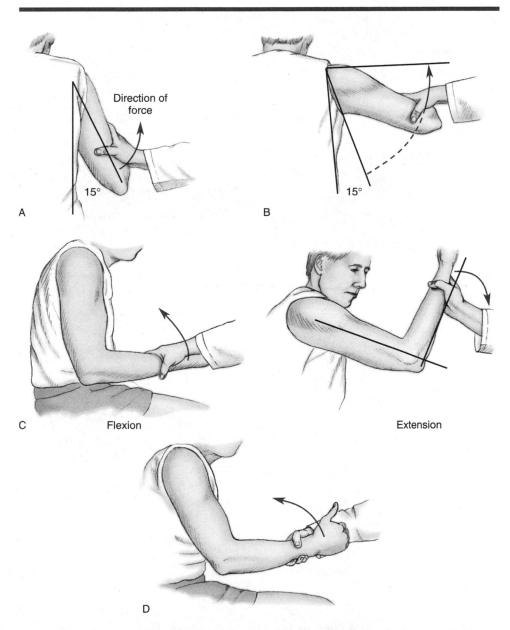

Figure 5-2 Examination of arm movements: movement, muscle, **primary root(s)**, and nerve. *A*. Arm abduction, first 15 degrees: Supraspinatus, **C5**, C6, suprascapular nerve. *B*. Arm abduction, 15 degrees through 90 degrees: Deltoid, **C5**, C6, axillary nerve. *C*. Elbow flexion, forearm supinated: Biceps, **C5**, C6, musculocutaneous nerve. Elbow extension: Triceps, C6, **C7**, C8, radial nerve. *D*. Elbow flexion, semi-pronated: Brachioradialis, C5, **C6**, radial nerve.

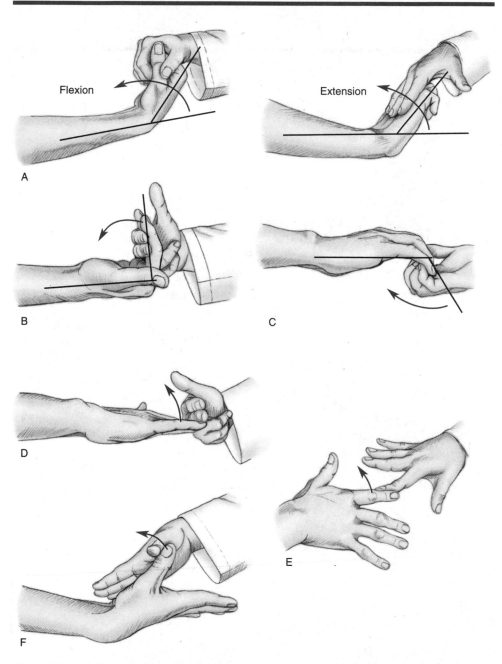

Figure 5-3 Examination of hand movements: movement, muscle, **primary root(s)**, and nerve. *A.* Wrist flexion: Anterior forearm muscles, **C7, C8,** T1, median nerve (flexor carpi ulnaris via ulnar nerve). Wrist extension: Extensor carpi radialis and ulnaris, **C6, C7,** C8, radial and posterior interosseous nerve (branch of radial). *B.* Finger flexion (proximal interphalangeal joints): Flexor digitorum superficialis, **C8,** T1, median nerve. *C.* Finger flexion (distal interphalangeal joints: Flexor digitorum profundus, C7, **C8,** median nerve (digits 2 and 3), and ulnar nerve (digits 4 and 5). *D.* Finger extension: Extensor digitorum, **C7,** C8, posterior interosseous nerve (branch of radial). *E.* Index finger abduction: First dorsal interosseous, C8, **T1,** ulnar nerve. *F.* Thumb abduction, abductor pollicis brevis, C8, **T1,** median nerve.

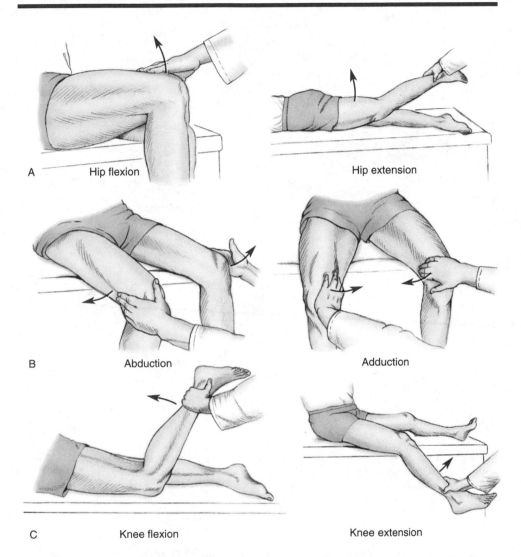

Figure 5-4 Examination of leg movements: movement, muscle, **primary root(s)**, and nerve. *A.* Hip flexion: Iliopsoas, **L1, L2**, femoral nerve. Hip extension: Gluteus maximus, L5, **S1**, inferior gluteal nerve. *B.* Hip abduction: Gluteus medius, minimus, **L4, L5**, superior gluteal nerve. Hip adduction: Adductor group, **L2, L3**, L4, obturator nerve. *C.* Knee flexion: Hamstring group, L5, **S1**, sciatic nerve. Knee extension: Quadriceps, L2, **L3, L4**, femoral nerve.

Spontaneous Activity

While observing the muscle at rest, you may see spontaneous muscle discharges. The most common are *fasciculations*: spontaneous discharges of an anterior horn cell leading to contraction of all the muscle fibers it innervates, producing visible partial muscle twitches. This is in contradistinction to *fibrillations*: spontaneous discharges of single

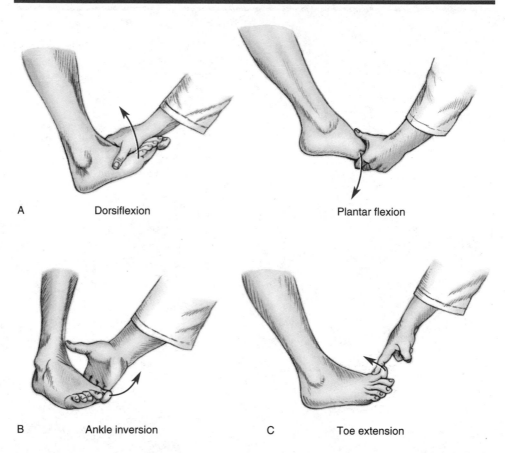

A   Dorsiflexion   Plantar flexion

B   Ankle inversion   C   Toe extension

Figure 5-5 Examination of foot movements: movement, muscle, **primary root(s)**, and nerve. *A.* Ankle dorsiflexion: Tibialis anterior, **L4**, **L5**, peroneal nerve. Plantar flexion: Gastrocnemius/soleus, **S1**, **S2**, tibial nerve. *B.* Ankle inversion: Tibialis posterior, **L4**, **L5**, tibial nerve. *C.* Great toe extension: Extensor hallucis longus, **L5**, S1, peroneal nerve.

muscle fibers usually present after denervation that can be detected only by needle electromyography. *Myokymia* refers to more prolonged, irregular longitudinal contractions of muscle segments that cause the skin to appear like a "can of worms." It is less common than fasciculations and is better detected during needle electromyography.

Resistance to Passive Manipulation (Tone)

Muscle tone is the term used for the resistance you feel when you move a patient's joint passively with the muscles of the limb relaxed. Tone is a combination of the intrinsic viscoelastic properties of the joint and surrounding muscles and the activation of muscles. Even when relaxed, all muscle groups and joints possess a certain amount of intrinsic resistance to passive manipulation. Neurologic disease produces both increases (hypertonia) and decreases (hypotonia) in muscle tone.

Initiate the examination of tone by asking the patient to relax and then gently move the joint. You can assess resistance to passive manipulation only in the absence of significant musculoskeletal abnormalities. Almost any joint can be examined, but the most common maneuvers include flexion and extension of the elbow, rotation of the wrist, rotation of the thumb, flexion and extension of the knee joint, flexion and extension or rotation of the ankle, and rotation of the neck. Examine tone in all patients as part of a general neurologic examination and make the examination extensive in all patients with suspected motor system disorders. Rather than examining tone in all muscle groups, you should focus the examination on the most pertinent areas. Examination of the neck, elbow, wrist, and thumb joints is straightforward. Examine the lower extremities by seating the patient on a high table or chair so that the legs dangle above the floor. With the legs relaxed, the knee and ankle joints can be manipulated. Alternatively, place the patient in the supine position, ask the patient to relax the legs, place your hands in the popliteal fossae, and lift the patient's knees off the examination surface. Similarly, ankle tone can be examined in the supine position by placing your hands on top of the thigh and passively rotating the entire limb at the hip joint while observing the ensuing movements of the foot. With experience, you can estimate the tone around the ankle joints from the amplitude of foot movements. Hypertonia is easier to detect than is hypotonia, but with experience you will be able to detect diminished tone. In patients with hypotonia, you can move a limb to the limit of its range of motion more easily than you can in a normal individual. Other maneuvers may be useful in detecting hypotonia. Instruct the patient to hold the forearms vertically above the head and then observe the angle between the hand and forearm at the wrist. In a hypotonic arm, the angle of the hand will be closer to or even below the horizontal. This maneuver is most useful in patients with asymmetries in tone. You can detect abnormal tone when testing the tendon reflexes. Patients with hypotonia have "pendular" reflexes; the limb shows a greater number of oscillations than normal after tendon stretch.

When you find increased tone, you should classify it as spasticity or rigidity. Certain types of neurologic pathology cause characteristic patterns of hypertonia, and detecting those patterns is useful in the anatomic localization of pathology. Hypotonia cannot be classified further, and localization of pathology depends on the evaluation of other clinical signs.

SPASTICITY Spasticity is a form of hypertonia resulting from injury to the corticospinal system and represents the unmodulated activity of local spinal neurons and sensory afferents at this level of the spinal cord. The principal feature of spasticity is that resistance is velocity-dependent and varies with the extent of tendon stretch. In a spastic limb, resistance will be normal when you manipulate the joints passively at slow velocities and will be enhanced when you increase the velocity of passive movement. Examine resistance to passive movement at both low and relatively fast velocities of movement. It is particularly useful to examine elbow flexion and knee flexion. For elbow flexion, support the patient's arm to facilitate relaxation of the arm and flex the forearm at the elbow at a slow velocity and then at a faster velocity. In normal individuals, you will find no difference in resistance between the two velocities. In spastic patients, resistance increases with higher velocity of movement and spastic elbow joints exhibit the "clasp-knife" phenomenon, in which resistance increases and then diminishes as maximum flexion or extension is achieved. This finding is analogous to the sensation of closing or opening a pocket-knife blade and reflects the dynamics of spinal reflex arcs controlling muscle activity. To evaluate tone about the knee joint, a useful maneuver is to examine the patient in a supine position and flex the knee joint by lifting it from the surface of the bed or examination table. In spastic individuals, no abnormalities occur as the knee is lifted slowly and the heel will slide along the top of the table or bed. When you lift the knee quickly, tone will increase, the leg distal to the knee will "catch," and the heel will be lifted off the bed or examination table.

RIGIDITY   Rigidity occurs with lesions of the basal ganglia (see below). In contrast to spasticity, you encounter increased resistance throughout the range of motion of the joint regardless of the velocity of passive movement. Rigidity has a "plastic" or "lead pipe" quality, with the latter term connoting the feeling of bending a lead pipe. A closely related or coincident property is "cogwheeling." In many patients with rigidity, particularly those with Parkinson disease, examination of the wrist or other joints reveals rigidity as defined above accompanied by intermittent, brief increases in resistance that are akin to cranking a ratchet (hence the term cogwheel). Cogwheeling is related to the resting tremor expressed in many Parkinson disease patients who have involuntary tremulous movements intruding into the otherwise relaxed muscle groups. Rigidity, including cogwheeling, may be absent when the patient is relaxed but can be brought out by reinforcing maneuvers. The most commonly used maneuver consists of having the patient move one hand in a rotatory fashion ("screwing a lightbulb") while you examine tone in the contralateral arm.

PARATONIA   Paratonia, also called gegenhalten, is not strictly an abnormality of tone but can be confused with spasticity and sometimes with rigidity. When you examine muscle tone in a patient with paratonia, you get the sense that the patient is pushing back when you move a limb about a joint. The harder or faster you move the limb, the greater the degree of response from the patient is. Paratonia is associated with diffuse forebrain impairment and occurs in patients with degenerative disorders with frontal lobe dysfunction, where it may be analogous to "frontal release" signs.

Posture

Evaluate posture by observing the patient while sitting, standing, or walking. Watch the patient walk into the examination room and observe posture during the interview. Note whether the patient is erect, bent forward, or leaning to either side when standing, sitting, or walking and whether changes in position alter posture. During the examination, ask the patient to stand unassisted and observe the position of the patient's head, shoulder, pelvis, and body and note how far apart the feet are placed. Inability to maintain the upright stance will be obvious. While patients are standing, ask them to place the feet together and close the eyes and observe their ability to maintain normal posture. Difficulty in postural maintenance with marked swaying, loss of balance, or falling (Romberg's sign) may indicate a significant sensory disturbance.

Postural reflexes serve to maintain posture after displacement and are characteristically abnormal in some motor system disorders, notably basal ganglia pathology. Assess these postural reflexes by standing behind the patient, placing your hands on the patient's shoulders, and gently but firmly pulling the patient backward. Individuals with normal postural reflexes will sway backward but maintain their position without moving their feet or only take one step back. Patients with impaired postural reflexes will take steps backward to maintain their position or may fall backward. Stand behind the patient and be prepared to prevent a fall.

Gait

Evaluation of gait is one of the most important aspects of the neurologic examination. Walking is a highly demanding activity that requires the coordinated activity of the entire nervous system. Evaluating gait provides information about many aspects of motor and sensory function. Begin the examination by watching the patient walk from the waiting room into the examination room.

During the examination, ask the patient to ambulate in a straight line for 15 to 20 ft while observing the patient's gait. Observe posture, lateral spacing of feet, stride length, regularity of stride, coordination of leg movements, arm swing, and ability to turn smoothly. Ask the patient to walk on the toes and then on the heels to assess balance, coordination, and the power of ankle plantar flexion and dorsiflexion. Ask the patient to walk in tandem, attempting to walk in a straight line by placing the heel of one foot directly in front of the toe of the other foot. Remind the patient to walk in tandem slowly; some normal individuals have difficulty executing this task rapidly. Ask a patient with suspected basal ganglia disease to walk on the outsides or insides of the feet to elicit involuntary arm postures or movements.

Gait disorders have stereotyped patterns reflecting injury to different components of the motor system.

HEMIPARETIC GAIT Patients with unilateral weakness and spasticity resulting from corticospinal tract injury hold the affected leg stiffly in an extension at the hip and knee with internal rotation and plantar flexion of the foot at the ankle. With ambulation, the affected leg swings away from the axis of the body in a circular motion, with the toes often striking or scraping along the floor. This is known as circumduction. The affected arm is held adducted at the shoulder and flexed at the elbow and wrist, with the fist closed. The arm will not swing when the patient is walking.

SPASTIC DIPLEGIA Patients with bilateral injury to the corticospinal system maintain both legs in tonic extension. With walking, the legs show "scissoring," which consists of short steps with the striding leg placed in front of the stationary leg and the toes often scraping the floor.

ATAXIC GAIT Disorders of coordination caused by impaired sensation or cerebellar function often cause gait ataxia (incoordination of movement). The distance between the feet (base) is often broadened, stride length and placement of the feet are irregular, and the gait has a lurching quality. In ataxia from suspected sensory deficits, the ataxia is worsened markedly by ambulation with the eyes closed. In ataxia from cerebellar dysfunction, tandem walking elicits or exacerbates ataxia.

NEUROPATHIC GAIT   Disease of the peripheral nervous system causes gait disorders that reflect weakness in the distribution of the affected root, plexus, or nerve(s). Bilateral involvement of the distal portions of the legs occurs commonly. Because of weakness of ankle dorsiflexion, a high-stepping (steppage) gait occurs, with the foot slapped down on the floor.

MYOPATHIC GAIT   Most primary disorders of muscle cause weakness of proximal limb muscles. Weakness of the gluteal and other proximal lower extremity muscles results in a broadened base for greater stability and waddling with an exaggerated pelvic dip as patients attempt to compensate for the proximal weakness that causes pelvic instability. These patients have particular difficulty with activities involving proximal muscle function, such as climbing stairs and rising from a chair without using the arms. Ask the patient to lie on the floor and arise without assistance to evaluate proximal lower extremity function. Patients with proximal lower extremity weakness will use their hands to "climb up their legs" (Gowers' sign) to compensate for trunk extensor weakness.

PARKINSONIAN GAIT   In Parkinson disease and some other basal ganglia disturbances, posture is stooped, the base is narrow, and patients take many small steps. Normal arm swing is lost, and the arms are held close to the sides of the body. Many short steps are required for a turn, and the whole body moves as a rigid object (en bloc turning). These patients often take increasing numbers of short steps (festination) and cannot stop or change directions quickly.

HYSTERICAL GAIT   Gait disturbances occur commonly in patients with conversion (hysterical, somatization) disorders, and at times these disorders are difficult to diagnose. Three points are helpful in the diagnosis. First, the abnormality must make sense; significant motor system disturbances do not cause difficulties with gait alone, and other neurologic examination abnormalities should be consonant with the gait abnormalities. Second, the diagnosis should be based on positive findings in the neurologic examination. Third, hysterical disorders are notoriously inconsistent. Careful observation of patients when walking into the examination room, during the recording of the history, or while responding to other parts of the examination usually reveals discrepancies with the abnormalities of gait. Similar inconsistencies can be seen as the patients walk. They may report difficulty walking, but when walking in tandem, they may execute movements normally while exhibiting impressive contortions of the torso and flailing movements of the arms. Patients who walk abnormally may walk on the heels or toes relatively normally or hop on one foot without difficulty. Such inconsistencies provide positive evidence of hysterical gait disorders. Hysterical gaits usually do not resemble any of the typical gait disturbances resulting from neurologic disease.

Coordination

Abnormalities of coordination are common in motor system disorders, and the pattern of abnormality provides information for the localization and characterization of pathology.

Several maneuvers assessing coordination should be incorporated into the examination. Ask the patient to tap the index finger against the first joint of the thumb and observe the speed, amplitude, and regularity of the tapping movements. If you cannot determine whether tapping movements are regular, ask the patient to tap a tabletop with an index finger in concert with your index finger. The tapping should be firm enough to produce a readily audible sound. Normal individuals match precisely the rate and rhythm that you establish, and deviations from your rhythm can be detected aurally. Test alternating pronation and supination of the hands (rapid alternating movements). Ask patients to slap the palm and back of one hand against the palm of the other hand with alternating gentle movements. Note the speed, amplitude, and regularity of the movements. Ask the patient to tap the heels rapidly against the floor in a sitting position. A patient in the supine position can slap the soles of the feet against your palm.

Test finger-nose-finger movements by holding your index finger about 1 m from the patient's face and ask the patient to use an index finger to touch repeatedly and alternately your index finger and then the patient's own nose. Observe the accuracy of finger movements to the targets, whether movements between targets show a smooth trajectory, and the presence of any tremor or involuntary movements that interrupt performance. Cerebellar system disorders often cause side-to-side movements as the finger approaches the target. To evaluate the legs, employ the heel-knee-shin test. Ask the patient to place the heel of one foot on the knee of the opposite leg and run the heel down the shin across the dorsum of the foot to the great toe. Observe the accuracy of heel placement, the smoothness and trajectory of movement, and the intrusion of involuntary movements. This test should be done with the patient in the supine position because in the seated position, a patient may be able to let the leg fall down the shin. You can also ask the patient to touch your outstretched index finger with the patient's great toe. Assess the accuracy and smoothness of movements.

Subtle alterations of coordination from a corticospinal tract injury can be detected by asking the patient to roll his or her forearms around each other. Normally, the forearms rotate equally about a common axis of rotation. A patient with a subtle unilateral corticospinal injury will hold the affected forearm stationary and rotate the unaffected arm around the affected forearm. A better known but harder to interpret test of mild corticospinal injury is pronator drift. Ask the patient to extend the arms, palms held upward, in front of the patient and close the eyes. The affected arm pronates and drifts downward from the original position.

THE CORTICOSPINAL SYSTEM

Anatomy

The conception and formulation of movement plans take place within the neocortex. As with the rest of the motor system, the motor components of the neocortex are organized in a hierarchy of specialized regions. Motor areas are within the frontal lobes, and there is an anterior to posterior gradation in specialization for motor function. Moving from the frontal pole to the central sulcus, there are three vertically oriented belts of neocortex with broadly different roles in motor function (Fig. 5-6A). The most anterior neocortical regions, the prefrontal cortices, perform executive functions in the overall selection and planning for motor acts. These cortical regions are not specialized for motor function and participate in many aspects of cognition and executive behavior. Moving posteriorly, the next belt of cortical regions are the premotor regions, which are relatively specialized for

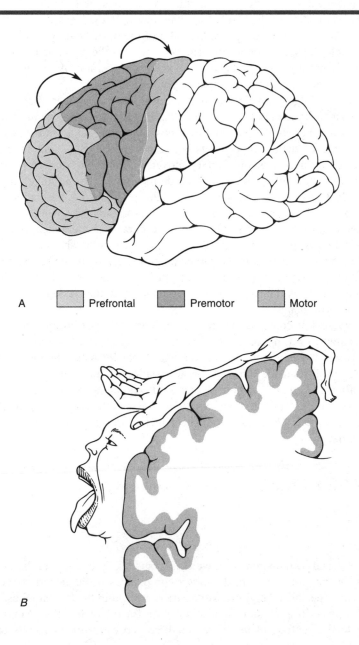

A   ☐ Prefrontal   ☐ Premotor   ☐ Motor

B

Figure 5-6   *Continued*

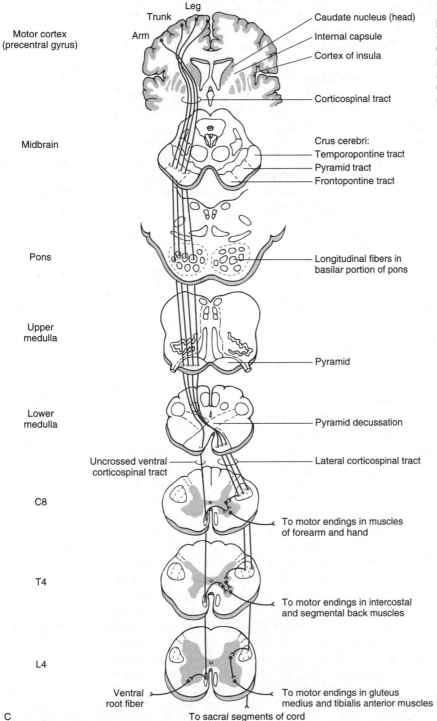

Motor cortex
(precentral gyrus)

Leg
Trunk
Arm

Caudate nucleus (head)
Internal capsule
Cortex of insula
Corticospinal tract

Midbrain

Crus cerebri:
Temporopontine tract
Pyramid tract
Frontopontine tract

Pons

Longitudinal fibers in
basilar portion of pons

Upper
medulla

Pyramid

Lower
medulla

Pyramid decussation

Uncrossed ventral
corticospinal tract

Lateral corticospinal tract

C8

To motor endings in muscles
of forearm and hand

T4

To motor endings in intercostal
and segmental back muscles

L4

Ventral
root fiber

To motor endings in gluteus
medius and tibialis anterior muscles

C

To sacral segments of cord

Figure 5-6 *A.* Anterior to posterior organization of the frontal cortex. *B.* Medial to lateral organization of the primary motor cortex represented as the motor homunculus. *C.* Organization of corticospinal tract.

the appropriate selection of motor acts. The final cortical belt is the primary motor cortex (PM), area 4 in the Brodmann classification, a strip of neocortex that occupies the anterior bank of the central sulcus. The PM is organized topographically with the face and arm represented laterally and the leg represented medially, forming the motor homunculus. The PM probably is responsible for the control of fine coordinated movements.

The three cortical belts are interconnected, though the predominant flow of information appears to be anterior to posterior: prefrontal to premotor to primary motor. These regions receive input from many neocortical, allocortical, and subcortical regions that affect motor performance by modulating frontal lobe neocortical neuron activity.

The motor neocortical regions give rise to the corticospinal tract, a collection of axons that convey information from neurons in neocortical regions to the spinal cord. The corticospinal tract arises from the primary motor, premotor, and primary somatosensory cortices (Fig. 5-6C). The axons forming the corticospinal tract emerge from the immediately subjacent white matter and gather together in a compact bundle in the posterior limb of the internal capsule. The topography of the primary motor cortex is preserved, but the orientation is rotated, with the posterior fibers directed at the lower extremity segments of the spinal cord, the anterior fibers directed at the facial motor neurons, and fibers in between directed at the upper limb segments of the spinal cord. The corticospinal tract continues ventrally, forming a good portion of the cerebral peduncles of the midbrain, where the facial fibers are most medial, the leg fibers are lateral, and the arm fibers are in between. Within the pons, the corticospinal tract breaks into smaller discrete bundles within the basis pontis and finally collects again into a ventrally located compact bundle on the surface of the medulla. Within the pons, fibers innervating the motor nuclei of the eighth cranial nerve cross the midline to innervate the contralateral seventh cranial nerve nuclei. The triangular appearance of the medullary bundle inspired the name *pyramidal tract*, which is a common synonym for the whole corticospinal pathway. Throughout the forebrain and brainstem, the corticospinal tract maintains the topography of the primary motor cortex. At the cervicomedullary junction, most corticospinal axons cross the midline (decussate) and migrate laterally to form the lateral corticospinal tract, which is located lateral to the dorsal horn of the spinal gray matter. With decussation, the topography of the corticospinal tract changes. The axons innervating lumbar segments become the most lateral component of the corticospinal tract, while the axons innervating the cervical segments take up the most medial position. A minority of corticospinal axons, probably less than 10 percent, do not decussate and continue their course along the ventral surface of the spinal cord, forming the uncrossed ventral corticospinal tract. At their level of termination, the axons of the ventral corticospinal tract cross the midline in the anterior commissure of the spinal cord to synapse on spinal neurons. In deducing the location of corticospinal tract lesions, consider the lateral corticospinal tract to be the predominant pathway.

Most corticospinal axons terminate within the intermediate laminae of the spinal cord, synapsing on interneurons that project to other neurons within the spinal cord, including the anterior horn neurons that give rise to axons that innervate muscles. A minority of corticospinal axons synapse directly on the anterior horn cell motor neurons. There is a phylogenetic variation in the volume of corticospinal axons terminating on primary motor neurons. In rodents and carnivores, virtually no corticospinal axons terminate on primary motor neurons. In monkeys and to a greater extent in apes, a significant number of corticospinal axons terminate on primary motor neurons. The extent of direct innervation of primary motor neurons by the neocortex is clearly correlated with the ability of different species to perform finely coordinated hand (paw) and wrist movements.

Clinical Abnormalities and Examination

Corticospinal system dysfunction evokes a specific constellation of weakness, incoordination, hypertonicity, and reflex changes. Characteristic findings occur with chronic disease. The extent and distribution of these findings depend on where in the rostral to caudal axis of the tract the injury occurs, but the character of the clinical findings is identical whether the corticospinal system is injured in the forebrain or in the spinal cord.

Decreased power from corticospinal system injury evokes characteristic patterns of weakness in the face, arm, and leg. The face shows weakness of the lower two-thirds of the muscles with at least relative sparing of the upper third. At rest, a patient with a corticospinal system lesion above the level of the seventh nerve nucleus has a slack lower face *contralateral* to the locus of injury, with downward deflection of the corner of the mouth and widening of the palpebral fissure on the affected side. When asked to smile, the patient does not elevate the corner of the mouth or activate the muscles in the lower face. With mild corticospinal impairment, when the patient smiles, the corner of the mouth on the affected side does not rise as quickly as does the corner on the unaffected side. Slight asymmetries in mouth configuration should not be overinterpreted, as many normal individuals have one corner of the mouth slightly higher than the other. Assess the movements with smiling on command rather than spontaneous smiling. Spontaneous or reflexive smiles often do not show the motor impairment seen with voluntary smiling elicited on command. Ensure that patients make a sustained vigorous effort to smile. Ask them to grimace or grit their teeth to activate these motor pathways fully. In contrast to the weakness apparent in the lower two-thirds of the face, the muscles of the upper third of the face are spared. You can demonstrate this by asking a patient to wrinkle the forehead or push the eyebrows upward. In a patient with a corticospinal system injury, the forehead wrinkles symmetrically. With lesions of the seventh cranial nerve nucleus or axons, the entire half of the face ipsilateral to the site of injury becomes weak. The explanation for the dissociation of upper and lower facial movement after a corticospinal tract injury is that motor neurons innervating upper facial muscles receive relatively little direct corticospinal input.

In the arm, corticospinal system injury results in weakness of extensor muscles with relative sparing of flexor muscles. The arm is adducted at the shoulder and flexed at the elbow and wrist, and the fingers tend to curl into a fist. All affected muscle groups show spasticity. In the leg antigravity muscle (extensor) power is relatively spared, but leg flexors are weak. The leg is extended at the hip, knee, and ankle, and the foot is rotated internally. The limb is spastic. Rapid finger and foot movements are slowed but rhythmic. Finger-nose-finger and heel-knee-shin maneuvers may be limited in power, but if sufficient power remains, these movements will be performed accurately. Gait testing reveals evidence of weakness and spasticity in the affected limbs, and walking may disclose a hemiparetic or spastic diplegic gait. The tendon reflexes are increased in affected muscle groups, and clonus may occur. The reflexes may spread to affect muscles across joints other than those tested. Tendon reflexes that are normally difficult to elicit, such as the pectoralis and internal hamstrings, may be elicited readily on the affected side. An extensor plantar reflex, the Babinski sign, will appear on the affected side.

These findings result from chronic corticospinal system injury. Spasticity and increased tendon reflexes are often absent immediately after acute lesions. At this time, profound weakness (plegia) often is accompanied by hypotonus (flaccidity) and diminished tendon reflexes. The typical pattern then emerges gradually over the course of several days to weeks. The distribution of weakness and the presence of extensor plantar reflexes will not vary with time.

The specific patterns of weakness, spasticity, hyperreflexia, and extensor plantar reflexes identify corticospinal system injury almost anywhere along its axis. The rostral-caudal level of the injury can be judged by assessment of which body parts are affected and which are spared. Involvement of the lower limbs alone indicates a spinal cord process caudal to the primary motor neurons innervating the arms and rostral to the lumbar primary motor neurons of the leg muscles. Since the corticospinal tract decussates at the level of the cervicomedullary junction, the lesion must be ipsilateral to the affected leg. If both legs are affected, the corticospinal tract must be affected bilaterally. Processes producing ipsilateral impairment of arm and leg function must be located above the level of the cervical primary motor neurons innervating arm muscles, while involvement of the face, arm, and leg indicates impairment of the contralateral corticospinal system above the level of the seventh cranial nerve nucleus in the lower pons. A process sparing the face but causing arm and leg involvement must be between the cervical motor neurons and the seventh nerve nucleus. Because the corticospinal tract decussates at the cervico-medullary junction, if the lesion is in the brainstem, it will be contralateral to the affected limbs, and if it is in the high cervical cord, it will be ipsilateral to the affected limbs. For processes affecting the corticospinal tracts in the spinal cord, more precise rostral-caudal localization can be achieved by using the "root levels" of the affected muscle groups.

The topographic organization of the corticospinal tract can be useful. Some forebrain lesions, such as middle cerebral artery strokes, affect lateral cortex more than medial cortex and thus cause face and arm impairment with relative sparing of the leg. Midline pathology, such as parasagittal meningiomas and bilateral anterior cerebral artery strokes, preferentially involves the legs. As the corticospinal tract becomes compact, as at the level of the internal capsule or midbrain, even small lesions will affect all corticospinal fibers, and the face, arm, and leg are involved equally. In the cervical cord, central lesions affect the medial arm and hand fibers within the lateral corticospinal tracts, causing preferential hand weakness.

THE BASAL GANGLIA

The basal ganglia consist of a group of interconnected subcortical nuclei. Lesions of these nuclei produce a remarkably disparate array of clinical phenomena, varying with injury to the different nuclei.

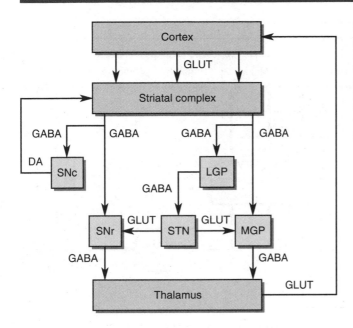

Figure 5-7 Basal ganglia schematic. LGP = lateral globus pallidus; STN = subthalamic nucleus; MGP = medial globus pallidus; SNr = substantia nigra pars reticulata; SNc = substantia nigra pars compacta; GABA = γ-aminobutyric acid; GLUT = glutamate; DA = dopamine.

Anatomy

The basal ganglia consist of the stratum, globus pallidus, substantia nigra, and subthalamic nucleus. Most of these nuclei have more than one component. The striatum consists of the medial caudate nucleus and lateral putamen, which are separated by the fibers of the internal capsule, and the ventral nucleus accumbens. These striatal elements merge into one another. The globus pallidus contains two discrete components: the external (or lateral) globus pallidus and the internal (or medial) globus pallidus. Likewise, the substantia nigra consists of two segments: the pars compacta and the pars reticulata. The cell morphology and connectivity of the substantia nigra pars reticulata are similar to those of the internal globus pallidus, and these two structures should be regarded as a single unit divided anatomically by fibers of descending pathways from the cortex.

The basal ganglia are a component of a corticobasal ganglionic-thalamo-cortical loop (Figs. 5-7 and 5-8). The striatum receives massive excitatory innervation from the whole cortical mantle and allied regions. The striatum in turn projects to both segments of the globus pallidus and both segments of the substantia nigra. These striatal outputs are inhibitory. The internal globus pallidus and substantia nigra pars reticulata are the output stations of the basal ganglia; they send inhibitory projections to a restricted set of thalamic nuclei that in turn send excitatory projections to the primary motor, premotor, and prefrontal cortices. The basal ganglia receive information from virtually all neocortical and allied regions and funnel information back to the neocortical fields involved in motor function. Within this corticobasal ganglionic-thalamo-cortical loop are two important intrinsic basal ganglia circuits. In one circuit, substantia nigra pars compacta neurons receive striatal input and send a prominent dopaminergic projection back to the striatum.

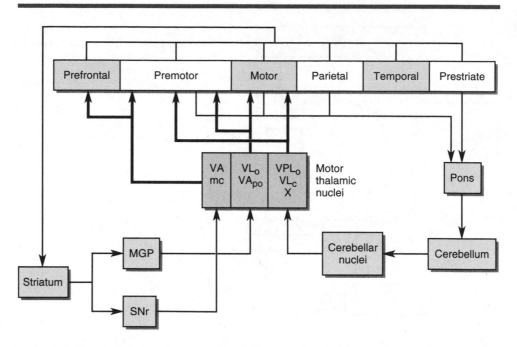

Figure 5-8   Organization of basal ganglia and cerebellar system interconnections with the motor thalamus and neocortex. MGP = medial globus pallidus; SNr = substantia nigra pars reticulata; VA = ventral anterior; VL = ventral lateral; VPL = ventral posterolateral; X = area X.

The other circuit begins with the projection from the striatum to the external globus pallidus, which provides inhibitory projections to the subthalamic nucleus. Neurons within the latter structure give rise to excitatory projections to both segments of the globus pallidus and the substantia nigra. The excitatory subthalamic efferents are crucial modulators of substantia nigra pars reticulata and internal globus pallidus neurons projecting to the thalamus.

The striatum can thus influence basal ganglia output to the thalamus via two pathways: projections to the substantia nigra pars reticulata and internal globus pallidus (the direct pathway) and projections via the external globus pallidus and subthalamic nucleus (the indirect pathway). Basal ganglia regulation of thalamocortical neuron activity is the major final common pathway of basal ganglia modulation of motor function.

Clinical Abnormalities and Examination

Basal ganglia disorders can be classified into three major categories on the basis of clinical phenomenology, clinical pharmacology, and currently known pathophysiology. These categories are parkinsonism, hyperkinetic movement disorders, and dystonia (Table 5-2).

PARKINSONISM   The syndrome of parkinsonism is a reflection of impaired dopaminergic neurotransmission in the basal ganglia. This can result from degeneration of the substantia nigra pars compacta [idiopathic Parkinson disease or 1-methyl-4-

TABLE 5-2. Clinical Features Differentiating Several Movement Disorders

Disorder	Clinical Phenomenology	Clinical Pharmacology	Probable Pathophysiology
Parkinsonism	Bradykinesia Rigidity Tremor Impaired postural reflexes	Caused or worsened by dopamine antagonists; improved by dopamine agonists	Impaired striatal dopaminergic neurotransmission
Hyperkinetic movement disorders	Choreoathetosis Ballism Tics	Improved by dopamine antagonists; exacerbated by dopamine agonists	Intrinsic striatal neuron dysfunction; subthalamic nucleus destruction or underactivity
Dystonia	Fixed posturing of affected body parts	Little effect of dopaminergic manipulations; sometimes improved by anticholinergics	Unknown

phenyl-1, 2, 3, 6-tetrahydropyridine (MPTP) intoxication], pharmacologic depletion of dopamine within substantia nigra pars compacta terminals in the striatum (reserpine, alpha methyl tyrosine), or blockade of striatal dopamine receptors (antipsychotics, antiemetics) or degeneration of striatal neurons (multiple system atrophy). The loss of normal striatal dopamine function results in a strikingly stereotyped constellation of symptoms and signs.

The hallmarks of parkinsonism are bradykinesia, rigidity, impaired postural reflexes, and tremor. Patients often give a history of decreased speed of movement, especially walking, and the initiation of movement becomes increasingly difficult. Rising from a chair and getting in and out of cars are often paticularly difficult. Patients complain of weakness, but questioning reveals not a loss of power but an impairment of coordination. Finely coordinated activities such as buttoning become increasingly difficult, and handwriting is visibly altered. Micrographia, or the tendency of letters to become smaller as writing progresses, is commonly reported and virtually pathognomonic for parkinsonism. Features often unnoticed by patients but commented on by family members and friends include stooped posture, loss of facial expression, and decreased voice volume and clarity.

On examination, power is normal but tone is increased with rigidity and cogwheeling. There is stooped posture, and postural reflexes are impaired. The gait consists of characteristic stooped posture, loss of associated movements of the arms, narrow base, short and often shuffling steps, and "en bloc" turning. Parkinsonian patients have difficulty initiating gait but after a few abnormal steps may be able to walk relatively normally. Ask the patient to arise from a chair with the arms crossed; parkinsonian patients will experience difficulty in standing or be unable to stand even though proximal muscle power is normal. Finger tapping is slow, and the amplitude of movements is diminished. The rhythm of movements is usually relatively normal, though severely affected patients exhibit arrest of movement. Finger-nose-finger and heel-knee-shin maneuvers are slow but otherwise intact. Romberg testing shows no abnormalities. Evaluation of handwriting can be rewarding. Dictate a simple sentence to a patient and observe the handwriting sample for evidence of incoordination and micrographia. Do not ask patients to write only their names because such strongly overlearned acts can be insensitive to motor impairment. Ask the patient to draw the Archimedean spiral, which is a spiral that gradually widens outward. Observing patients during the interview will reveal masked facies (hypomimia) with reduced blinking and diminished voice amplitude (hypophonia). The tendon reflexes are normal, and plantar responses are downgoing.

Many of these patients have a tremor, which is characteristically a low-frequency (4 to 6 Hz) distal resting tremor that improves or vanishes with use of the limb. Common sites include the hands, where it may have a "pill-rolling quality," the legs, and the chin.

Early in the course, idiopathic Parkinson disease often presents with unilateral tremor, rigidity, bradykinesia, and incoordination. Unilateral loss of associated arm movements when walking is a particularly sensitive sign of early parkinsonism.

HYPERKINETIC MOVEMENT DISORDERS   The hyperkinetic movement disorders encompass a variety of phenomenologically disparate movement disturbances (Table 5-3). These disorders have two common elements: they consist of involuntary movements intruding into normal motor behavior, and they are reduced by dopamine antagonists. These disorders have a common pathophysiology involving abnormalities of striatal and/or subthalamic function. The most common of these disorders are chorea and/or athetosis and ballism. Chorea, derived from the Greek word for *dance*, refers to brief, relatively rapid involuntary movements that flow from one muscle group to another randomly. Ballism is a rare and dramatic exaggeration of chorea with many of the same characteristics plus large-amplitude flinging movements of the limbs about proximal joints. Athetosis, which has a sinuous quality, lies on a spectrum between chorea and ballism. These disorders result from destruction of the subthalamic nucleus or striatal dysfunction leading to diminished subthalamic nucleus activity.

TABLE 5-3.   Hyperkinetic Involuntary Movements

Movement	Characteristics	Common Etiologies
Chorea	Brief, randomly distributed, and relatively rapid movements that flow from muscle group to muscle group; may involve any body part	L-dopa excess Huntington disease
Athetosis	Continuous writhing and/or sinuous movements somewhat slower than chorea that also flow from muscle group to muscle group; may involve any body part	L-dopa excess Huntington disease
Ballism	Violent, high-amplitude, often "flinging" movements of limbs with a proximal quality	L-dopa excess Huntington disease Subthalamic nucleus destruction
Tics	Stereotyped and often repetitive movements, sometimes relatively complex; grimacing, blinking, shrugging, and involuntary vocalizations are common	Tourette syndrome Simple tics

Tics are a related hyperkinetic movement disorder that is thought to have some of the same underlying pathophysiology. Tics have a stereotyped quality and may be relatively complex, coordinated motor acts. Typical tics include head turning, shoulder shrugging, eye blinking, grimacing, and involuntary vocalizations.

Characterization of hyperkinetic movement disorders depends almost entirely on observation, with relatively little contribution from the formal examination. Since patients can suppress these movements, observation during the interview as well as the examination is important. Ask the patient to extend the arms in front of himself or herself with the fingers curled slightly, close the eyes, and perform a distracting task such as counting backward from 100 while you observe the digits of the hands and feet for involuntary movements.

A combination of chorea and athetosis that is commonly termed choreoathetosis occurs as a side effect of numerous drugs, with metabolic disturbances, and in a variety of neurodegenerative conditions. Two relatively common causes of choreoathetosis account for the great majority of choreoathetosis seen in practice. The most common cause is L-dopa–induced dyskinesias, a common side effect of treatment in patients with advanced Parkinson disease. Rarer is Huntington disease, an autosomal dominant neurodegeneration with prominent striatal pathology. Occasional patients will be seen with acute unilateral onset of chorea and/or ballism. In these individuals, acute destruction of the contralateral subthalamic nucleus, usually caused by stroke, is the most common etiology.

DYSTONIA   Dystonia is an involuntary movement disorder defined by the assumption of fixed postures by affected muscle groups. These movements are generally sustained for at least seconds and often for longer. Unlike parkinsonism and hyperkinetic movement disorders, which respond to manipulations of dopaminergic neurotransmission, dystonias are not reliably affected by dopaminergic agents. Dystonia is classified on the basis of its anatomic distribution. Generalized dystonia involves the whole body, hemidystonia one side of the body, segmental dystonia the muscles innervated by discrete sets of spinal and/or branchial segments, and focal dystonia specific muscle groups. Dystonia may be classified as primary, with no inciting cause, or secondary, in which case it is due to another neurologic disorder, and other symptoms and/or findings may be present. Secondary dystonia occurs in a variety of childhood-onset metabolic disorders and Wilson disease. Dystonia is presumed to be of basal ganglia origin, though primary dystonias show no pathologic changes in these structures. The clearest connection between dystonia and basal ganglia dysfunction comes from studies of symptomatic hemidystonia after lesions of the forebrain. The most common site of injury in this situation is the putamen. The association of dystonia with basal ganglia dysfunction is strengthened by the occurrence of dystonia in other disorders involving the basal ganglia, such as advanced Huntington disease, progressive supranuclear palsy, dystonic cerebral palsy, and Wilson disease.

In adults, the great majority of dystonias are idiopathic and focal and/or segmental. Common adult dystonias include torticollis (wryneck) with involuntary turning, flexion, or extension of the head; blepharospasm (involuntary eye closure); spasmodic dysphonia (involuntary laryngeal movement); and writer's cramp (involuntary posturing of the hand when writing). Generalized dystonias are common in childhood, and in this age group they usually are inherited or secondary to metabolic disorders.

Evaluation of dystonia requires careful observation during the interview, at times when patients are unaware that you are watching them, and during the examination. Eliciting a history of factors that precipitate, exacerbate, or relieve dystonia is useful. Be cautious about labeling a dystonia as hysterical because of inconsistent involuntary movements. Some dystonias are task-specific; for example, a patient with writer's cramp may have dystonia when writing and not when typing, and patients with lower extremity dystonia may have difficulty walking forward but not backward. Many patients describe apparently bizarre maneuvers that alleviate dystonia. One example is the "geste antagoniste" in patients with torticollis; these patients will be seen holding the head in the midline by placing a finger on the side of the face ipsilateral to the direction of rotation. These individuals are not pushing the head into the midline; the cutaneous stimulation mitigates their torticollis.

TARDIVE DISORDERS   Tardive disorders have a unified etiology but present with diverse manifestations. These involuntary movements develop after long-term use of dopamine antagonists such as antipsychotics and antiemetics. Any type of hyperkinetic movement or dystonia may be seen as a tardive phenomenon. This includes dystonias, tics, and choreoathetosis. The most common tardive disorder is tardive dyskinesia, which consists of repetitive, usually stereotyped oral-buccal-lingual movements. These involuntary movements are not choreic; they are stereotyped and not random. These movements result from long-term changes in striatal dopaminergic function after chronic blockade of dopamine receptors.

MYOCLONUS   Myoclonus is an involuntary movement characterized by rapid, random, lightning-like movements of the limbs, trunk, or head. Myoclonus is not specifically associated with disorders of the basal ganglia and can follow injuries at any level of the central nervous system from the neocortex to the spinal cord.

THE CEREBELLAR SYSTEM

The cerebellar system (Fig. 5-9) is particularly important in the coordination of movement but also may participate in higher-level nonmotor functions. In the motor sphere, the cerebellum is responsible for piecing together the individual muscle and muscle group acts that form a movement. Injury to the cerebellum leads to a stereotyped set of symptoms and findings that vary in anatomic distribution depending on the parts of the system affected. The cerebellar system functions as a modulator of corticospinal system function by providing inputs to the motor and premotor areas. The cerebellum also provides outputs that affect spinal and brainstem nuclei by influencing descending pathways that originate from the red nuclei, reticular nuclei, and vestibular nuclei.

Anatomy

The cerebellum has two major components: the cortex and the deep nuclei. Both of these components receive cerebellar afferents, and the cortex projects to the deep cerebellar

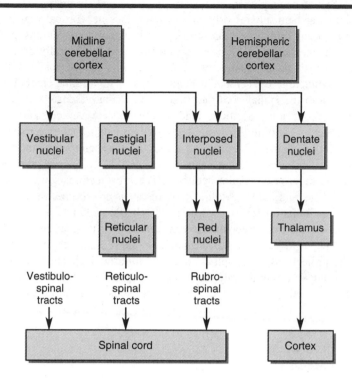

Figure 5-9   Schematic of cerebellar system.

nuclei, which serve as the output sites of the cerebellum. The one exception is the direct projection from the cerebellar cortex to the vestibular nuclei. The portions of the cerebellar cortex projecting to the vestibular nuclei, mainly in the midline cerebellum and the small and phylogenetically ancient floccular and/or modular cerebellar cortex, also receive vestibular input. For these parts of the cerebellar cortex, the vestibular nuclei can be considered to be a homolog of the deep cerebellar nuclei. The cerebellar cortex and deep nuclei form a series of sagittally arranged units. The midline cerebellum (vermis) projects on the most medial of the deep cerebellar nuclei, the fastigial nuclei, and the lateral cerebellar cortex (hemispheres) projects to the large and most lateral deep cerebellar nuclei, the dentate nuclei. An intermediate zone between the vermis and the hemispheres projects to the interposed nuclei: the globose and emboliform nuclei. The cerebellum is connected to the rest of the central nervous system by the superior, middle, and inferior cerebellar peduncles. With a few exceptions, the superior peduncle contains cerebellar efferents, while the middle and inferior peduncles contain cerebellar afferents.

For purposes of clinical localization, the cerebellar cortex and nuclei can be viewed as being organized roughly into two major functional units—the midline cerebellum and the cerebellar hemispheres—which are differentiated on the basis of afferent and efferent targets.

The cerebellar hemispheres are neocortically related structures. The primary afferents to the cerebellar hemispheres originate in numerous neocortical regions, including both primary motor and primary somatosensory cortices, premotor regions, parietal association areas, and visual cortices. These projections synapse ipsilaterally on neurons within the nuclei of the basis pontis. Pontocerebellar projections project ipsilaterally via the middle cerebellar peduncle to the cerebellar hemispheres. The midline cerebellum receives input principally from the spinal cord and brainstem. Primary sensory afferents that transmit information about joint position, tendon and muscle stretch, and muscle activation synapse on neurons within the spinal cord and brainstem that give rise to spinocerebellar and trigeminocerebellar afferents that enter the cerebellum via the inferior cerebellar peduncle. The only exception to this is the ventral spinocerebellar projection, which enters via the superior cerebellar peduncle. These projections synapse within the midline cerebellum. The midline cerebellum also receives projections from brainstem reticular nuclei and vestibular nuclei via the inferior cerebellar peduncle.

The anatomy of the cerebellar efferents mirrors that of afferents. The midline deep cerebellar nuclei project to brainstem nuclei—the red and reticular nuclei—which send descending projections to the spinal cord. The midline deep cerebellar nuclei also project to thalamic nuclei that innervate the motor and premotor cortices. The lateral cerebellar cortex projects to the dentate nuclei, which send substantial outputs to the thalamic nuclei innervating primary motor and premotor cortices (see Fig. 5-9).

Clinical Abnormalities and Examination

The cerebellum can be separated into two clinically useful divisions: the midline cerebellum, which is concerned mainly with head position, maintenance of posture, and oculomotor function, and the lateral cerebellum, which is involved more with limb use and execution of fine coordinated movements. These distinctions are somewhat arbitrary, and because of the indistinct borders between the midline and hemispheric divisions, localization of cerebellar dysfunction is imprecise. Patients with cerebellar pathology may exhibit dysfunction of both divisions.

MIDLINE CEREBELLAR DYSFUNCTION Midline cerebellar disease causes impairment of posture, head position, gait, and oculomotor function. Gait disorders are common; patients with midline cerebellar dysfunction complain of stumbling, falling, or incoordinated walking. Evaluation discloses an ataxic gait with a broadened base, irregular stride length, and stumbling. Performance of tandem gait is especially difficult. The heel-knee-shin test and analogous maneuvers are abnormal. Marked midline cerebellar impairment may cause great difficulty in maintaining a normal erect standing or sitting posture. Romberg's test is negative in that balance is poor but does not worsen greatly with the eyes closed. The head may be tilted or rotated. Limb power is generally normal, and arm and hand coordination is relatively normal. Hypotonia may be found in the legs. Oculomotor abnormalities are common but variable in nature and do not possess precise localizing value. Gaze-evoked nystagmus, dysmetric saccades, abnormalities of pursuit, and optokinetic nystagmus are all seen with midline cerebellar disease. Perhaps the only oculomotor disturbance unique to the cerebellum is rebound nystagmus, in which the fast component begins in the direction of laterally evoked eye movements and then reverses direction. This finding does not, however, distinguish midline from hemispheric cerebellar disease.

HEMISPHERIC CEREBELLAR DYSFUNCTION Hemispheric cerebellar dysfunction results in abnormalities of coordinated limb movements, especially the arms and hands, out of proportion to gait or postural abnormalities. Symptoms and findings are mainfest ipsilateral to the affected cerebellar hemisphere. These patients complain of loss of coordination without loss of power or changes in sensation. On examination, power is normal but resistance to passive manipulation may be reduced. Hypotonia may allow stretching of a joint to its extreme range of motion, and pendular deep tendon reflexes may be found. Coordination invariably is affected with irregular amplitude and dysrhythmic movements with finger to thumb tapping or alternating pronation and supination of the hands. The finger-nose-finger maneuver exhibits dysmetria (disturbed trajectory of movements) and decomposition (breaking down of a smooth integrated movement into several components). Placement of the finger on the examiner's finger or the patient's nose is inaccurate and may include a side-to-side tremor from the shoulder. Impaired check and rebound are also manifestations of impaired coordination in cerebellar disease. They can be assessed by asking patients to extend the limbs in front of them, with the hands pronated and the eyes closed. The examiner gently but firmly taps a hand to displace it vertically. Normally, a modest excursion occurs from the original position with return to the starting position after a mild overshoot; in patients with hemispheric cerebellar disease, the excursion and overshoot are much larger. Many oculomotor disturbances occur, including all those seen with midline cerebellar disease. Gaze-evoked nystagmus may be of some localizing value, as the amplitude of the fast component may increase with gaze in the direction of the hemispheric lesion. Dysarthria is common with hemispheric cerebellar lesions and usually has a distinct pattern with disturbed rhythm, poor articulation, and variations in pitch and volume (ataxic speech).

Frontal lobe injury, presumably because of damage to the frontopontocerebellar pathway, sometimes results in unilateral limb ataxia. Patients with this localization of pathology do not show the extraocular movement or speech abnormalities characteristic of cerebellar disease.

TREMOR Tremor consists of a regular and rhythmic involuntary movement that is defined on the basis of when it occurs and which body parts are affected. Resting tremor occurs only when the body part is relaxed, postural tremor develops when the body part maintains posture, kinetic tremor occurs when the body part is in motion, and task-related tremor becomes manifest only during the performance of specific tasks. Observe the patient with the limbs relaxed and then ask the patient to place the affected limb in a fixed posture (for the arms, this is with them extended forward), then perform a simple motor task (generally the finger-nose-finger or heel-knee-shin maneuver), and finally direct the patient to execute the specific task associated with tremor.

All individuals have a mild physiologic tremor that can be seen by extending the arms in front of the body. This tremor results from the intrinsic viscoelastic properties of the limbs and increases with sympathetic activation. Resting tremors are associated strongly with parkinsonism. Many drugs cause tremor, probably by enhancing the normal physiologic tremor.

Cerebellar disease often causes tremor that is usually ipsilateral to the lesions in unilateral cerebellar hemisphere disease. These tremors are usually postural and kinetic, but in severe cases resting tremor may occur. In midline cerebellar dysfunction, titubation, a coarse truncal tremor, may be manifest with sitting or standing and may be severe enough to cause falls. Titubation is a postural tremor that is alleviated by resting in a supine or prone position. With hemispheric cerebellar disease, postural and kinetic limb tremors often occur during maintenance of fixed limb postures and with the finger-nose-finger and heel-knee-shin tests. Cerebellar tremor often is manifest in the proximal muscle groups, in contrast to the distal tremor seen in parkinsonism. Tremor consists of regular movements and can be distinguished from the decomposition of limb movements that leads to dysmetria. Patients with cerebellar disease have inaccurate placement of the distal limb during finger-nose-finger and heel-knee-shin maneuvers in addition to tremors. Rubral tremor occurs with contralateral lesions of the midbrain in the region of the red nucleus. This tremor is often severe, can occur both at rest and with limb use (both postural and kinetic tremor), and is associated with typical cerebellar disturbances of coordination. The red nucleus is closely adjacent to the superior cerebellar peduncle, and rubral tremor may stem from interruption of cerebellar output.

The most common pathologic tremor is benign essential tremor or benign familial tremor, a very slowly progressive disorder seen commonly in the elderly. Age-related alterations in cerebellar system function are part of the pathophysiology of this tremor. This type of tremor usually affects the arms and hands, often the head, and occasionally the voice. Postural and kinetic in nature, this tremor is exacerbated by certain tasks, such as eating, drinking, and writing. These patients show no other signs of cerebellar or other motor system dysfunction.

THE PERIPHERAL NERVOUS SYSTEM: SPINAL CORD AND ANTERIOR HORN CELLS, ROOTS, PLEXUSES, AND PERIPHERAL NERVES

Anatomy

The anterior horn cells, or "lower motor neurons," are the large alpha motor neurons in the anterior gray horn of the spinal cord and are the final component of the central nervous system motor pathways and the first element of the peripheral nervous system. Activation of motor neurons induces muscle contraction and produces movement organized by descending motor fibers, afferent information, and spinal interneurons. One anterior horn cell, along with all the muscle fibers it innervates, constitutes a motor unit. The number of muscle fibers innervated ranges from 3 in extraocular eye muscles, which require fine increments of movement, to over 100. Thousands of inputs reach motor neu-

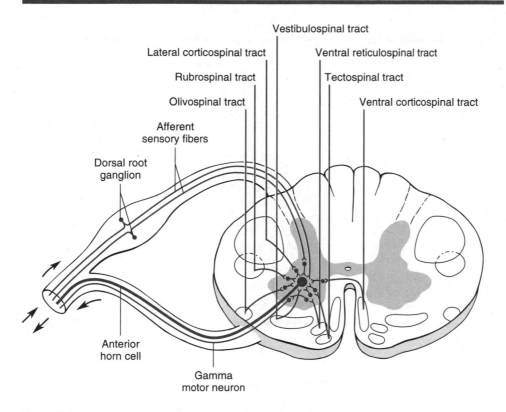

Figure 5-10   Spinal cord, cross section. Anterior horn cell integrates many different motor and sensory system inputs ("final common pathway").

rons derived from incoming sensory fibers, descending motor fibers, and interneurons synapsing onto these neurons (Fig. 5-10). Depending on the sum of these inputs, the action of the anterior horn cell may be facilitated or inhibited. As the extremities require many anterior horn cells to innervate the limb muscles, the number of anterior horn cells and the size of the anterior horns vary at different spinal levels; the largest populations are at the cervical and lumbosacral levels. The features of individual motor units vary with the characteristics of the individual muscles. Muscles used for fine coordinated movements have a relatively high ratio of anterior horn cells to muscle fibers, and this permits fine control of movement. Muscles used for grosser tasks have a lower ratio of anterior horn cells to muscle fibers.

The anterior horn cell axons exit the spinal cord as ventral root filaments at the anterior lateral sulcus, joining with dorsal root filaments (see Fig. 5-10) to form the 31 mixed spinal nerve roots (8 cervical, 12 thoracic, 5 lumbar, 5 sacral, and 1 coccygeal) (Fig. 5-11). The spinal nerve roots contain not only alpha but also gamma motor neuron axons, whose cell bodies also occupy the anterior gray matter with input to muscle spindles. At many levels the spinal nerve roots also contain autonomic fibers.

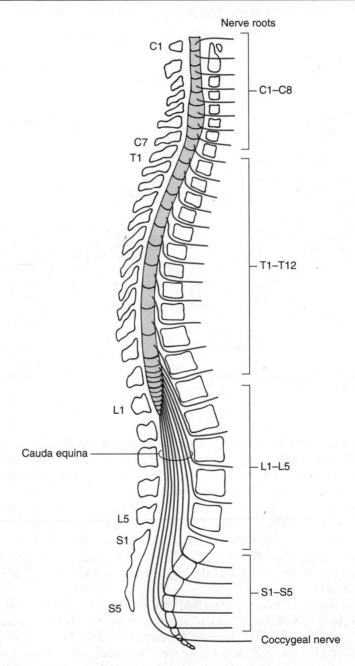

Figure 5-11   Spinal cord, longitudinal with 31 mixed spinal nerve roots. Note "cauda equina" formed by long course of lumbar and sacral roots.

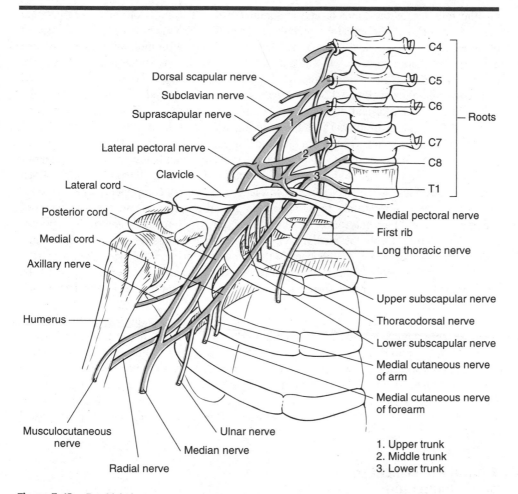

Figure 5-12   Brachial plexus.

The spinal roots exit the spine through the neural or intervertebral foramen; in the cervical region they emerge *above* the correspondingly numbered vertebral body (i.e., the fifth cervical root exits from above the fifth cervical vertebra). The eighth spinal root emerges below the C7 vertebral body, and the spinal roots caudal to the C8 spinal root (thoracic, lumbar, etc.) emerge *below* the corresponding vertebral body. As a result of different growth rates during development, the spinal column is longer than the spinal cord, with the distal portion of the spinal cord (conus medullaris) remaining at level of the L1 or L2 vertebra. Thus, the nerve roots at the lumbar and sacral levels are considerably longer than those at the cervical and thoracic levels, passing from the spinal cord to their neural foramina within the spinal canal. This intraspinal collection of nerve roots is termed the cauda equina (horse's tail) (see Fig. 5-11). After exiting the neural foramina, the spinal nerves divide into posterior rami, innervating the paraspinal muscles, and anterior rami. The thoracic anterior rami form the intercostal and subcostal nerves, innervating the muscles of the thoracic and abdominal walls. The anterior rami form cervical (along with T1) and lumbosacral segments and then fuse into the brachial and lumbosacral plexuses, respectively, which branch into the nerves innervating the limb muscles. All the muscles that share innervation by the anterior horn cells in one spinal nerve segment are termed a *myotome*. Most muscles receive innervation from more than one spinal segment.

The brachial plexus (Fig. 5-12) is formed from the C5–C8 and T1 anterior rami in the lateral neck and axilla and consists of a complex interlacing of axons that creates the nerves of the upper extremity. These five anterior rami form three trunks, with C5 and C6 forming the upper trunk, C7 the middle, and C8 and T1 the lower. The brachial plexus travels between the anterior and middle scalene muscles, then below the clavicle anterior to the first rib, and then through the roof of the axilla surrounding the axillary artery. Each trunk divides into an anterior component and a posterior component. The posterior components of all three trunks fuse to form the posterior cord, the anterior component of the upper and middle trunk forms the lateral cord, and the remaining anterior component of the lower trunk forms the medial cord. Groups of axons emerge from the trunks and cords, forming the nerves. As this occurs, the remaining portions of the lateral, posterior, and medial cords become the musculocutaneous, radial, and ulnar nerves, respectively. The median nerve is formed from the fusion of some components of the lateral and medial cords.

The lumbosacral plexus is somewhat less complex. This plexus travels through the pelvis, within the psoas muscle, and then along the sacrum and the posterolateral pelvic wall. A lumbar plexus is derived from the anterior rami of L1 through L4, forming the femoral and obturator nerves, with motor branches directly to the iliopsoas. The sacral plexus is formed from the anterior rami of S1 to S3, with components from L4 and L5 carried by the lumbosacral trunk. This gives rise to the sciatic nerve (which later divides into the peroneal and tibial nerves) as well as the superior and inferior gluteal nerves.

Clinical Abnormalities and Examination

Loss of power, muscle wasting, diminished tendon reflexes, and fasciculations represent hallmarks of *peripheral* motor system (anterior horn, nerve root, plexus, or nerve) disease. Immediately after axons are injured or stop conducting action potentials (conduction block), fewer muscle fibers are depolarized and decreased maximal strength can be generated. With acute nerve injury, weakness is roughly proportional to the number of fibers involved. With gradually progressive injury, 50 to 75 percent of axons must be involved before weakness becomes apparent. The reason for the difference is the active reinnervation by remaining axons in gradual injury, with increased numbers of muscle fibers innervated by each functioning anterior horn cell. Muscle wasting, or loss of muscle bulk, is apparent weeks after axonal interruption. Weakness without eventual wasting suggests that the weakness is due to motor nerve *conduction block* (e.g., myelin dysfunction, with continuity of the axon to muscle), pain inhibition, limited effort, or a central nervous system disorder. Fasciculations indicate axonal hyperexcitability caused by nerve compression, axonal degeneration, muscle fatigue, or metabolic derangement (e.g., excessive caffeine, thyrotoxicosis, hypocalcemia). Tendon reflexes are diminished

TABLE 5-4. Pattern of Weakness and Reflex Change After Nerve Root Injury

Nerve Root	Expected Weakness	Diminished or Absent Reflex
Upper extremity		
C5, C6	Shoulder abduction, elbow flexion	Biceps, brachioradialis
C7	Elbow extension, wrist extension	Triceps
C8	Wrist flexion, finger flexion	Triceps
T1	Finger abduction, thumb abduction, adduction, opposition	
Lower extremity		
L3, L4	Knee extension	Patellar
L5	Ankle dorsiflexion, inversion, eversion	Internal hamstring
S1	Ankle plantar flexion	Achilles

when peripheral nervous system disease affects the sensory or motor components (or both) of the reflex arc.

The principal means of determining the region of the peripheral nervous system affected is the distribution of the abnormality. With careful clinical examination and attention to peripheral nervous system anatomy, one can determine the precise localization of peripheral nervous system abnormalities.

In diffuse anterior horn cell diseases (motor neuron diseases), many or all anterior horn cells degenerate, causing *diffuse* weakness, wasting, and fasciculations. Abnormalities are not limited to the distribution of one nerve root, division of plexus, or nerve. Sensory and autonomic functions are spared. If you detect these abnormalities along with increased deep tendon reflexes, you should suspect motor neuron disease affecting both the corticospinal tract and the lower motor neuron [e.g., amyotrophic lateral sclerosis (ALS)].

Injury of a single nerve root causes weakness, eventual wasting, and fasciculations in several or all of the muscles innervated by axons exiting the spinal cord within that root. If the injured root contains fibers that are components of a reflex arc, tendon reflexes may be diminished or absent. Although a single ventral nerve root carrying motor fibers can be injured in isolation, most often both dorsal and ventral roots are involved, producing pain, dermatomal sensory loss, and weakness. Common patterns of weakness and reflex change

TABLE 5-5. Distribution of Weakness in Brachial Plexopathy

Trunk	Clinical Findings
Upper	Weakness of arm abduction, elbow flexion; diminished biceps reflex
Middle	Weakness of elbow, wrist, and finger extension; diminished triceps reflex
Lower	Weakness of intrinsic hand muscles

TABLE 5-6. Commonly Encountered Mononeuropathies

Nerve	Common Sites of Involvement	Distribution of Weakness	Distribution of Sensory Loss	Clinically Useful Muscle(s)	Other Considerations
Facial	Stylomastoid foramen	Face	None	Face	Exclude more diffuse involvement on examination
Median	Wrist	Thumb abduction, opposition	Digits 1 and 2	Abductor pollicis brevis	Weak hand intrinsics suggest C8–T1 radiculopathy or lower trunk plexopathy
Ulnar	Wrist, elbow	Hand intrinsic muscles (wrist), deep finger flexors, digits 4 and 5 (elbow)	Digits 4 and 5	First dorsal interossei (abduct index finger)	Weak median innervated hand muscles (thumb abduction) suggests trunk or root localization
Radial	Spiral groove (lower humerus)	Extensors of wrist and fingers	Dorsal arm and hand	Weak brachioradialis, wrist extensors, normal triceps (innervated above spiral groove)	Weak deltoid muscle suggests plexopathy; weak wrist flexors suggest radiculopathy
Long thoracic	Brachial plexus	Scapula stabilizers	None	Serratus anterior	Scapular winging may be due to trapezius weakness (spinal accessory nerve)
Femoral	Inguinal ligament, retro-peritoneal space	Knee extension, hip flexion	Anterior thigh	Quadriceps	Thigh adduction spared in femoral nerve lesions, weak with plexus or lumbar root lesions
Sciatic		Leg flexor (hamstring), all muscles below the knee	Lower leg and foot		
Peroneal	Fibular head (knee)	Foot dorsiflexion, eversion	Lateral leg, dorsum of foot	Ankle dorsiflexors	Foot inversion involved in L5 radiculopathy, spared in peroneal neuropathy

are listed in Table 5-4. The clinical findings after nerve root injury can be limited, as most muscles receive innervation from more than one nerve root and usually multiple muscles move a joint in a given direction. Many root injuries are partial, and variable amounts of reinnervation occur, maintaining strength and minimizing the clinical findings. The methods of testing individual muscle groups are described in Figs. 5-2 to 5-5.

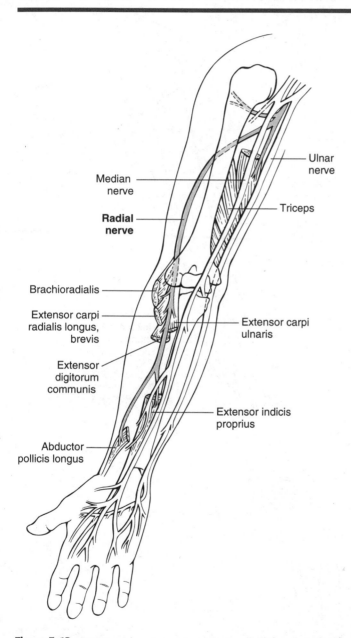

Figure 5-13 Radial nerve, course and muscles innervated.

In lesions of the brachial plexus, the pattern of weakness, wasting, fasciculation, and reflex loss and/or diminution varies, depending on the region of plexus injured. A simplified scheme of patterns of abnormality in brachial plexopathy is outlined in Table 5-5. Differentiating plexopathy from multiple radiculopathies or mononeuropathies

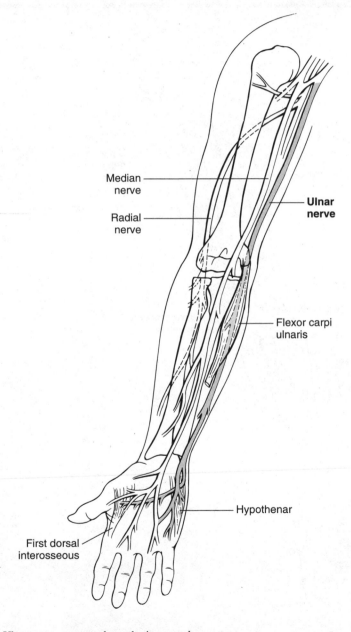

Median nerve

Radial nerve

Ulnar nerve

Flexor carpi ulnaris

Hypothenar

First dorsal interosseous

Figure 5-14 Ulnar nerve, course and muscles innervated.

can be difficult, requiring electrodiagnostic testing (electromyography and nerve conduction studies, as described in Chap. 10). Patterns of sensory loss and pain are useful in localization.

Lumbosacral plexus lesions cause weakness outside the distribution of one nerve or root. You should consider a plexopathy when you find weakness in sciatic innervated muscles plus the gluteal muscles, which are innervated by separate branches of the plexus. Consider a plexopathy also when there is weakness in femoral innervated muscles as well as obturator innervated (adductor) muscles.

The "named" nerves are formed from branching of the brachial and lumbosacral plexuses. These nerves travel through relatively well defined routes, innervating muscles of the limbs. These nerves are commonly entrapped or injured in predictable areas. Nerve injury causes weakness, wasting, and fasciculations in the muscles innervated by the nerve distal to the site of injury. Knowledge of muscle innervation helps you identify diffuse lesions (multiple mononeuropathies, plexopathy) and localize specific nerve involvement. Some of the nerves of the extremities that are commonly injured are listed in Table 5-6.

RADIAL NERVE   The radial nerve (Fig. 5-13), a continuation of the posterior cord of the brachial plexus, winds around the humerus in the spiral groove, between the heads of the triceps muscle. This nerve innervates extensor muscles of the arm, wrist, and fingers. With lesions in the spiral groove, triceps function remains normal, as the triceps muscle is innervated above the spiral groove. A complete radial nerve lesion causes wrist drop and apparent grip weakness. Grip weakness occurs because the finger flexors are placed at a mechanical disadvantage with the wrist flexed. The wrist should be supported during the examination to ensure that the radial nerve is affected without superimposed median or ulnar nerve injury. The radial nerve gives rise to the posterior interosseous nerve in the proximal forearm, supplying wrist and finger extensors but not the extensor carpi radialis, which the radial nerve innervates. Weakness of these muscles with normal radial sensory function suggests involvement of the posterior interosseous nerve.

ULNAR NERVE   The ulnar nerve (Fig. 5-14), a continuation of the medial cord, travels in the medial upper arm without innervating the muscles of the arm. It then travels

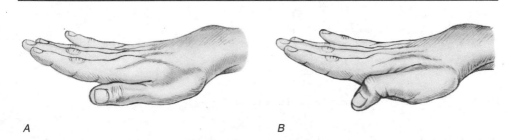

A   *B*

Figure 5-15   Froment's sign. *A*. Normal adduction of thumb. *B*. Adduction of thumb with adductor pollicis weakness after ulnar nerve lesion. Note activation of flexor pollicis longus, which flexes distal phalanx while also adducting the thumb.

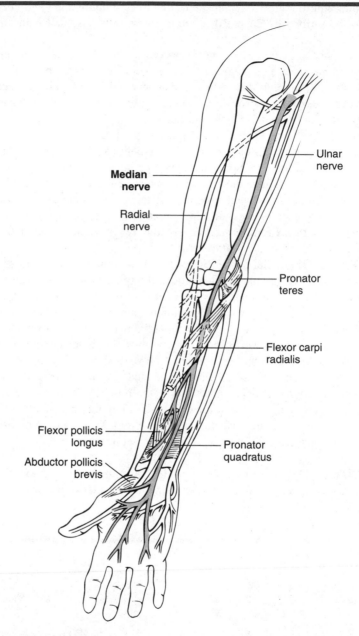

Figure 5-16   Median nerve, course and muscles innervated.

through the ulnar groove and cubital tunnel and along the medial forearm to the hand, there innervating forearm and hand intrinsic muscles. Ulnar nerve injury causes weakness of hand intrinsic muscles and numbness with sensory loss over digits 4 and 5. You can detect weakness most easily in first dorsal interosseus, which abducts the index finger, and the abductor digiti quinti, which abducts the little finger. Adductor pollicis involvement results in weakness of thumb adduction and overaction of the flexor pollicis longus, which is innervated by the anterior interosseous branch of the median nerve, producing flexion of the distal phalanx of the thumb with attempted thumb adduction (Froment's sign) (Fig. 5-15). Weakness of the ulnar innervated forearm muscles suggests localization at the elbow or more proximally. The flexor carpi ulnaris often is innervated by a branch above the elbow and may be spared in lesions at the elbow. Weakness of the hand intrinsic muscles also can result from C8–T1 radiculopathy and lower trunk or medial cord brachial plexopathy. Involvement of median innervated hand muscles supports these latter localizations.

MEDIAN NERVE   The median nerve (Fig. 5-16), which is formed from portions of the medial and lateral cords, travels medially in the upper arm, crosses the elbow anteriorly, and runs through the antecubital fossa and pronator teres. It innervates most of the wrist and finger flexor muscles and the thumb abductors. A motor branch, the anterior interosseous nerve, separates off just as the nerve exits the pronator teres. This nerve innervates the deep flexors of the thumb, the second and third digits, and the pronator quadratus. Injury to the anterior interosseous nerve causes weakness of flexion at the distal phalanges of the thumb and the second and third digits and failure to form a round "O" as part of the "OK" sign, producing a "pinch" sign instead (Fig. 5-17).

FEMORAL NERVE   The femoral nerve (Fig. 5-18) originates in the lumbar plexus and then passes beneath the inguinal ligament lateral to the femoral artery, innervating the quadriceps muscles. Femoral nerve injury causes weakness of knee extension, an absent quadriceps reflex, and diminished sensation over the anterior thigh and leg. Thigh adductors, which are innervated by the obturator nerve, are spared in patients with femoral nerve lesions but may be weak in patients with plexus or lumbar root lesions.

SCIATIC NERVE   The sciatic nerve (Fig. 5-19) exits the pelvis through the sciatic notch, travels posterior to the hip joint, and forms the tibial and peroneal nerves in the

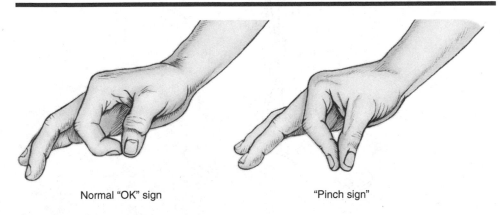

Normal "OK" sign   "Pinch sign"

Figure 5-17   Pinch sign (see text).

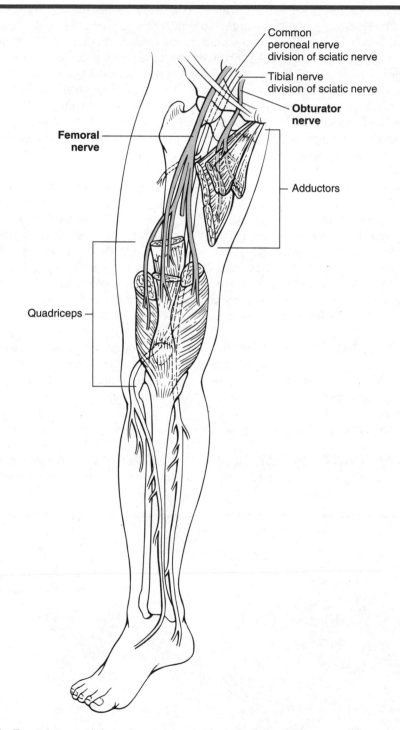

Figure 5-18   Femoral nerve and obturator nerve, course and muscles innervated.

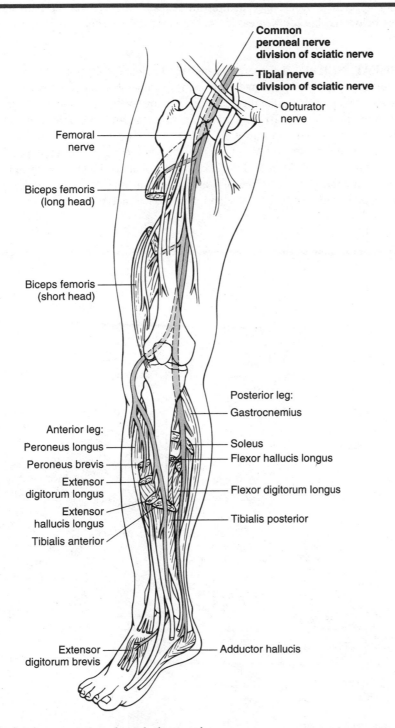

Figure 5-19   Sciatic nerve, course and muscles innervated.

posterior upper leg. Sciatic mononeuropathy causes weakness in the hamstrings and all muscles below the knee, a decreased ankle reflex, and sensory loss in the lower leg and foot.

PERONEAL NERVE   The peroneal nerve, the lateral division of the sciatic nerve, innervates the foot dorsiflexors and evertors. It is vulnerable to compression at the head of the fibula, which causes inability to dorsiflex or evert the foot or extend the toes, thus resulting in foot drop. To distinguish a peroneal mononeuropathy from an L5 radiculopathy, both of which can cause foot drop, examine foot inversion, which requires the action of the posterior tibial muscle. This action is spared in a peroneal mononeuropathy but is involved in an L5 radiculopathy. This is the case because the L5 nerve root innervates the posterior tibial and anterior tibial muscles, whereas the tibial nerve innervates the posterior tibial muscle and the peroneal nerve innervates the anterior tibial muscle.

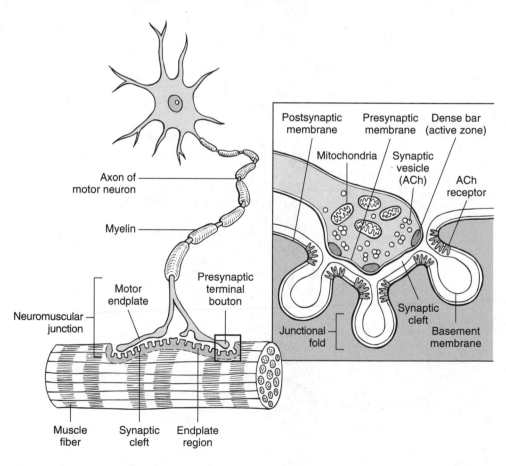

Figure 5-20   Neuromuscular junction.

THE NEUROMUSCULAR JUNCTION

Anatomy

All skeletal muscle contains the neuromuscular junction (Fig. 5-20), which is the site of neuromuscular transmission. Depolarization of the presynaptic motor nerve increases the entry of calcium ions through voltage-gated calcium channels, causing fusion of acetylcholine (ACh)-containing vesicles with the presynaptic membrane. The nerve terminal releases ACh into the synapse. ACh diffuses across the synapse, activating the postsynaptic ACh receptor (AChR), thus opening sodium channels with resultant depolarization of muscle membrane, release of calcium from the sarcoplasmic reticulum, and muscle contraction.

Normally the ACh released is more than is needed for activation of all the AChRs, providing a margin of safety in neuromuscular junction transmission. Disease-related loss of the safety margin provides the basis for clinical testing of neuromuscular junction function.

Clinical Abnormalities and Examination

The signature of neuromuscular junction dysfunction is fatigable weakness. Other aspects of the examination are generally normal, including tone, deep tendon reflexes, and coordination. Evaluate neuromuscular junction function by testing for fatigable skeletal muscle weakness that improves with rest. The most common cause of neuromuscular junction dysfunction is myasthenia gravis, an autoimmune disorder in which circulating autoantibodies to muscle AChRs cause loss of AChRs from the postsynaptic membrane. This leads to loss of the safety margin. In this situation, when an anterior horn cell depolarizes, the ACh released is insufficient to depolarize all the muscle fibers, and muscle weakness occurs. Repeated testing of muscle strength in the same muscle group or repeated firing of the nerve during a nerve conduction study further reduces the available presynaptic ACh, with worsening of weakness or a decremental response in nerve conduction recordings.

The weakness in myasthenia gravis most commonly involves extraocular, bulbar, and proximal limb muscles. Ptosis or ocular malalignment (with complaints of diplopia) may be produced during sustained upgaze or lateral gaze. Attempts by the patient to reduce ptosis by contraction of the frontalis muscle produce a wrinkled brow. Resting the lid by extreme downgaze (causing inhibition of the levator palpebrae) often results in transient correction of ptosis on upgaze. According to Hering's law of equal innervation (described in Chap. 4), unilateral ptosis may be associated with contralateral eye lid retraction or may be enhanced by manually elevating the contralateral lid (which reduces the oculomotor nerve firing rates to *both* lids).

Weakness of the lower facial muscles can cause a transverse smile owing to loss of the usual elevation of the lateral corners of the mouth with smiling. Dysarthria or hypernasal speech may occur and worsen with prolonged speaking. Proximal weakness can be provoked by repeatedly testing the muscle or asking the patient to maintain sustained postures (e.g., arms abducted while sitting, leg or neck flexed while supine). In conducting this examination, note the rapidity of exhaustion. Owing to pelvic girdle weakness, patients with neuromuscular junction dysfunction may exhibit a waddling and/or myopathic gait. Weakness may vary from hour to hour and day to day and usually improves with rest.

Weakness resulting from neuromuscular junction dysfunction may be improved transiently by anticholinesterase medication, forming the basis for the Tensilon test. This involves using intravenous edrophonium, a short-acting anticholinesterase medication, to identify reversible weakness. Measure strength in easily tested weak muscles before and after the administration of edrophonium. Unequivocal improvement in strength (e.g., resolution of ptosis or diplopia) within 60 s, lasting several minutes, supports neuromuscular junction localization. To properly evaluate patients while they are using anticholinesterase medications, you need to know when they took the last dose of medication. Fatigable weakness may be improved substantially shortly after the administration of these medications, only to worsen markedly as the medication is metabolized.

Although neuromuscular junction dysfunction usually results from *postsynaptic* disorders, you need to be aware that dysfunction can occur at the *presynaptic* region in a minority of patients with fatiguing weakness. Presynaptic neuromuscular junction dysfunction causes muscle weakness as well as diminished deep tendon reflexes and autonomic dysfunction. Lambert-Eaton myasthenic syndrome (LEMS) is an immune-mediated disorder of neuromuscular junction transmission, but unlike myasthenia gravis, the immune response affects the presynaptic voltage-gated calcium channel. This damages calcium channels, decreasing calcium entry during depolarization and diminishing ACh release, again leading to loss of the safety margin. Brief activation by asking the patient to contract the weak muscle or the muscle involved in the diminshed reflex may increase the presynaptic concentrations of calcium, leading to facilitation with transient improvement immediately after the contraction. This improvement and the incremental responses during nerve conduction studies (Chap. 10) result from similar physiologic mechanisms.

MUSCLE

Clinical Abnormalities and Examination

The primary function of muscles is to contract, causing movement or stabilizing joints. As weakness is the principal manifestation of muscle disease, the focus of the examination is assessment of muscle and muscle group power. Most muscles can be seen easily. Hence, you should employ visual inspection of muscles at rest, with contraction, and with muscle percussion.

Careful observation of patients' posture and gait is helpful. Observation of atrophy can be difficult, though when it is severe, muscles may be decreased in bulk or flattened. Larger than expected muscle bulk relative to other muscles is termed *pseudohypertrophy* and suggests muscle replacement by fibrosis. Watch the patient walk. Decreased stability of the pelvis produces a "waddle" or myopathic gait, with the pelvis dipping to the opposite side when each foot hits the ground. Weak hip and back extensor muscles cause a compensatory excessive lumbar lordosis, with abdominal protuberance, to place the center of gravity behind the weak extensor muscles. Weak quadriceps muscles lead to "throwing back" of the knees to lock them in a hyperextended position, and these patients use the joint's mechanical strength to compensate for muscle weakness. Patients with weak hip extensors may be unable to arise from a low chair or may need to push with their arms against their thighs to compensate for leg and trunk extensor (proximal) muscle weakness. Weak shoulder muscles allow anterior rotation at the joint, causing the hands to be held palm backward during ambulation.

Ask the patient to step onto a step or stool to look for weakness of the hip stabilizers, with excessive dip toward the leg that was on the floor or inability to lift the body weight with the hip extensors. Ask the patient to arise from the floor or attempt to execute a deep knee bend to look for hip extensor weakness. The patient may need to push with the arms against the thighs to extend the trunk (Gowers' sign). Scapular winging, which is backward protrusion of the scapula, occurs with either serratus anterior weakness (noted during forward arm abduction) or trapezius weakness (noted during lateral arm abduction). Bilateral scapular winging suggests underlying muscle disease, while unilateral winging is more likely to be due to mononeuropathy or brachial plexopathy.

Muscle percussion may cause the sustained contraction known as myotonia, suggesting persistent muscle fiber depolarization. This can occur in several muscle disorders. Myotonia can be seen after sustained muscle contraction (squeezing the eyes or fist tightly shut) as manifested by slow opening. Myotonia should be distinguished from myoedema—local transient muscle swelling after percussion—which is seen in patients with hypothyroidism.

Manual muscle testing is crucial in examining patients with suspected muscle disease. Proximal weakness occurs in most myopathies. Examine the neck flexors and extensors and shoulder girdle and pelvic girdle muscles when you suspect muscle disease. Specific patterns of weakness may be diagnostic of certain myopathies, which are often named according to the distribution of the abnormality (e.g., facioscapulohumeral dystrophy with weakness of the facial, scapular, and humeral muscles).

Observe physical findings associated with muscle weakness such as skin rash, skeletal abnormalities, and dysmorphic features. These findings can be important factors in determining the specific type of myopathy. A rash, for example, may suggest dermatomyositis.

CONCLUSION: INTEGRATING THE MOTOR EXAMINATION

Examination of the motor system is one of the most reliable and useful aspects of the neurologic examination. The motor examination provides information about pathways traversing the entire neuraxis and local and segmental levels of function. Information gleaned from the motor examination complements information derived from other aspects of the neurologic examination. Careful motor system examination frequently rewards a competent examiner with invaluable information for the diagnosis and management of neurologic disease.

DAVID M. DAWSON/FRISSO A. POTTS CHAPTER

REFLEXES

6

HISTORICAL ASPECTS

In the mid-seventeenth century, René Descartes introduced the concept of a reflex as a more or less involuntary motor response to external stimuli. In his schema, external stimuli were carried by nerves, which he thought were hollow tubes, into the brain. There they bounced or "reflected" off the ventricles or the pineal gland and reached an effector organ. It was not until the mid-eighteenth century that Robert Whytt and others carried out experiments in decapitated and spinalized frogs and hypothesized that central connections (or, as Whytt put it, a "sympathy") existed between motor and sensory nerves. Whytt's contemporary, Johann Augustus Unzer, introduced the term *reflex* in the modern sense. He proposed that a specific afferent impulse would be converted into a stereotyped efferent impulse by a process of reflexion in the brain or spinal cord. Subsequent investigators contributed to the further understanding of reflex action. It was not, however, until the work of Sir Charles Scott Sherrington in the late nineteenth and early twentieth centuries that a clear concept of the circuitry of reflex activity and the role of the central nervous system in modulating this activity was developed.

The end of the nineteenth century also saw the description of most of the reflexes used in the clinical examination today. Careful methods for eliciting and quantitating reflexes in the clinical examination were described by Sir William Gowers, Felix Babinski, Jean M. Charcot, Weir Mitchell, Hermann Oppenheim, and others. During this time there was little knowledge of the physiology or pathophysiology underlying the elicited normal or abnormal reflexes. In many instances, clinical reflex abnormalities were considered specific for a single disease entity rather than indicating a pathologic mechanism.

The correlation between observed clinical phenomena and pathophysiologic mechanisms proceeded slowly in the twentieth century. In the English literature, its greatest expression came in the works of Sir Henry Head, Hughlings Jackson, and Gordon Holmes, among others.

DEFINITION AND CLASSIFICATION OF REFLEXES

The term *reflex* has wide application in neurology and is used to describe many types of phenomena. The core meaning of the term, however, is that a stimulus results in a barrage of impulses that are carried toward the central nervous system by the *afferent limb* of the reflex. After a connection is made in the central nervous system, the *efferent limb* of the reflex carries impulses to an effector organ whose response can be observed. Usually, both the stimulus and the response can be quantitated and analyzed. This analysis allows inferences about the pathways and central modulation of the reflex.

We classify reflexes on the basis of their relevant pathways and central connections as follows:

Segmental Reflexes

In these reflexes the stimulus and the response have a fixed spatial relationship. The stimulus activates a barrage of impulses that enter the central system, where they activate motor neurons monosynaptically (a single synapse) or polysynaptically (more than one synapse before reaching a motor neuron). The afferent impulse then reaches an effector organ that is in the neighborhood of the stimulus. Segmental reflexes can be characterized as follows:

1. Monosynaptic reflexes: the stretch reflex, also known as deep tendon reflex.
2. Polysynaptic and oligosynaptic reflexes: the plantar response (sign of Babinski) and the blink reflex. These reflexes are also known as *superficial reflexes.*

Polysegmental Reflexes

In these reflexes, the stimulus produces a response that involves organs far removed from the stimulus site. Polysegmental reflexes can be characterized as follows:

1. Patterned behavioral reflexes
2. Postural and balance reflexes
3. Autonomic reflexes

The clinical examination relies almost exclusively on the observation of segmental reflexes and patterned behavioral reflexes; only these reflexes will be covered in depth in this chapter.

In clinical practice, examination of reflexes offers the following advantages:

1. The reflex responses of a patient are mostly involuntary, or only slightly under conscious control. They do not require volition on the part of the patient, only relaxation. Many reflexes can be elicited in a comatose or stuporous patient and provide information when other means are unavailable.

2. Many reflexes can be quantitated, minimizing interobserver variation.

3. Reflexes can provide information about focal disorders of the nervous system. The disorder may be in the afferent limb, central connections, or efferent limb of the reflex arc. For example, an absent patellar tendon reflex (knee jerk) clearly indicates pathology in the lumbar spinal cord, lumbar nerve roots, or femoral nerve provided that the other reflexes are in the normal range. Similarly, a pupil that does not constrict to bright light points to a lesion in the optic nerve, the tectum of the midbrain, or the oculomotor nerve.

4. In a few instances, a change in reflexes may be the harbinger of pathology that has not yet become clinically obvious. For example, the discovery of an extensor plantar response (Babinski sign) in a patient who has only a complaint of blurred vision often means that the patient has a second lesion in the nervous system and may prove to have multiple sclerosis.

5. Many reflexes provide anatomic specificity. Discovery of a decerebrate posture (extension of the extremities) in response to a noxious stimulus indicates dysfunction at the level of the upper pons or midbrain. The cause of the lesion may be unknown, but the localization is certain.

CLINICAL EXAMINATION OF REFLEXES

The Stretch Reflex

This is the most common reflex tested in clinical practice. *Myotatic reflex* is an equivalent term, though it is rarely used. *Deep tendon reflex* (DTR) is a term that should be avoided. There are no deep tendons that we use and no reflexes that are conversely superficial. This reflex is elicited by applying a brief stretch to a muscle, and the normal response is a contraction. In clinical practice, you give a quick rap to the muscle's tendon, and this results in the desired stretch. Of course, the tendon is not part of the reflex; it merely provides a convenient way to stretch the muscle. The stretch also could be produced by striking the muscle belly, but this would depolarize muscle fibers, and the resulting muscle contraction would not be "reflex" in nature. Figure 6-1 gives a diagrammatic and highly simplified view of the stretch reflex. Its components are described in the following section.

ANATOMY AND PHYSIOLOGY OF THE STRETCH REFLEX   Once the proper stimulus has been delivered, the following structures are concerned in completing the reflex arc.

Muscle Spindles.   These are stretch-sensitive structures located in most skeletal muscles (the muscles of facial expression do not have them). They are made up of short, thin muscle fibers (intrafusal fibers, i.e., inside the spindle) enclosed in a connective tissue capsule. These structures are a few millimeters long and lie embedded within the muscle mass (extrafusal fibers).

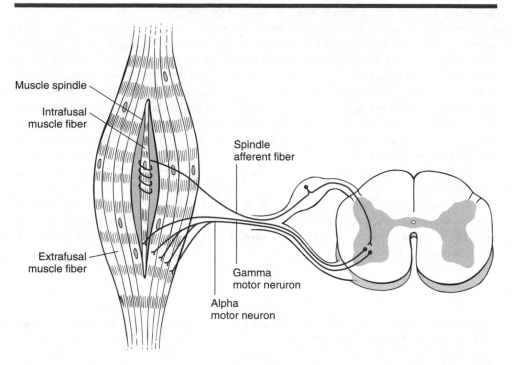

Figure 6-1 Muscle spindle apparatus. The alpha motor neurons innervate the extrafusal fibers, while the gamma motor neurons innervate the intrafusal fiber. By tonic firing, through a wide range of muscle lengths, the gamma motor neurons maintain contraction of the intrafusal fibers and maintain their responsiveness to stretch.

Spindle Afferents. These are dendritic terminals whose cell bodies lie in the dorsal root ganglia or cranial nerve sensory ganglia. These terminals are connected to the intrafusal fiber in such a way that muscle stretch causes mechanical deformation of the terminals, resulting in depolarization and subsequent conduction of nerve action potentials toward the central nervous system. The fibers primarily responsible for carrying the impulses are large, heavily myelinated group I fibers. Thinner, more lightly myelinated group II fibers also participate in the stretch reflex, however. The impulse volley originating in the spindle afferent enters the cord and synapses with alpha motor neurons that innervate extrafusal fibers of the stretched muscle. In some instances a single afferent may innervate all motor neurons supplying its muscle of origin. It also synapses directly with synergistic muscles. In addition, the same afferent supplies inhibitory input to antagonist muscles by way of interneurons. Consequently, as the agonist contracts, the antagonist will be relaxed in the process of *reciprocal inhibition*. By means of this complexity of connections, each alpha motor neuron receives excitatory as well as inhibitory input from many spindle afferents (Fig. 6-2).

Alpha Motor Neuron. Synapses between spindle afferents and alpha motor neurons take place in the dendritic tree of the alpha motor neurons. As impulses arrive, they generate excitatory postsynaptic potentials (EPSPs) in the motor neuron. If enough of these

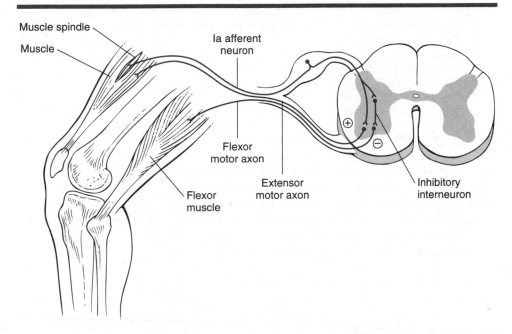

Muscle spindle

Muscle

Ia afferent neuron

Flexor motor axon

Extensor motor axon

Flexor muscle

Inhibitory interneuron

Figure 6-2 Reciprocal inhibition. In this example, a IA afferent from an extensor muscle excites the extensor motor neurons, while inhibiting the flexor motor neurons via an interneuron. In this way unimpeded contraction of the extensor muscle during a stretch can occur. Reciprocal inhibition also is found outside the reflex arc. Voluntary contraction of an agonist muscle requires inhibition of its antagonist. Even if the agonist muscle is deafferented it can be inhibited reciprocally. Loss of reciprocal inhibition, with resulting co-contraction of agonist and antagonist, is found with lesions of either the pyramidal or extrapyramidal motor systems.

impulses arrive within a brief interval, they summate; that is, each EPSP occurs before the previous one has decayed, and this summation brings the cell to the firing threshold. The closer the cell is to its firing threshold (the higher is its resting membrane potential), the fewer impulses it takes to cause the cell to fire. Conversely, a motor neuron whose state of excitability is low enough will not be brought to threshold regardless of the number of afferent impulses it receives.

Alpha Motor Neuron Efferent and Extrafusal Muscle Fiber. Once the motor neuron fires, its axon conducts impulses to its extrafusal muscle fibers, causing them to depolarize and contract. If enough motor units are activated, the muscle contracts visibly. Many spindles must discharge to depolarize a single motor neuron, and many motor neurons must fire to generate a clinically observable muscle contraction.

The Gamma Efferent. Just as a alpha motor neuron innervates extrafusal fibers, a gamma motor neuron supplies the intrafusal fibers. Each spindle receives its nerve supply from a single neuron located in the anterior horn of the motor pool of a given muscle. This neuron, by increasing or decreasing its firing rate, can cause contraction or allow relaxation of intrafusal fibers. Contrary to earlier views (Granit, 1955; Merton, 1972), gamma motor neurons do not initiate muscle activation; during voluntary movements, both the alpha and gamma motor neurons fire (*alpha-gamma coactivation*), resulting in

TABLE 6-1.   Segmental Levels Mediating Muscle Stretch Responses

1. Jaw: cranial nerve V, pons
2. Biceps: **C5**, C6
3. Triceps: C6, **C7**, C8
4. Brachioradialis: C5, C6, C7
5. Quadriceps: L2, **L3**, L4
6. Achilles: L4, L5, **S1**, S2

Note: Letters and numbers in bold type indicate the spinal segment with the greatest contribution.

contraction of both extrafusal and intrafusal fibers (Valbo, 1971). The principal role of gamma efferent innervation of muscle spindles may be to prevent "unloading" of the spindle during extrafusal muscle contraction. The effect of shortening of the muscle spindle (unloading) is to stop the flow of excitatory impulses to alpha motor neurons. Firing of gamma motor neurons increases spindle sensitivity, causing the barrage of impulses from spindles to continue during extrafusal muscle contraction.

CLINICALLY USEFUL STRETCH REFLEXES   The standard clinical examination now includes elicitation of four stretch reflexes, two in the upper limbs and two in the lower: biceps, triceps, patellar, and Achilles reflexes. Sometimes they are titled biceps, triceps, knee, and ankle; naming them for their tendons is a bit more precise. Table 6-1 lists individual reflexes and their segmental innervation.

Other stretch reflexes are used less frequently. These reflexes include the following:

1. Deltoid reflex. Tapping the insertion of the deltoid muscle at the humerus evokes contraction of the deltoid muscle.
2. Pectoralis reflex. The tendon of the pectoralis group is accessible just before it attaches to the humerus in the axilla.
3. Brachioradialis reflex. Tapping on the exposed surface of the radius 10 cm proximal to the wrist elicits contraction of the brachioradialis muscle. Usually the biceps, brachialis, and supinator muscles also participate; this results in flexion and supination of the forearm.
4. Finger flexor reflex. You evoke this reflex by placing two of your fingers against the slightly flexed fingers of the subject and tapping to elicit a stretch reflex of the long flexors of the fingers.
5. Hoffman's sign and Trömner's sign. These are variations of the finger flexor reflex. Rather than tapping on the partially flexed fingers, you stretch the flexor tendons by tapping the tip of the middle finger (Trömner) or flicking the fingernail of this digit (Hoffman). The response consists of flexion of the thumb.
6. Adductor reflex. With the patient in the seated position and the knees flexed, a tap on the medial side of the distal femur elicits an adduction movement of the legs. This reflex is absent in normal subjects.
7. Biceps femoris (hamstring) reflex. The tendon is accessible on the lateral side of the leg, with the knee in 30 to 40° of flexion. This reflex is absent in normal subjects.
8. Tibialis posterior reflex. The tendon of this muscle is located just above and behind the medial malleolus; this reflex is difficult to elicit and consists of foot inversion.

9.   Jaw jerk. You elicit this reflex by gently tapping the subject's relaxed jaw, causing masseter stretch; the response is masseter contraction.

HYPERACTIVITY OF THE STRETCH REFLEX   You should judge the reflexes to be hyperactive (hyperreflexia) on the basis of one or more of the following criteria:

1.   Reduction in threshold. A slight tap produces a brisk response. You can observe this best in the patellar and biceps reflexes.
2.   Spreading or irradiating reflex. Here a tap produces a response in one or more adjacent muscles; for example, a knee jerk elicits leg extension and adduction. Similarly, a tap of the biceps tendon causes pronation and finger contraction in addition to the expected forearm flexion.
3.   Large motor response. A large movement occurs after a normal or slight stimulus. This is probably the least reliable indicator of hyperreflexia, especially if it is seen in all the muscles tested. Anxiety, electrolyte disturbances, and other nonneurologic causes can increase the size of the muscular response. Often, large responses vary from stimulus to stimulus. It is easiest to determine that stretch reflexes are hyperactive if you find them on one side of the body only or in the legs but not in the arms. In many normal patients, the reflexes can be hyperactive. Only a 4+ reflex (a reflex with clonus) can be viewed as definitely abnormal.

MECHANISMS OF HYPERACTIVE STRETCH REFLEXES   In global terms, the finding of increased reflexes indicates a disorder of descending inhibitory pathways. This results in enhanced excitability of the lower motor neuron pool. Clinically, this usually is taken to indicate a corticospinal or pyramidal tract disorder, but this is inaccurate. The *pyramidal tract* consists of fibers arising from precentral and postcentral regions of the cerebral cortex that pass through the medullary pyramids to make monosynaptic or polysynaptic connections with lower motor neurons. These fibers account for only 2 to 5 percent of the entire corticospinal outflow.

Many other tracts provide suprasegmental input to lower motor neurons, particularly reticulospinal and vestibulospinal. The use of the term *pyramidal tract disorder* to describe hyperreflexia is well established. A more accurate and more inclusive term is *upper motor neuron disorder*. In fact, hyperreflexia is only one component of upper motor neuron disorders and is the least likely to result from a lesion affecting only the corticospinal tract. The other components include weakness, spasticity, postural abnormalities, and extensor plantar responses.

Here is an example of the usefulness of stretch reflex testing. A patient reports that he has weakness, dragging, and stiffness of the right leg. The reflexes in that extremity are increased. Tapping on the patellar tendon produces knee extension and adduction. You surmise that the problem is one affecting the descending motor pathways (perhaps a stroke in the left hemisphere) and test the other extremities. The reflexes are normal in both arms, while the reflexes in the asymptomatic left lower extremity are increased. Immediately, your attention shifts to the spinal cord, not the contralateral hemisphere.

HYPOACTIVE (REDUCED) STRETCH REFLEXES   As was noted earlier, every stretch reflex has an afferent limb, central connections, and an efferent limb, and the reflex requires muscular activity to be visible clinically. A disorder of any of these components could produce hyporeflexia or areflexia. For example, a patient in the middle of an attack of periodic paralysis will have intact efferent, afferent, and central connections yet will demonstrate no tendon reflexes, since the muscles cannot contract. In clinical practice, the most common cause of hyporeflexia is a disorder of the afferent limb of the reflex arc, the sensory fibers; however, you need to consider other possibilities.

You need to distinguish between reduced and truly absent reflexes. Young and healthy people, particularly trained athletes, often have reduced reflexes. Reduced reflexes sometimes can be increased by *reinforcement*. You can use a number of techniques to reinforce or heighten stretch reflexes. One of these is the Jendrassik maneuver, in which you ask the patient to link the fingers of each hand and pull one hand forcefully against the other as you percuss a tendon in the leg. A useful means of reinforcing the reflexes in the upper limbs is to ask the subject to clench the jaws as you percuss the tendon. A useful technique for the patellar reflex is to ask the patient to extend the knee very slightly, maintaining a background contraction as you elicit the reflex. These maneuvers increase the number of postsynaptic potentials in the alpha motor neuron pool, enhancing the excitability of these neurons.

A segmentally absent tendon reflex usually indicates a disorder of the peripheral nervous system at that level. The most common example encountered in a clinical setting is an absent ankle jerk caused by an S1 radiculopathy (see Table 6-1).

Nevertheless, segmental loss of a reflex can have other causes. Table 6-2 lists a few representative peripheral nerve trunks which, when damaged, may cause segmental reflex deficits.

The segmental loss of a tendon reflex may be due to intrinsic spinal cord disease. The best example of this is *syringomyelia,* in which tendon reflex loss results from interruption of the central connections of the reflex arc. Since this lesion may spare the anterior horn gray matter, the reflex loss may occur without weakness, atrophy, or fasciculations of the corresponding muscle groups and therefore can be an important early finding. Usually, decreased pin and temperature sensation in a segmental pattern indicates the location of the pathologic process.

Other intrinsic spinal cord diseases may be accompanied by reflex loss. Some patients with *multiple sclerosis* lose one or more reflexes, often because of demyelination of afferent fibers in the root entry zone. The afferent limb in the root exit zone also may be affected. Spinal cord neoplasms, trauma, hemorrhage, or infarction also can cause reflex loss.

TABLE 6-2.   Peripheral Nerves and Muscles Involved in Stretch Reflexes

Nerve	Reflex	Muscle Group
Radial	Triceps	Elbow extensors
Musculocutaneous	Biceps	Elbow flexors
Femoral	Patellar	Knee extensors
Sciatic	Achilles	Ankle flexors

MECHANISMS OF HYPOACTIVE STRETCH REFLEXES Diminished stretch may be caused by inadequate conduction of afferent volleys, decreased excitability of the motor neuron pool, loss of central connections, decreased excitability of efferent fibers, a block of the neuromuscular junction, primary muscle disease, or a combination of all these. Inadequate conduction of afferent impulses may be due to a *complete block* in conduction as a result of severing or stretching a peripheral nerve or root or to severe root compression by a herniated intervertebral disk or another tissue abnormality in the spinal canal. These conditions are rare in clinical practice; much more common is conduction disturbance secondary to *partial block* in conduction as a result of entrapment or partial injury to a peripheral nerve or root. In such cases, only the fibers spared injury will conduct afferent impulses. Since fewer fibers are activated, fewer alpha motor neurons respond, and the resulting muscle contraction will be weak or absent.

Axonal peripheral neuropathies also interfere with impulse transmission to the spinal cord. In this instance, the pathologic process prevents adequate propagation of impulses along the nerve fiber. This results in slowing of nerve conduction velocity in some of the fibers that carry the afferent volley, leading to desynchronization of the impulses arriving at the cord and failure of the EPSPs to summate and bring the neuron to threshold. These neuropathies may be associated with axonal loss, thus decreasing the number of available fibers carrying impulses to the cord.

A similar abnormality may occur in *demyelinating peripheral neuropathies*. The loss of myelin blocks afferent impulses or desynchronizes the afferent volley as a result of slowing of nerve conduction, and the EPSPs generated are insufficient in number or fail to occur synchronously enough to make the motor neuron reach threshold.

Afferent volleys entering the spinal cord can be diminished by *presynaptic inhibition* within the cord. The clinical significance of presynaptic inhibition in clinical situations is not clear.

Hyporeflexia caused by decreased excitability of alpha motor neurons occurs most commonly after acute injury to descending motor pathways, most notably lesions to the corticospinal tract. The most extreme example of this is *spinal shock* after major spinal cord transection. In these circumstances, the motor neuron becomes hyperpolarized and the afferent volleys cannot generate sufficient numbers of EPSPs to bring the motor neurons to threshold. The mechanism for this hyperpolarization is not known, but it may be due to inhibitory effects of propriospinal intersegmental neurons. Ordinarily, the long descending pathways such as the corticospinal tract provide a balancing influence, preventing domination by these circuits.

Superficial Reflexes

Scratching, pinching, or squeezing the skin evokes responses termed the superficial reflexes or nociceptive reflexes. The response usually consists of withdrawal, since these reflexes protect the organism from injury. The response shows a distinct topographic relationship between the stimulus and the muscle groups involved in withdrawal. This close relationship between stimulus and response is called the *local sign*. The most widely studied superficial reflex is the *flexor reflex*. Figure 6-3 demonstrates a typical withdrawal response with simultaneous facilitation of flexor muscles and inhibition of extensors on the side of the stimulus: the *flexor reflex*. The effect in the contralateral limb is facilitation of extensors and inhibition of flexors, resulting in the *crossed extensor reflex*. These

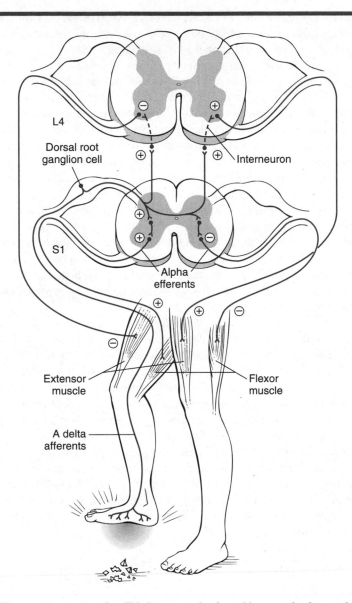

Figure 6-3　The crossed extensor reflex. This is an example of a multisegmental polysynaptic nociceptive reflex. As a noxious stimulus is applied to the foot, the contralateral extensor muscles contract, and the flexor muscles relax, *before* the ipsilateral flexor muscles withdraw the limb. Propriospinal tracts mediate this reflex. Pain afferents, polysynaptically, excite alpha motor neurons and produce a contraction of agonist muscles, and excitation of interneurons to produce relaxation of antagonists.

reflexes are normally present, as they protect people from injury. Withdrawing a leg from a sharp prick to a foot and quickly removing a finger from a source of heat are examples of nociceptive reflexes. Apart from the responses to strong stimuli, these reflexes normally are suppressed. The presence of these reflexes under circumstances in which they should be absent makes them abnormal.

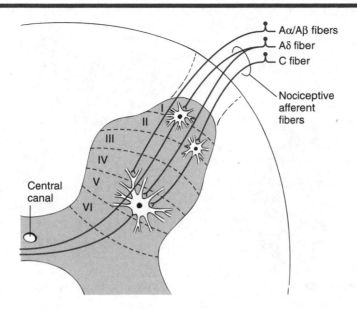

Figure 6-4   Dorsal horn of the spinal cord. The synaptic connections of small nociceptive afferents, (C and A delta), and of large fibers (A beta) carrying epicritic sensation, are shown. Superficial layers of the dorsal horn receive input primarily from nociceptive fibers, and are responsible for initiating flexor reflexes. The deeper layers receive input primarily from A delta and A beta fibers. Both types of fibers converge in layer 5 of the dorsal horn. Under normal circumstanses, tracts from hihger levels of the nervous system, via inhibitory interneurons, regulate the response of second-order neurons derived from the dorsal horn. When these tracts are disrupted, as they are in spinal cord lesions, input from large fibers may generate flexor reflexes.

The extensor plantar response (Babinski sign) is a form of flexor reflex. Many other superficial reflexes have been described previously but abandoned because they have not furnished new or useful clinical data. Those that have survived include the *abdominal reflex*, the *cremasteric* and *bulbocavernosus reflexes*, and some alternative means of testing the plantar response.

ANATOMY AND PHYSIOLOGY OF SUPERFICIAL REFLEXES   Nociceptive afferent fibers (A-δ and C) mediate most of the superficial reflexes. In the spinal cord, these afferents synapse on neurons located in layers I and V of the dorsal horn (Fig. 6-4). From here, polysynaptic connections with propriospinal arcs form connections for discrete, reflex withdrawal. For nociceptive reflexes mediated by the cranial nerves, the same afferents, central connections, and efferent pathways are involved, depending on the segment implicated.

The *blink reflex* is a special form of the nociceptive reflex since it can be elicited by cutaneous or visual stimulation. With cutaneous stimulation, the pathway requires the fifth cranial nerve as the afferent limb. With visual stimulation, the visual system is the afferent limb. The efferent limb remains the seventh cranial nerve in both cases.

CLINICALLY USEFUL SUPERFICIAL REFLEXES   The Babinski sign is the single most meaningful clinically evoked reflex. It is sensitive, specific, and reproducible.

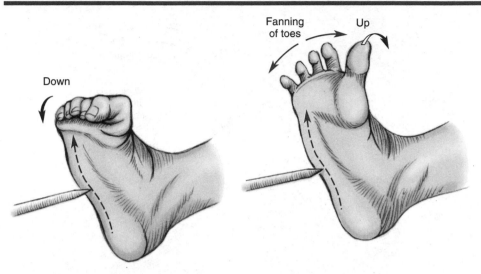

A. Normal plantar reflex   B. Extensor plantar reflex (Babinski's sign)

Figure 6-5   The plantar response. The normal response *(A)* is plantar flexion, or no movement, of the toes. The abnormal response *(B)* consists of dorsiflexion of the great toe, often with fanning of the other toes. This is called the sign of Babinski. It is a partial flexor reflex, and is correlated with dysfunction in the descending corticospinal systems.

When it was described a hundred years ago, the plantar reflex included two components that Babinski described in separate papers. One is dorsiflexion of the great toe, and the other fanning (*l'eventail*) of the toes. (Fig. 6-5).

Most clinicians use the term *dorsiflexion* rather than *extension* to describe the abnormal response to plantar stimulation. This avoids the confusion that may occur between anatomic and physiologic extensors in the legs. Anatomic extension (dorsiflexion) is physiologic flexion, since this movement does not oppose gravity. The reverse is true of plantar flexion. When the extensor plantar response is pronounced, it may be accompanied by dorsiflexion at the ankle, flexion of the knee and hip, and visible contraction of the tensor fascia lata. The opposite extremity may extend, a form of the crossed extensor reflex described above, or the opposite toe also may dorsiflex, a response termed *crossed extensor plantar*.

Currently, neurologists consider the direction of the movement of the great toe as the crucial sign; fanning of the other toes is not required.

In testing the plantar response, use a mildly noxious or unpleasant stimulus in an awake patient, such as a key, the tip of a reflex hammer, a tongue blade, or the end of a tuning fork. Few examiners have access to a goose quill, said to be Babinski's choice for the test. Apply the stimulus to a 5- to 10-cm-long strip of plantar skin near the lateral edge of the sole. Move the stimulus from the heel toward the little toe at a deliberate pace. If you evoke no response, carry the stimulus across the metatarsal heads to the base of the great toe. When you perform the test correctly, the patient may wince slightly but will not voluntarily withdraw. The proper amount of stimulation is that which produces toe movement only. Too strong a stimulus will cause the patient to withdraw the extremity, and too light a stimulus produces no response, a common error of the beginner.

You should be able to detect a delay between stimulus and response. You should expect this delay and sometimes can detect a factitious response by dorsiflexion of the great toe with no delay. This delay is due to the polysynaptic path of the reflex.

The plantar response depends partly on the position of the patient; it is easiest to do and more consistently elicited when the patient is lying supine. Carrying out the test on a seated patient may produce factitious dorsiflexion. This position causes a bias toward activation of physiologic flexors.

Various substitutes for direct plantar stimulation have been described, and some occasionally are useful. An extensor plantar response may be obtained by squeezing the calf (Gordon's sign), applying pressure to the tibia (Oppenheim's sign), or stroking the lateral margin of the foot (Chaddock's sign). In Rossolimo's sign, great toe dorsiflexion is elicited by the examiner's forced abduction of the patient's little toe. Fick's sign brings about great toe dorsiflexion by scratching the dorsal surface of the toe. The last two signs are of historic interest only.

An extensor plantar response carries the strong implication that the descending motor pathways, particularly the corticospinal tract, are abnormal. Apart from this, the sign has little localizing value. Although we expect the plantar response to be extensor in patients with corticospinal tract lesions, important clinical inferences may be made when it is unexpectedly unreactive or flexor. The following are some of the circumstances in which it may occur:

1. An absent plantar response can occur with paralysis of the muscles controlling dorsiflexion, loss of the afferent pathway from severe sensorimotor polyneuropathy, lesions in the cauda equina, or sensory mononeuropathy.

2. Focal weakness of the extensor hallucis longus muscle, which is innervated by the L5 root and the deep peroneal nerve, can result in an absent response. If you observe a correctly timed contraction of knee flexors, hip flexors, or tensor fascia lata muscles, you can infer that upper motor neuron pathology exists.

3. A tonic foot response, or foot grasp, occasionally occurs in patients with frontal lobe pathology. You can evoke tonic plantar flexion of all toes by pressure over the skin covering the metatarsal heads. The tonic foot response may interfere with the plantar response and convert an extensor plantar response into a flexor response.

4. Some hemiplegic patients have hyperactive stretch reflexes and spasticity but a flexor plantar response. This occurs with lesions in the parietal lobe.

5. Acute lesions of the corticospinal tract often depress the reflex responses, superficial as well as stretch reflexes.

Occasionally you will encounter an extensor plantar response in the absence of corticospinal tract pathology, a false-positive response. This finding may remain unexplained, but you should seek two possible explanations: First, voluntary withdrawal can include extension of the great toe. In an exceptionally ticklish or anxious patient, you will find it difficult to reduce the stimulus to the point where only toe movement is visible. Second, imbalance of muscle weakness in the foot can produce an extensor toe response, as occurs when the plantar flexors are weaker than the extensor hallucis longus. Patients with hereditary axonal neuropathy or demyelinating neuropathy may show this.

Superficial reflexes other than the plantar response also may aid in localization. You can elicit the *abdominal reflexes* by stroking the skin of the abdomen with a mildly sharp object, taking care not to injure the skin. The expected response is contraction of the underlying abdominal muscles. Deliver the stimulus separately to all four abdominal quadrants and the response will be restricted to the stimulated quadrant. As with the plantar response, acute corticospinal tract lesions may obliterate the reflex, while a chronic lesion may enhance the response. Spread of the reflex contraction beyond the stimulated quadrant indicates enhancement. Radiculopathy and spinal lesions may interrupt the afferent or efferent pathways and decrease or abolish this reflex. For example, patients with multiple sclerosis may be expected to have enhanced abdominal reflexes because of corticospinal tract pathology but may have absent reflexes as a result of failure of central transmission in the cord.

PATHOLOGIC APPEARANCE OF SUPERFICIAL REFLEXES Although present in normal newborns, the Babinski sign disappears by the end of the first year. Corticospinal tract development is the likely reason for the physiologic suppression of this reflex. The reflex returns upon damage to the corticospinal tract, probably resulting from loss of presynaptic inhibition. The corticospinal tract maintains flexor reflex afferents, and after loss of this inhibition, these afferents have unimpeded access to the alpha motor neuron pool. The enhancement of the extensor response with time after corticospinal tract lesions probably is due to collateral sprouting of afferent terminals, thus increasing the effective number of excitatory synapses in the motor neuron pool.

Small lesions affecting the corticospinal tract produce a limited form of the flexion reflex. Larger or more widespread lesions yield a more full expression of the uninhibited flexor reflex. This is most striking in chronic lesions of the spinal cord, which result in loss of input from rubrospinal, reticulospinal, and vestibulospinal tracts in addition to the corticospinal tract. The enhancement of flexor reflexes can be so marked that a stimulus as innocuous as blowing a gentle puff of air on the skin of the foot may trigger strong withdrawal of both limbs, sometimes accompanied by autonomic responses that include sweating, tachycardia, increased peristalsis, and bladder contraction. The term applied to this is *mass flexion reflex.*

In the intact nervous system, nociceptive afferents (A-δ and C) fibers mediate the flexor reflex. After loss of the major descending pathways with small cord lesions, A-α and A-β fibers become the mediators, since they carry this sort of innocuous sensation into the dorsal horn. These larger fibers have input into dorsal horn layers concerned with nociceptive stimuli (Fig. 6-5). This input is normally inhibited, allowing only nociceptive afferents to have access to the flexor reflex mechanism. With loss of the suprasegmental influences, the specificity of the system fails. The systems responsible for maintaining this specificity probably arise in the medullary reticular formation and the adjacent raphe nuclei.

PATHOLOGIC LOSS OF SUPERFICIAL REFLEXES Abnormally present or "released" superficial reflexes are a common feature of chronic lesions of the descending tracts, while their absence is a feature of acute lesions of these tracts. The most common example of this is the immediate decrease or loss of segmental and multisegmental reflexes after spinal cord transection. In severe cases, not even the flexor reflex can be elicited.

Spinal cord transection decreases the resting potential of the alpha motor neuron pool, although this level of decrease is insufficient to account for the motor neuron refractoriness to stimuli. This indicates that there are systems in the spinal cord acting both pre- and post-synaptically to maintain this refractoriness. Spinal shock resolves with time and is replaced by the enhanced reflex activity associated with chronic upper motor neuron disorders.

Patterned Behavioral Reflexes

A number of reflex responses to tactile stimuli occur in association with dementia and disorders of the frontal lobes. Most of these are generated by lightly touching or stroking the face or hand, and the behavioral response seen is often complex and relatively slow and resembles a behavior pattern. These responses occur most often in older patients with diffuse or poorly localized dysfunction of the cerebral hemispheres, often involving the frontal lobes. These responses have been described in patients with pathology localized to the frontal lobes from neoplasms, infarctions, and abscesses but more commonly occur with multi-infarct dementia, Pick disease, or Alzheimer disease.

Patients with focal frontal lobe pathology often present with more subtle deficits that are helpful in localization. Patients with orbitofrontal disease present with slowness of thought and movement, abulia, and concrete thinking. Those with lateral frontal disorders demonstrate imitative behavior, disinhibited or labile emotional states, and difficulty changing or inferring sets (executive dysfunction). If the basic pathology progresses, these disorders may evolve to produce the primitive reflexes described below.

GRASP REFLEX OF THE HAND The instinctive or orienting grasp reflex is evoked by a light tactile stimulus to the lateral margin of the ulnar or radial side of the hand. The response is automatic turning of the hand and gripping of the stimulating object. The grasp reflex is evoked by a light tactile stimulus to the palm of the hand. The response is gripping of the stimulating object. The grasp reflex can be confused with the traction response, a sign of spasticity. This reflex is evoked by flexion of the fingers with forceful movement of the interphalangeal joints.

A grasp reflex of the hand is most common in patients with diffuse disorders such as Alzheimer dementia and toxic encephalopathy. Occasionally, a unilateral grasp reflex will indicate contralateral hemispheric disease, especially of the lateral convexity.

GRASP REFLEX OF THE FOOT This reflex is elicited by firm pressure on the metatarsal heads, which evokes a slow, sustained flexion of all the toes that may outlast the stimulus by many seconds. Both the quick response and the slow, tonic sustained contraction may interfere with the Babinski sign.

SUCK REFLEX The stimulus consists of a light stroking of the lips with a tongue blade or finger; the response is pursing the lips and opening the mouth. There may be an orienting of the lips or following of the stimulus if it is moved away or toward one side. This reflex resembles the sucking behavior of infants.

SNOUT REFLEX This response, a pursing or pouting of the lips, follows a tap with the reflex hammer or fingers over the width of both lips. This reflex relies entirely on cutaneous afferents and is not a stretch reflex.

ROOTING REFLEX   Pressure along the corner of the mouth produces opening of the mouth and turning of the lips and head toward that side.

BULLDOG REFLEX   If a tongue blade (not a finger) is inserted between the teeth, the patient will bite it, and efforts to extract the tongue blade are met by firm and increasing resistance. This response is seen most often in patients with dementia, rigidity, and paratonic rigidity.

SUGGESTED READINGS

Babinski J: Du phénomène des orteils et sa valeur sémiologique. *Sem Med* 18:321, 1898.

Brain R, Wilkinson M: Observations of the extensor plantar response and its relationship to the functions of the pyramidal tract. *Brain* 82:297, 1959.

Daroff RB: Book review: The Babinski Sign: A Centenary by J van Gijn. *Neurology* 48:1749, 1997.

Granit R: *Receptor and Sensory Perception.* New Haven, Yale University Press, 1955.

Huff FJ, Growdon JH: Neurological abnormalities associated with severity of dementia in Alzheimer's disease. *Can J Neurol Sci* 13:403, 1986.

Koller WC, Glatt S, Wilson RS, Fox JH: Primitive reflexes and cognitive function in the elderly. *Ann Neurol* 12:302, 1982.

Matthews PBC. The 1989 James A. Stevenson Memorial Lecture: The knee jerk: Still an enigma? *Can J Physiol Pharmacol* 68:347, 1989.

Merton PA: How we control the contraction of our muscles. *Sci Am* 226(5):30, 1972.

Valbo AB: Muscle spindle response at the onset of isometric voluntary contractions in man: Time difference between fusimotor and skeletomotor effects. *J Physiol* 218:405, 1971.

KENNETH L. CASEY

CHAPTER 7

THE SOMATOSENSORY SYSTEM

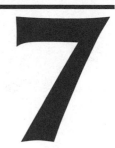

ANATOMY AND PHYSIOLOGY

Peripheral Nervous System

CUTANEOUS

Tactile Receptors and Afferents　Tactile stimuli excite discharges in the largest diameter fibers innervating the skin. These fibers, classified as "A beta" (A-β) afferents, are the most heavily myelinated and have the highest conduction velocities of all cutaneous afferents (70 to 50 m/s). These fibers innervate a variety of specialized corpuscular endings in both hairy and glabrous skin as well as simple, undifferentiated endings associated with hair follicles (Fig. 7-1). Some tactile afferents innervating corpuscular endings maintain constant rates of discharge during constant intensity stimulation (slowly adapting) and are capable of encoding pressure or indentation maintained on the skin. Other fibers discharge only during the onset of skin stimulation (rapidly adapting) and may encode the rate of skin indentation. The afferent fibers innervating pacinian corpuscles, for example, are among the most sensitive and most rapidly adapting of cutaneous afferents and respond most effectively to vibratory stimulation (100 to 300 Hz). Pacinian corpuscles may also be found in deep tissues, including the periosteum. Hair follicle afferents are activated by the bending of hairs and may show directional specificity.

Thermoreceptors　Thermal stimuli below the noxious range activate finely myelinated afferents, most of which are not associated with unique corpuscular endings. These fibers have conduction velocities of 3 to 30 m/s and are classified as "A delta" (A-δ) afferents. Warmth and cold activate separate groups of fibers. Warm afferents respond within the range of innocuous heat (35 to 44°C; 95 to 111°F) and stop discharging at skin temperatures above 45°C (113°F; approximate heat pain threshold). Cold afferents are active in the innocuous range (5 to 30°C; 41 to 86°F) and most are silent below the approximate noxious level of 2°C (36°F).

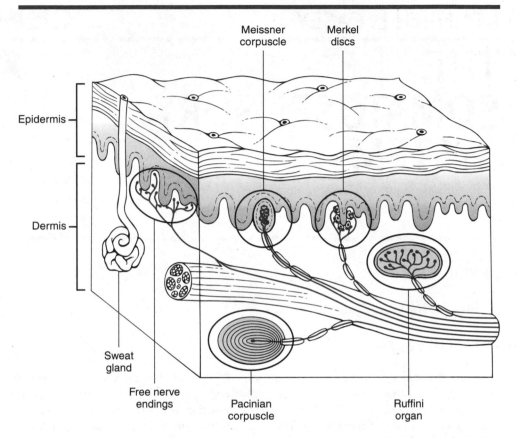

Figure 7-1 The location of corpuscular and other types of sensory endings in the skin. (From Purves D, et al, 1997, with permission.)

Nociceptors   Painful stimuli activate afferent fibers that innervate nociceptors. The activity of these fibers is correlated with the intensity of pain sensation. The nociceptive fibers include both finely myelinated A-δ afferents and unmyelinated afferent fibers (C fibers), both without corpuscular endings. A-δ fibers innervate primarily high threshold mechanoreceptors and some heat nociceptors. C fibers innervate receptors that respond to either heat (above 45°C; 113°F), cold (below 2°C; 36°F), mechanical, or chemical stimuli that are painful. Some of these nociceptive afferents respond only to one type of stimulus, such as noxious heat or noxious cold, but others are "polymodal," responding to all noxious stimulation, regardless of the physical agent. Some C fibers respond to tactile stimuli or to chemical or mechanical stimuli that produce itching. C polymodal nociceptors respond to substances produced during inflammation, such as H^+, K^+, bradykinin, prostaglandin, leukotrienes, cytokines, and other compounds produced in response to tissue damage.

SUBCUTANEOUS (LIGAMENTS, PERIOSTEUM, JOINT CAPSULES, TEETH)
A-δ and C afferent fibers innervate joint capsules and ligaments. Most of these afferents are nociceptors that respond to extremes of joint position or stretch. Some are "silent" nociceptors that never discharge unless they are sensitized by inflammation and tissue damage. Joint capsule afferents provide little or no information about the movement of a limb about the axes of a joint. Some myelinated afferents with pacinian corpuscles innervate periosteum and ligaments; these respond to tactile (vibratory) stimuli. Most tooth pulp afferents are unmyelinated and have undifferentiated endings in the dentinal canals. These afferents innervate polymodal nociceptors, which are activated by inflammation or by mechanical, thermal, or chemical stimuli. Periodontal tissues, like the skin, receive innervation from sensory afferents that cover the range from large-diameter tactile to small-diameter nociceptive fibers.

MUSCLE   Large-diameter myelinated afferents (CV of 70 to 100 m/s) innervate the muscle spindle apparatus and encode information about muscle length. Although muscle spindle afferents are under central nervous system control through the action of gamma motor neurons, these afferents are the primary source of information about limb movement and position (see below). Muscle spindle afferents also form the afferent limb of the monosynaptic muscle stretch reflex. Nociceptive A-δ and C fiber afferents innervate the contractile portion of the muscle and the surrounding muscle fascia. These afferents respond to extremes of stretch, ischemia, chemical stimuli, and inflammation. The intense, acute pain of muscle cramping may be caused by the shearing forces developed on nociceptors between contracted and noncontracted muscle fibers. The delayed muscle tenderness that appears 12 to 24 h after unaccustomed exercise probably results from nociceptor sensitization and activation by an inflammatory response to microscopic muscle damage (Mense, 1993).

VISCERA AND INTERNAL ORGANS   A-δ and C fibers provide the major innervation of the internal organs. These afferents travel in sympathetic nerves with projections to the central nervous system (CNS) via the autonomic rami communicantes to the dorsal root. Some of these afferents serve regulatory functions that are specific to the innervated organ (e.g., gut motility, urinary bladder reflexes, baroreceptor functions), but others serve a nociceptive function during extremes of distention or stretch, or during ischemia. Still other afferents are active at lower stimulus intensities—as when there is a sensation of fullness in a viscus.

Innervation Patterns of Nerves and Roots

The sensory component of peripheral nerves is composed principally of fibers that arise from the ganglion cells of more than one dorsal root. Consequently, the cutaneous sensory abnormality that follows peripheral nerve damage is usually limited to a proximal or distal portion of the limb or trunk and often extends across the cutaneous boundaries innervated by a single dorsal root (dermatome). In addition, the sensory loss caused by transection of a peripheral nerve is usually severe because the overlapping cutaneous innervation territory of nearby peripheral nerves is restricted. In contrast, there is a

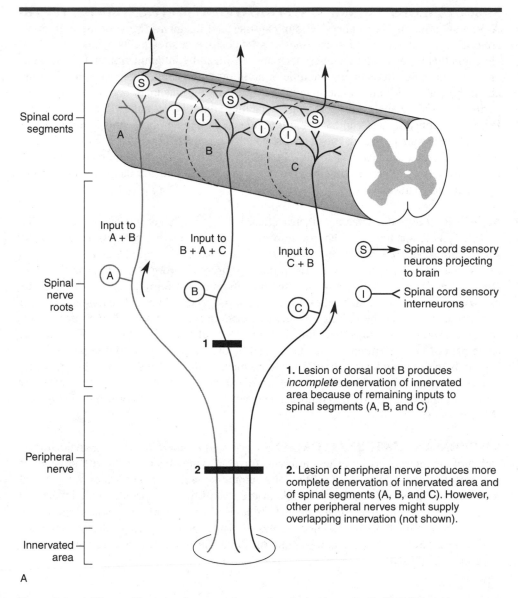

Figure 7-2   *A.* Diagram illustrating the sensory innervation of spinal segments (A, B, C) by spinal nerve roots and peripheral nerves. Each nerve root innervates more than one spinal segment, and a peripheral nerve contributes fibers to more than one spinal root. *B* to *E.* Cutaneous fields of peripheral nerves. (Reproduced with permission from Figures 51 to 54 in *Clinical Examinations in Neurology*, 2d ed. Philadelphia, Mayo Clinic, Saunders, 1963.)

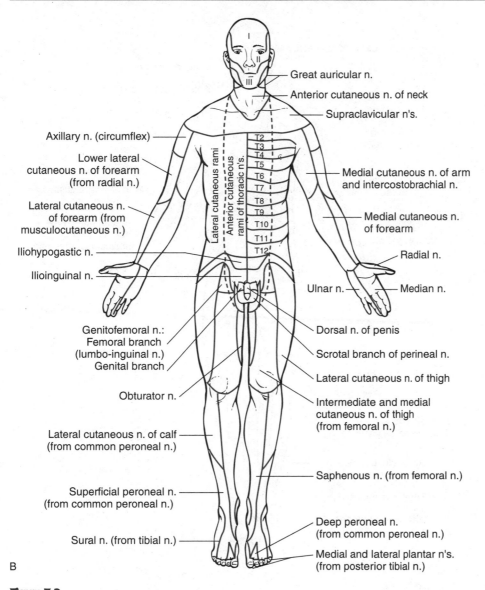

Great auricular n.

Anterior cutaneous n. of neck

Supraclavicular n's.

Axillary n. (circumflex)

Lower lateral cutaneous n. of forearm (from radial n.)

Lateral cutaneous n. of forearm (from musculocutaneous n.)

Iliohypogastic n.

Ilioinguinal n.

Lateral cutaneous rami

Anterior cutaneous rami of thoracic n's.

T2
T3
T4
T5
T6
T7
T8
T9
T10
T11
T12

Medial cutaneous n. of arm and intercostobrachial n.

Medial cutaneous n. of forearm

Radial n.

Ulnar n.

Median n.

Genitofemoral n.:
Femoral branch (lumbo-inguinal n.)
Genital branch

Obturator n.

Lateral cutaneous n. of calf (from common peroneal n.)

Superficial peroneal n. (from common peroneal n.)

Sural n. (from tibial n.)

Dorsal n. of penis

Scrotal branch of perineal n.

Lateral cutaneous n. of thigh

Intermediate and medial cutaneous n. of thigh (from femoral n.)

Saphenous n. (from femoral n.)

Deep peroneal n. (from common peroneal n.)

Medial and lateral plantar n's. (from posterior tibial n.)

B

Figure 7-2 *(continued)*

substantial overlap between spinal cord sensory inputs from adjacent dorsal root afferents. This is because interneurons in each segment of the spinal cord dorsal horn interconnect with three to four other spinal segments (via Lissauer's tract) so that impulses transmitted over one dorsal root can affect spinal sensory neurons in several spinal segments (Willis and Coggeshall, 1978). As a result, sensory loss caused by injury to a dorsal root may be minimal, depending on the degree of dermatomal overlap. The distribution of the

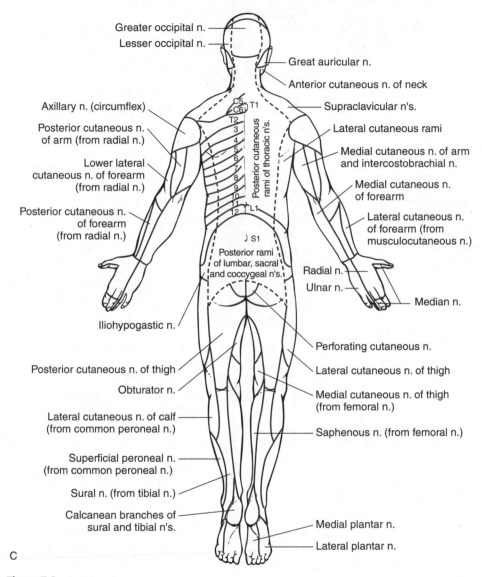

Greater occipital n.
Lesser occipital n.
Great auricular n.
Anterior cutaneous n. of neck
Axillary n. (circumflex)
Posterior cutaneous n. of arm (from radial n.)
Supraclavicular n's.
Lateral cutaneous rami
Medial cutaneous n. of arm and intercostobrachial n.
Lower lateral cutaneous n. of forearm (from radial n.)
Medial cutaneous n. of forearm
Posterior cutaneous n. of forearm (from radial n.)
Lateral cutaneous n. of forearm (from musculocutaneous n.)
Posterior cutaneous rami of thoracic n's.
Posterior rami of lumbar, sacral and coccygeal n's.
Radial n.
Ulnar n.
Median n.
Iliohypogastic n.
Perforating cutaneous n.
Posterior cutaneous n. of thigh
Lateral cutaneous n. of thigh
Obturator n.
Medial cutaneous n. of thigh (from femoral n.)
Lateral cutaneous n. of calf (from common peroneal n.)
Saphenous n. (from femoral n.)
Superficial peroneal n. (from common peroneal n.)
Sural n. (from tibial n.)
Calcanean branches of sural and tibial n's.
Medial plantar n.
Lateral plantar n.

C

Figure 7-2   *(continued)*

sensory loss will, however, extend beyond the sensory innervation boundaries of a peripheral nerve.

Figures 7-2 and 7-3 depict the cutaneous innervation patterns of peripheral nerves and spinal sensory roots. Each diagram was developed from a limited amount of information

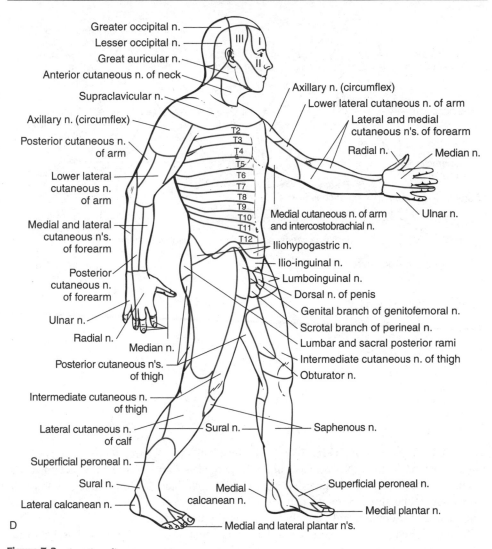

Greater occipital n.
Lesser occipital n.
Great auricular n.
Anterior cutaneous n. of neck
Supraclavicular n.
Axillary n. (circumflex)
Posterior cutaneous n. of arm
Lower lateral cutaneous n. of arm
Medial and lateral cutaneous n's. of forearm
Posterior cutaneous n. of forearm
Ulnar n.
Radial n.
Median n.
Posterior cutaneous n's. of thigh
Intermediate cutaneous n. of thigh
Lateral cutaneous n. of calf
Superficial peroneal n.
Sural n.
Lateral calcanean n.

Axillary n. (circumflex)
Lower lateral cutaneous n. of arm
Lateral and medial cutaneous n's. of forearm
Radial n.
Median n.
Medial cutaneous n. of arm and intercostobrachial n.
Ulnar n.
Iliohypogastric n.
Ilio-inguinal n.
Lumboinguinal n.
Dorsal n. of penis
Genital branch of genitofemoral n.
Scrotal branch of perineal n.
Lumbar and sacral posterior rami
Intermediate cutaneous n. of thigh
Obturator n.
Sural n.
Saphenous n.
Medial calcanean n.
Superficial peroneal n.
Medial plantar n.
Medial and lateral plantar n's.

T2
T3
T4
T5
T6
T7
T8
T9
T10
T11
T12

D

Figure 7-2   *(continued)*

obtained primarily from clinical pathologic cases rather than by direct experiment. Moreover, neither diagram reflects the degree of overlapping innervation (functional or anatomic) that adjacent nerves or roots provide. Consequently, these diagrams serve only as general guides to the pattern of cutaneous sensory innervation.

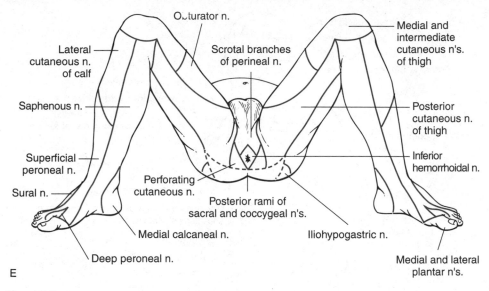

Obturator n.

Lateral cutaneous n. of calf

Scrotal branches of perineal n.

Medial and intermediate cutaneous n's. of thigh

Saphenous n.

Posterior cutaneous n. of thigh

Superficial peroneal n.

Inferior hemorrhoidal n.

Sural n.

Perforating cutaneous n.

Posterior rami of sacral and coccygeal n's.

Medial calcaneal n.

Iliohypogastric n.

Deep peroneal n.

Medial and lateral plantar n's.

E

Figure 7-2   *(continued)*

Central Nervous System

TACTILE SENSATION (Fig. 7-4)   The sense of touch is frequently preserved following lesions of the CNS because multiple pathways carry tactile information to the brain. The tactile information carried by the large, myelinated afferent fibers is immediately routed into three different pathways for transmission to the brain: (1) the dorsal columns, (2) the dorsolateral funiculus, and (3) the spinothalamic tract.

Tactile afferents from the body enter the dorsal spinal cord via the medial aspect of the dorsal root. One branch of each afferent fiber is added to the dorsal columns, which relay tactile information to the brain after one synapse. The other branch courses medially to the medial aspect of the dorsal horn gray matter. From the dorsal horn, tactile information reaches the brain via the dorsolateral funiculus and the spinothalamic tract.

Dorsal columns: Afferent fibers are added to the lateral aspect of the dorsal columns in rostral succession (caudal to rostral) at each spinal cord segment, producing a laminated pattern with fibers from more caudal segments positioned medially and fibers from rostral segments laterally. Thus, the body map is represented dermatotopically within the dorsal columns. As they ascend the spinal cord, dorsal column fibers give off collateral branches to the dorsal horn gray matter for several segments. Ascending dorsal column branches synapse in the dorsal column nuclei (DCN) of the medulla. The medial branches, which

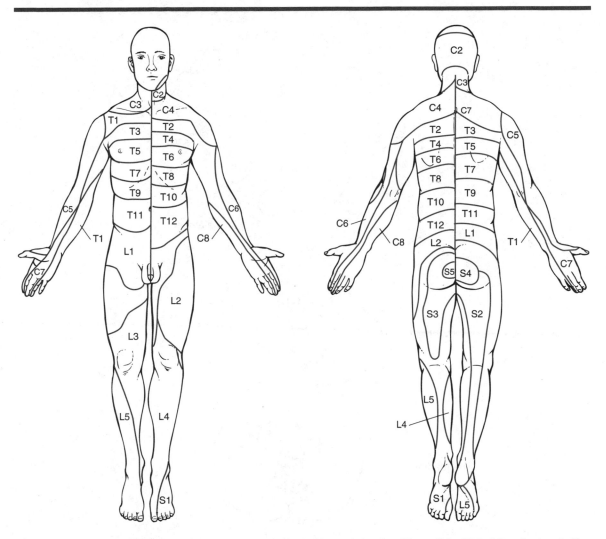

Figure 7-3   Distribution of the spinal dermatomes. (Reproduced with permission from Figure 49 in *Clinical Examinations in Neurology*, 2d ed. Philadelphia, Mayo Clinic, Saunders, 1963.)

form the fasciculus gracilis, end in the nucleus gracilis, and the lateral branches (fasciculus cuneatus) in the nucleus cuneatus. Within the DCN, the body map is reorganized somatotopically so that adjacent body areas have adjacent neural representations. Transection of the dorsal column fibers permanently impairs the ability to determine the direction of movement of cutaneous stimuli but does not affect the ability to simply detect touch or tactile movement (Makous and Vierck, 1994; Ross et al, 1979). The axons of the postsynaptic neurons in the DCN form the medial lemniscus, which projects to the ventral posterior lateral thalamus, the major thalamic relay to the primary somatosensory cortex in the anterior parietal lobe.

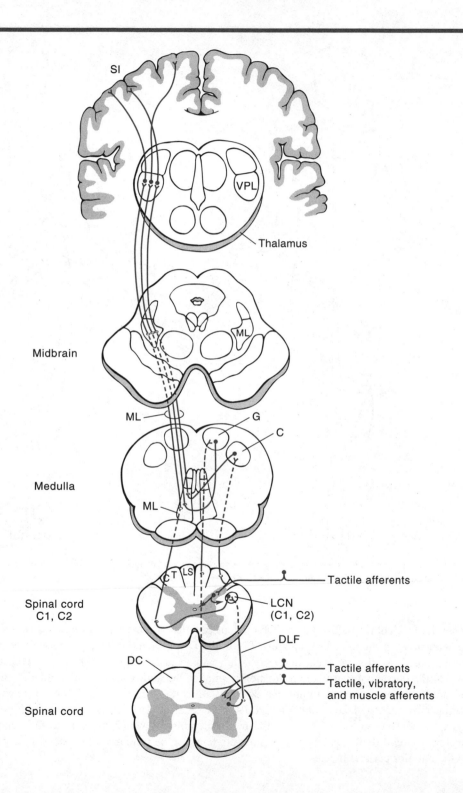

Dorsal horn: Tactile afferents form synapses on neurons in the neck and ventral part of the dorsal horn. The axons of these second-order neurons then ascend in the spinal cord either ipsilaterally or contralaterally. Axons ascending *ipsilaterally* travel primarily within the dorsolateral spinal cord white matter where they form synapses with cells of a lateral cervical nucleus (just ventral to the dorsal horn) at the most rostral cervical levels. (Some fibers may also travel in the ipsilateral ventral spinal cord.) The neurons within this pathway are somatotopically organized and probably contribute significantly to somesthetic discriminative functions. The postsynaptic cells from the lateral cervical nucleus immediately cross the midline to join the medial lemniscal projections to the ventral posterior lateral thalamus. Axons ascending *contralaterally* cross the midline via the anterior spinal commissure within two to four spinal segments to join the direct spinothalamic projections to the lateral and medial thalamus. Transection of the lateral spinothalamic tract results in a loss of tactile erogenous sensations caudal and contralateral to the lesion, but tactile threshold and discriminative capacity are not affected.

Thalamus: The medial lemniscus and portions of the spinothalamic tract terminate in the ventral posterior lateral (VPL) thalamus. Medial lemniscal and spinothalamic fibers form synapses on the dendrites and cell bodies of thalamocortical neurons, which send projections to the somatosensory cortex of the postcentral gyrus. There is a detailed somatotopic organization of the body map within VPL, and many neurons within this nucleus respond to light tactile or hair stimulation of skin surfaces only a few millimeters or centimeters in area. Neurons in the medial (and intralaminar) thalamus also receive input from tactile-responsive spinothalamic tract neurons.

Cerebral cortex: The thalamus transmits tactile information to the (primary or S1) somatosensory cortex of the postcentral gyrus where the somatotopic map becomes more elaborate and detailed, especially for those cutaneous surfaces used for tactile exploration, such as the lips, tongue, and finger pads (Fig. 7-5). The S1 cortex sends projections to the posterior parietal association cortex for the integration of tactile with other sensory information and with mechanisms mediating attention and sensory awareness. The body map in S1 cortex has as many as five representations, each with slightly different physiologic properties. Many of the cortical neurons in S1 discharge most rapidly when a cutaneous stimulus moves in a particular direction. Thus, if subcortical and peripheral pathways are intact, an impairment of cutaneous direction sense points to an abnormality within the postcentral gyrus.

Figure 7-4 Diagram of central pathways mediating tactile, vibratory, and kinesthetic senses. Afferent fibers innervating pacinian (vibratory), muscle stretch, and tactile receptors excite spinal cord dorsal horn neurons with rostral projections through the dorsolateral funiculus (DLF) either directly or after a synapse in the lateral cervical nucleus (LCN) at spinal cervical segments C1 and C2. Tactile afferents also bifurcate, one branch forming the dorsal columns (DC) and the other contacting dorsal horn cells with rostral projections through the contralateral spinothalamic tract (not shown) or the DLF. Note the laminated representation of spinal segments within the DC (LS = lumbosacral; T = thoracic; C = cervical). Dorsal column fibers terminate in either the gracile (G; sacral and lumbar) or cuneate (C; thoracic and cervical) nuclei. The postsynaptic fibers cross within the medulla to form the medial lemniscus (ML), which terminates in the ventral posterior lateral (VPL) thalamic nucleus. Thalamocortical fibers from VPL project to the primary somatosensory cortex (S1) of the postcentral gyrus.

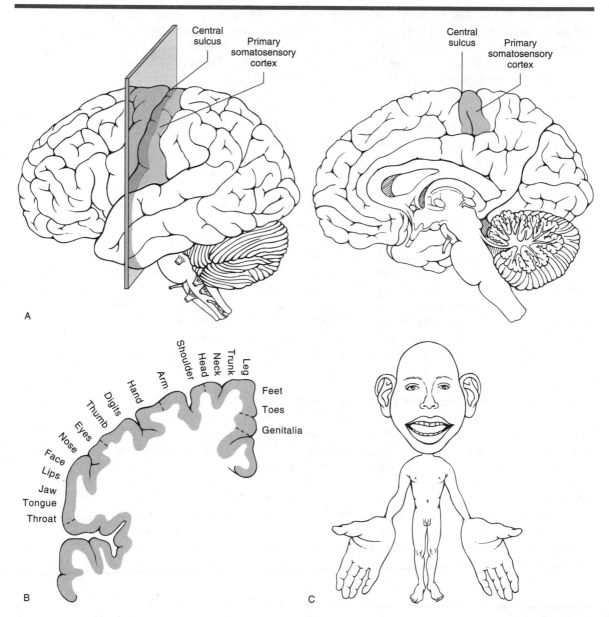

Figure 7-5 Location of primary somatosensory cortex (S1) on lateral and medial surfaces of the left hemisphere (*A*) and the somatotopic organization of the body surface (*B*). The figurine (*C*) indicates the relative amount of cortex devoted to each body area. (From Purves et al, 1997, with permission.)

In addition to the S1 cortex, tactile information reaches secondary somatosensory cortical areas adjacent to the lateral (sylvian) sulcus or folded within it (insular cortex). These areas are necessary for some forms of tactile learning.

Vibratory Sensation (See Fig. 7-4)

Testing the sense of vibration assesses the capacity of the somatosensory system to detect rapid mechanical changes in the skin or in underlying tissues. At the peripheral level, the largest diameter, most rapidly adapting, heavily myelinated afferent fibers mediate this function. These fibers innervate pacinian corpuscular endings in the skin, subcutaneous tissue, periosteum, and connective tissues of the gut. Cutaneous pacinian corpuscles are responsible for the rapid adaptation of these afferent fibers, giving them the ability to respond to each cycle of the vibration and thus help mediate the temporal analysis of tactile stimuli. The central processes of these fibers follow the pathway of tactile afferents, with one collateral ascending in the dorsal columns to the dorsal column nuclei and another branch sending terminal endings to the dorsal horn. From the dorsal spinal gray matter, second-order neurons form an ascending pathway in the dorsolateral funiculus. This dorsolateral pathway may be the major one mediating vibratory sense in humans (Ross et al, 1979). Dorsal column fibers synapse in the dorsal column nuclei of the lower brainstem, and fibers of the dorsolateral funiculus terminate in the lateral cervical nucleus of the cervical spinal cord. Both of these nuclei send postsynaptic projections to the VPL thalamus and thence to the somatosensory (S1) cortex to innervate vibratory responsive neurons (Willis, 1985).

Kinesthetic Sensation (Sensation of Limb Position and Movement) (See Fig. 7-4)

The term "kinesthesia" is preferred over the commonly used "position sense" or "proprioception" because it emphasizes the specific and dynamic aspect of the sense of the direction and amplitude of body movements. Afferent fibers innervating muscle spindles provide the principal afferent basis for kinesthesia (Matthews, 1982). Cutaneous afferent fibers, activated by skin stretch, also contribute significantly to the sense of movement and direction of movement. The myelinated afferents from muscle spindles travel with tactile afferents, forming synaptic terminals on second-order neurons within the deeper layers of the dorsal horn. Some of these neurons send axons through the dorsal columns to terminate in the dorsal column nuclei. However, it currently appears that the major ascending pathway for kinesthesia is the dorsolateral funiculus of the spinal cord rather than the dorsal columns. The postsynaptic pathways ascend within the medial lemniscus to innervate the VPL thalamus. Thalamocortical projection neurons terminate in the S1 cortex upon neurons encoding movement and position.

The Differentiation of Vibratory and Kinesthetic Senses

These sensory functions are often discussed together because of the similarity of their central pathways; however, they are separate at thalamic and cortical levels. Furthermore, afferent fibers that innervate distinctly different receptors mediate these sensations. In clinical practice, one of these sensory functions may be affected while the other is spared or relatively preserved.

Pain and Temperature Sensation

Both of these sensations are mediated by A-δ and C peripheral afferent fibers, and their central pathways overlap considerably. However, innocuous thermal sensations are processed differently and involve separate neural mechanisms at thalamic and cortical levels.

A-δ and C fibers are clustered within the lateral aspect of the dorsal root at their point of entry into the spinal cord. These afferents terminate within the substantia gelatinosa at the dorsal apex of the spinal cord dorsal horn. Some of these afferents branch for three to four spinal segments within the dorsolateral Lissauer's tract before making synaptic contact with dorsal horn neurons. Some postsynaptic substantia gelatinosa cells also distribute axons to three to four adjacent spinal segments. This wide distribution of nociceptive input may underlie the perceived spatial radiation of severe pain beyond the site of injury.

Thermal and nociceptive afferents activate two distinct types of dorsal horn neurons that contribute axons to the spinothalamic tract. The pattern of nociceptive processing described here is also found in the caudal portion of the trigeminal sensory nucleus (see Chap. 4). *Nociceptive specific* (NS) neurons are found within the substantia gelatinosa and receive input exclusively from A-δ and C fibers. These neurons respond only to noxious stimuli; thermal or mechanical stimuli may be differentially effective for some, but others respond to all forms of noxious stimulation. *Wide dynamic range* (WDR) neurons have their dendrites within the substantia gelatinosa, but their cell bodies are located ventrally. WDR neurons receive synaptic input from tactile, thermal, and nociceptive afferents and respond to both innocuous and noxious somatic stimuli. These neurons provide a frequency coding of noxious stimulation because their discharge increases progressively as the intensity of a somatic (or visceral) stimulus increases from innocuous to noxious levels.

Visceral afferent nociceptive fibers excite the same NS and WDR neurons that respond to somatic stimulation. Thus, stimulation of cardiac or gall bladder afferent fibers excites nociceptive dorsal horn cells that also respond to noxious cutaneous stimulation of upper thoracic or lower cervical dermatomes. This synaptic convergence of somatic and visceral nociceptive inputs is thought to underlie the phenomenon of referred pain (Table 7-1).

The axons of WDR and NS neurons cross the midline via the anterior spinal commissure ventral to the spinal canal. Some axons ascend ipsilaterally for three to four spinal segments before crossing. The axons ascend in the ventrolateral quadrant of the spinal cord to form the spinothalamic tract. In contrast with the pattern of fiber lamination

TABLE 7-1.   Common Patterns of Referred Pain

Spinal Segment	Organ	Somatic Reference
Cervical	Central diaphragm	Shoulder, neck
Thoracic	Heart	Medial arm, lower jaw
	Gall bladder	Upper back, shoulder, neck
Lumbar	Renal pelvis, ureter	Groin, genitals
	Hip joint	Knee
Sacral	Bladder (trigone)	Rectum, genitals, caudal leg

within the dorsal columns, the spinothalamic tract is formed "from the outside in" as fibers from rostral segments are added sequentially from the lateral ("outside") layers to the medial ("inside") layers of the tract. Consequently, sacral segments are represented most laterally, and cervical segments most medially; axons from lumbar and thoracic levels are situated sequentially between them. The axons of spinothalamic neurons that respond primarily to subcutaneous or visceral stimulation tend to be concentrated in the medial aspect of the spinothalamic tract (Fig. 7-6).

The spinothalamic tract sends axons directly to the VPL thalamus, where synaptic endings are found on neurons that also receive medial lemniscal fibers. The representation of NS and WDR encoding of noxious stimulation in the spinal cord is preserved at the thalamic level.

Thalamocortical neurons in the ventral posterior thalamus receive spinothalamic input and send axons to the S1 cortex, where both NS and WDR type neurons have been identified. The selective destruction of S1 cortex impairs the ability to discriminate different intensities of noxious stimulation, but does not eliminate the ability to perceive noxious stimuli as painful. There are at least two explanations for this. One is that neurons in the ventrolateral thalamus send axons to the second (S2) somatosensory and insular cortices adjacent to the lateral (sylvian) fissure. A second explanation is that neurons in the spinothalamic tract send collateral fibers and terminal endings medially into the brainstem reticular formation, hypothalamus, and medial thalamus. From these sites, nociceptive information is transmitted widely throughout the forebrain, particularly to prefrontal, premotor, posterior parietal, insular, and medial limbic cortical areas. These cortical structures mediate the cognitive, mnemonic, motivational, and emotional aspects of pain perception and prepare autonomic and somatomotor responses.

There is less information about the mechanisms of innocuous temperature sensation than about the encoding of pain and tactile sensations. Although some peripheral afferent A-δ and, possibly, C fibers respond differentially to innocuous warm or cool temperatures, most neurologic disorders that impair temperature discrimination, whether affecting the peripheral or central nervous system, are associated with hypoalgesia.

Neurotransmitters of the Peripheral Afferent and Central Ascending Sensory Pathways

Peripheral afferent fibers. The neurotransmitters of A-β tactile and other large-diameter myelinated afferents are amino acids, probably glutamate or aspartate. These amino acids activate postsynaptic receptors of the *N*-methyl-D-aspartate (NMDA) or alpha-amino methyl propionic acid (AMPA) type. These neurotransmitters are called excitatory amino acids (EEAs) because their release opens sodium channels in the postsynaptic membrane, leading to the generation of excitatory postsynaptic potentials (EPSPs) of relatively short duration (tens or hundreds of milliseconds). In addition to the EEAs, peptides such as substance P and calcitonin gene-related peptide (CGRP) are neurotransmitters for the small-diameter unmyelinated C fibers and, possibly, the finely myelinated A-δ afferent fibers. Afferent fibers from visceral organs contain a unique peptide neurotransmitter, vasoactive intestinal peptide (VIP). These peptide neurotransmitters produce EPSPs of very

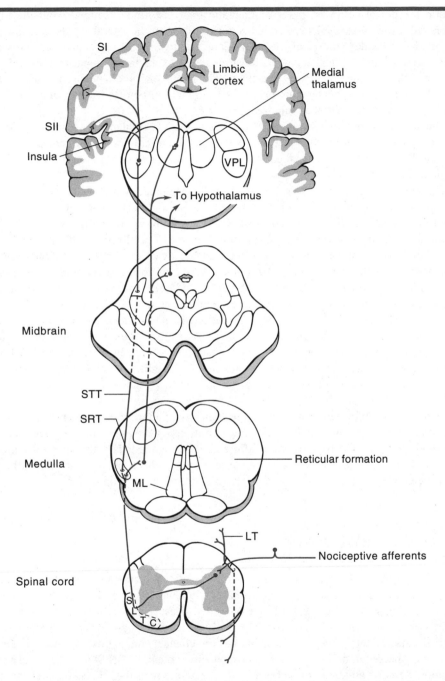

Figure 7-6 Diagram of ascending spinothalamic and spinoreticular pathways. Nociceptive afferents contribute intersegmental connecting fibers to Lissauer's tract (LT) and also excite spinal cord dorsal horn neurons with direct spinothalamic tract (STT) projections to the ventral posterior lateral (VPL) thalamus. Ascending fibers also activate neurons of the spinoreticular tract (SRT), which excites cells of the reticular formation of the medulla, midbrain, hypothalamus, and medial thalamus through direct monosynaptic or polysynaptic pahways. Thalamocortical neurons that receive nociceptive input project to both sensory and limbic cortical regions. Note the segmental lamination of the ascending fibers (S = sacral; L = lumbar; T = thoracic; C = cervical).

long duration (seconds), thus permitting prolonged excitatory effects of nociceptive afferent fiber activity.

Central ascending pathways. One or more of the EEAs are thought to be neurotransmitters for the ascending fibers of the medial lemniscus, the dorsolateral funiculus, and the spinothalamic tract.

Sensory Modulation in the Central Nervous System

Sensory function and experience is affected by CNS activities that mediate attention and—especially in the case of pain—fear, anxiety, and depression. CNS modulating functions can be impaired by drugs and disease that affect the central or peripheral nervous system.

AFFERENT MODULATION (Fig. 7-7A) It is a common experience that tactile stimulation, such as rubbing or scratching, relieves pain or itching. Innocuous or even near-noxious heating or cooling can have a similar effect. This is because the excitatory

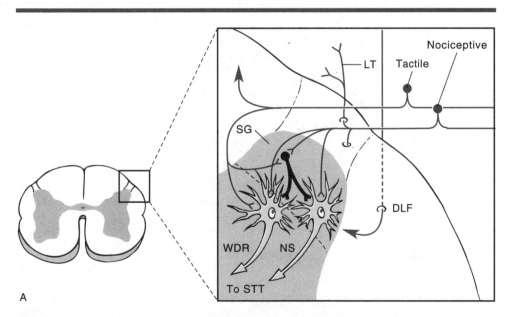

A

Figure 7-7 *A.* Diagram of inhibitory circuits in the dorsal horn. Wide dynamic range (WDR), but not nociceptive specific (NS) neurons, receive input from both tactile and nociceptive afferent fibers. Nociceptive afferents contribute intersegmental connecting fibers to Lissauer's tract (LT). Both tactile and nociceptive afferents excite substantia gelatinosa (SG) inhibitory interneurons (dark filled neuron) that mediate afferent sensory inhibition. Supraspinal neurons may augment or suppress sensory inhibition via descending axons in the dorsolateral funiculus (DLF). *B.* Diagram of descending sensory control pathways. Limbic and sensory (S1 and S2) corticofugal fibers modulate spinal cord sensory processing directly through corticospinal (CS) projections or indirectly through thalamic, midbrain periaqueductal gray (PAG), and lateral or midline medullary neurons with axons descending in the dorsolateral funiculus (DLF).

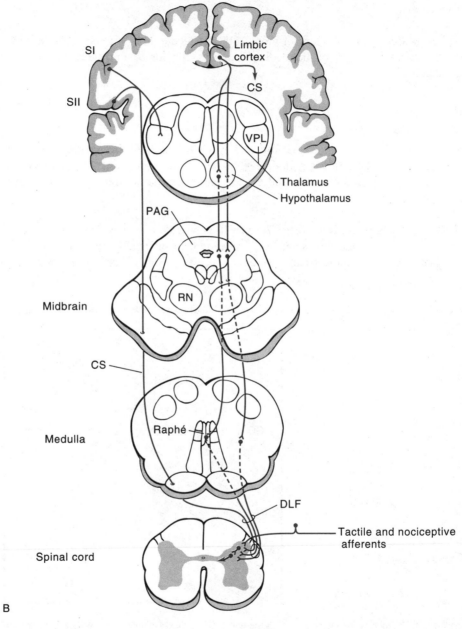

B

Figure 7-7   *(continued)*

effect of afferent activity is normally controlled by neuronal mechanisms that are activated by afferent activity. Both myelinated and unmyelinated afferent fibers excite inhibitory interneurons in the substantia gelatinosa of the spinal or trigeminal dorsal horn. These interneurons release GABA, glycine, or enkephalinergic neurotransmitters or neuromodulators that can pre- or postsynaptically suppress the excitatory effects of afferent input to WDR or NS spinal sensory neurons. Peripheral neuropathies, which affect the magnitude, composition, and temporal pattern of afferent activity, can reduce the effectiveness of this afferent inhibition, producing abnormal and sometimes painful spontaneous and evoked sensations.

SUPRASPINAL MODULATING SYSTEMS (Fig. 7-7B)   The transmission of somatosensory information is controlled by brainstem and cerebral neurons that can suppress or enhance sensory processing at each level of the central nervous system. Corticothalamic neurons of the S1 somatosensory cortex, for example, can enhance or, through GABAergic interneurons, suppress the responses of VPL thalamic cells. Electrical or chemical stimulation of the medial midbrain can activate noradrenergic, dopaminergic, and serotonergic medullary neurons with axonal projections to the spinal dorsal horn. These bulbospinal neurons can specifically attenuate the nociceptive responses of WDR and NS dorsal horn cells and may mediate the analgesic effects of drugs. These central modulatory systems are the neural mechanisms through which cerebral functions mediating "psychologic" states can profoundly affect somatic sensations. Furthermore, drugs or central nervous system diseases may activate or suppress these sensory control mechanisms, resulting in abnormal and sometimes painful spontaneous or evoked sensations.

EXAMINATION OF SENSORY FUNCTION

The sensory examination assists the interpretation of other aspects of the neurologic examination. Sensory abnormalities may be the only findings that provide evidence for neurologic disease. Sensory function can be tested reliably and quantitatively with simple instruments. Understanding the underlying anatomy and physiology and developing an examination strategy greatly facilitate the examination and its interpretation.

The History

The history usually provides the first evidence for disorders of sensory function. Sensory symptoms are categorized as positive, abnormal, or negative. All three types of symptoms may occur together. The most common *positive* symptoms include pain and paresthetic (abnormal) sensations usually described as "tingling" or as "pins and needles" or ". . . as if my arm has gone to sleep." Paresthesias may or may not be painful, but are usually unpleasant. Abnormal sensory symptoms often accompany positive symptoms and consist of unusual, altered sensations evoked by naturally occurring stimuli such as touch or temperature. The sensations are described as "electric," "funny," or "different" in which case the term *dysesthesia* is used. The term *allodynia* refers to pain elicited by normally innocuous stimuli. Negative sensory symptoms refer to the perceived loss of a sensory function, such as tactile discrimination, the sense of position and movement (kinesthesia), or the ability to detect temperatures or feel pain. Obtain the following information about each sensory symptom when taking the history:

- Location, spread, or radiation
- Onset
- Duration
- Intensity (consider using a rating scale*)
- Temporal pattern (steady, paroxysmal, duration of each paroxysm)
- Exacerbating factors (activity, position, emotional state, other stimuli)
- Relieving factors
- Other associated symptoms (nausea, weakness, visceral, or other sensations)

Strategy of the Examination

The history guides the examination by focusing on the chief complaint. Nonetheless, you should perform a screening examination to assess the general integrity of somatosensory function.

ASSESS THE PATIENT'S RELIABILITY   The mental status examination helps you assess the patient's ability to report sensory experiences reliably. Impaired cognitive or language functions, abnormal emotional states (depression or high levels of anxiety), or personality disorders degrade the validity and reliability of the examination. Begin with an initial screening, using several trials, of the patient's ability to detect and report differences between stimuli that are applied at widely different intensities to areas that may be presumed normal on the basis of the history or other aspects of the neurologic examination. Some patients will guess when asked to respond. You should acknowledge and discourage this behavior when you encounter it. If the patient continues to guess, you should judge the reliability of the examination accordingly.

DEVELOP A PERSONAL ROUTINE THAT IS BASED ON A PHYSIO-LOGIC AND ANATOMIC RATIONALE   The sensory examination helps to detect and localize the site of neurologic abnormalities. Accordingly, you should think about what you are testing and not perform the examination as a ritualistic exercise. Somatic sensation can be divided into large-fiber and small-fiber functions, so you can screen sensory function by sampling vibratory and pinprick or temperature sensations at cervical, thoracic, lumbar, and sacral dermatomes. The intensity of stimulation should be slightly but definitely suprathreshold for a normal person. Testing a few known nerve and dermatomal patterns should be sufficient and require only 2 to 3 min. You can follow this with a more focused examination based on the results of screening, the history, or other findings. Simple touch is not a good screening stimulus because multiple peripheral and central pathways can mediate this sensation.

EXPLAIN THE EXAMINATION TO THE PATIENT AND KEEP IT SIM-PLE   Tell your patients that you are going to test sensations and that you want them to relax, close their eyes, and concentrate on what they will be feeling. Ask the patient first to describe or identify the stimulation (pin, warm or cold object, touching with finger,

---

*Standardized visual analogue scales can be constructed or are commercially available in the form of pocket slide rules. These devices are especially useful in monitoring responses to treatment.

moving a toe, vibration) with eyes closed to enhance concentration. This avoids suggesting the "correct" response and gives some initial information about clinically significant abnormalities and the reliability of the patient's report. Next, use more detailed questioning about abnormalities such as lateralized differences in intensity or the direction of movement about a joint. Instructions should be simple, and unambiguous responses should be requested. For example: "Which feels sharper, (stimulus) 1 or 2, or are they the same?" rather than, "What is the difference, if any, between 1 and 2?" The former question forces a simple choice, but the latter invites an unfocused description, which is difficult for many patients and is usually difficult to interpret. When asking for subjective comparisons, you may need to apply the stimulus three to four times at the same intensity to assure adequate sensory sampling.

TEST SIMPLE FUNCTIONS FIRST, COMPLEX ONES LATER   There is little point in testing refined discriminative functions such as the ability to recognize palpated objects with eyes closed if the patient has an elevated threshold for tactile stimuli. Complex sensory functions require intact peripheral, spinal, and brainstem pathways, which you can best examine by determining the patient's ability to detect simple stimuli delivered at intensities that are easily detected by a normal subject.

Tactile Discriminative Functions

THRESHOLD FOR TOUCH   Tactile senses are mediated principally by A-β myelinated afferent fibers, but some A-δ and C fibers may also be activated by touch and pressure. Several central nervous system pathways mediate tactile sensations. Consequently, testing tactile detection or threshold has little localizing value compared to tests of other sensory functions. Normal individuals can detect the movement of hairs and, on the noncalloused glabrous skin of the finger pads or lips, displacements of about 6 μm and pressures of 8 mg as delivered with calibrated (von Frey type) hairs. Devices for measuring touch detection thresholds are commercially available but are used principally for research. In neuropathic pain states, tactile stimulation is necessary to detect mechanical allodynia.

TWO-POINT DISCRIMINATION   If peripheral afferent tactile fibers and subcortical tactile pathways are normal, mechanisms within the primary somatosensory (S1) cortex of the anterior parietal lobe determine the ability to detect the separation of two points on the skin. For screening purposes, apply this test to the tongue or the noncalloused glabrous skin of the lips and finger pads. These surfaces are specialized for somesthetic acuity and have the most extensive cortical representations of the body. Normal individuals can detect point separations of 1 mm on the tongue and 2 to 4 mm on the lips and finger pads. A compass or calibrated esthesiometer is the preferred instrument for this test, but the points of a bent paper clip can be used as a substitute if absolutely necessary.

DETECTION OF TACTILE MOVEMENT AND GRAPHESTHESIA   The ability to identify the direction of moving cutaneous tactile stimuli is perhaps the most sensitive test of anterior parietal (S1) cortical function, provided that peripheral and subcortical pathways are intact. A test of cutaneous direction sense can be used to detect the approximate segmental level of a spinal cord lesion affecting dorsal column function. When used for this purpose, patients should be instructed to close their eyes and indicate the direction of movement by pointing or by responding verbally when you move tactile stimuli in lateral or rostrocaudal directions. Apply movements of approximately 2 to 3 cm during 1 s at 2- to 3-s intervals. Apply a few test stimuli to presumably normal areas to determine test validity and reliability.

Graphesthesia is the ability to identify letters or numbers written on the skin. This complex ability requires an intact S1 and parietal association cortex, as well as enough language function to recognize and recite numbers and letters. Test this on the finger pads, using a fine, dull point to write single numerals or letters and ask the patients to identify them.

Vibratory Sensation

Pallesthesia refers to the ability to detect rapidly oscillating (usually 100 Hz or more) pressure applied to the skin, usually over bony prominences of joints such as the lateral or medial malleoli of the ankle. This sensation is mediated by nerve endings (primarily pacinian corpuscles) that are innervated specifically by A-β fibers, the largest diameter myelinated afferents of the somatosensory system. A mild impairment of pallesthesia can affect otherwise normal elderly subjects (over 70 years of age), but especially in younger patients, it may be the first sign of a demyelinating process affecting the peripheral or central nervous system. The critical ascending spinal pathways include the dorsal columns, but the dorsolateral funiculus is the major ascending pathway mediating vibratory sense. Both pathways converge within the medial lemniscus to form the afferent pathway to the VPL thalamus. Impairment of vibratory sensation usually results from subcortical, brainstem, or peripheral lesions even though the information reaches the S1 cortex.

Use a 128-Hz tuning fork and apply the stimulus to skin overlying bone instead of fat or muscle to transmit the vibration through a large volume of tissue. However, since pacinian corpuscles are distributed widely throughout the body, the stimulus can be applied to the skin overlying muscle or fat if necessary. When testing threshold initially, give the patient a choice of responding only "yes" or "no" to indicate the presence of vibration. By altering the force of the striking of the fork, you can begin with strong, and then progressively weaker, stimuli until the patient detects stimuli near normal threshold. If needed, you can assess the patient's threshold against your own by placing your finger on the side of the joint opposite the stimulation.

Kinesthesia

The term *position sense* is sometimes used incorrectly to refer to tests of the ability to sense the direction of movement about a joint. Kinesthesia, the more appropriate term, is mediated primarily by muscle spindle afferents, which are activated by muscle stretch. Cutaneous afferent fibers contribute to this sensory function. The spinal pathways ascend in the dorsolateral funiculus and probably also in the dorsal columns of the spinal cord. After a synapse in the dorsal column nuclei and the lateral cervical nucleus, postsynaptic fibers join the medial lemniscal projections to the VPL thalamus. If these subcortical pathways are intact, deficits in kinesthesia may be attributed to functional abnormalities within the S1 somatosensory cortex and/or the somatosensory association areas immediately posterior to the postcentral gyrus.

Kinesthesia is critical for the execution of nearly all motor functions (ocular movements excepted). Consequently, the first indication of a severe kinesthetic deficit may be a complaint of clumsiness in walking or in coordination of the hands. If gait ataxia is due to a kinesthetic deficit (*sensory ataxia*), and vestibular and cerebellar functions are normal, the patient may be able to stand with feet together and eyes open, but not with the eyes closed (positive *Romberg* test). If the hands are involved, fine, slow, writhing movements of the digits (*pseudoathetosis*) may be seen when the patient holds the arms outstretched with the eyes closed. These kinesthetic deficits can be confirmed and less severe deficits detected by passively moving a digit (or even a proximal joint) and asking the patient, with eyes closed, to indicate the direction of movement verbally ("up" or "down") or by pointing. Hold the digit (or limb) as lightly as possible and parallel to the plane of movement to avoid stimulation of tactile pressure receptors. Normal subjects can correctly identify movements of 1 degree or less across the interphalangeal joints of the fingers and of 2 to 3 degrees at the toes. The sensitivity of the test is inversely related to the velocity of the displacement, so it is best to attempt to execute the excursions over 1 to 2 s when testing each joint.

Contrary to earlier conceptions, kinesthesia and vibratory sense are mediated by different neural mechanisms. Consequently, one of these functions may be impaired while the other is spared. This is due to the fact that, although they share spinal pathways, each sensation is mediated by different receptors and afferent fibers, and each activates different forebrain mechanisms.

Temperature

Thermesthesia is mediated by finely myelinated A-δ and some unmyelinated C fibers that respond to cutaneous stimuli either in the warm (35 to 44°C; 95 to 111°F) or cool (5 to 30°C; 41 to 86°F) range. Temperatures above the warm or below the cool range will attenuate the activity of these fibers and begin to excite discharges in nociceptive afferents. Separate and distinct central neural mechanisms mediate the sensations of pain and temperature. Specific deficits of warm sensation, for example, occur following lesions within the parietal cortex. Nevertheless, thermanesthesia or thermhypesthesia accompanies analgesia or hypoalgesia in most clinical conditions.

Most examining rooms do not contain calibrated thermal devices, which makes routine thermal testing difficult. As a practical method for screening, you can use two glass test tubes or glass syringes filled alternately with warm and cool water within the proper temperature range as tested on your skin. The tuning fork is usually slightly below room temperature and may be cooled or warmed quickly with tap water. Because the metal quickly changes temperature, however, this method allows testing of only one temperature at a time. Calibrated devices are available commercially for more detailed quantitative testing. Ask the patient to identify, with eyes closed, the stimulus as either "warm" or "cool" after it has been applied to the skin for about 2 s. Hairy skin should be tested because thermal discrimination on glabrous skin is less sensitive. Three applications at each temperature in random order usually suffice to detect a deficit.

Pain

Some nociceptive cutaneous afferents are specialized to respond to noxious mechanical, thermal, or possibly chemical stimuli. All of these fibers, including the less specialized "polymodal" nociceptive afferents, are finely myelinated A-δ and unmyelinated C fibers that innervate the substantia gelatinosa and dorsal horn of the spinal cord. The postsynaptic neurons ascend ipsilaterally for three to four segments before crossing in the anterior spinal commissure to form the ventral and lateral spinothalamic tract in the ventrolateral quadrant of the spinal cord.

CUTANEOUS MECHANICAL STIMULATION Use noxious mechanical stimulation as an initial screening test for abnormalities of cutaneous pain. Apply mechanical stimuli at just above noxious intensities to the hairy skin with a safety pin. Do not use very sharp instruments, such as hypodermic needles, because they penetrate the skin easily and cause bleeding. To avoid spreading infection, the pin should be discarded between the examination of each patient. Pinching a fold of skin may be used as an alternative.

For initial screening, inform the patient about the stimulus and then ask the patient, with eyes closed, to choose between responding "sharp" or "dull" when you apply the pin or blunt end in approximately random sequence two to four times each to cervical, thoracic, lumbar, and sacral dermatomes. Keep the stimulus intensity at just above noxious levels and as uniform as possible. This procedure assesses the patient's reliability and discriminative capacity, familiarizes the patient with the stimulus, and may reveal unsuspected abnormalities. Then focus the examination on other areas of interest that may have been identified in the history or other parts of the examination. Ask patients who are capable of giving reliable responses to rate the intensity of pin stimuli that are applied alternately to normal and suspected abnormal sites. Ask the patient, "Which is sharper, 1 or 2?" while applying the stimulus first to one site and then to the other in alternate order. You can obtain more refined assessments by asking the patient to rate the relative intensity of one stimulus, which you establish as 100 or "one dollar," against the other stimulus, which the patient may rate as "50" or "50 cents," for example. If the patient's consistent responses reveal a sensory abnormality, determine the distribution of the deficit by asking the patient to indicate when the pinprick becomes sharp while you move repetitive, evenly applied stimuli from less sensitive to more sensitive areas. Patients usually recognize increases in intensity more readily than decreases. Accordingly, you can best define hypoalgesic areas by proceeding from within the affected area toward normal surfaces; the opposite is true of areas of hyperalgesia or allodynia. Occasionally, it is helpful, with the patient's permission, to outline the abnormal area with a few removable marks of a wax pencil.

NOXIOUS HEAT AND COLD The peripheral and central neural mechanisms mediating heat and cold pain are different from those mediating innocuous thermal sensations. Although most clinical abnormalities affect both of these sensory functions, you should examine thermal pain sensation specifically if you suspect a pain sensory deficit. Instruments for the quantitative testing of heat and cold pain are available commercially. Otherwise, you should conduct the examination as described above for innocuous thermal testing except that the test temperature must be in the noxious (but tolerable) range as tested on your skin. Warn the patient that slightly painful stimulation will be used and that, as each stimulus is applied, the patient should indicate whether it is painful. Occasionally, you will need to compare noxious with innocuous temperatures to clarify the distinction that is to be made. As in other aspects of the examination, the patient should be encouraged to choose between "painful" and "not painful" in this part of the examination.

SUBCUTANEOUS (DEEP) PAIN   This sensation is most likely to be affected selectively or differentially by intramedullary lesions of the spinal cord, such as a syrinx, tumor, granuloma, hemorrhage (hematomyelia), or arteriovenous malformation. Diseases that produce severe and extensive damage of the dorsal roots (tabes dorsalis, plexus avulsions) affect deep pain along with the superficial sensations. Deep pain is often spared in diseases that affect cutaneous nociceptive afferents or by central, particularly cortical, lesions that impair thermal or pinprick sensations. Loss of subcutaneous pain sensation is definite evidence for pathology involving the spinothalamic tract or its synaptic connections in the dorsal horn or thalamus.

Inform the patient that you are testing the ability to feel pain and to report when the stimulus first becomes painful. Place the patient's muscles, tendons (e.g., Achilles tendon), or bones (e.g., first metacarpal) between your flexed index finger and the interphalangeal joint of your thumb and slowly apply increasing pressure until the patient signals that the stimulus is painful. Another approach is to apply pressure to the finger or toenails with the handle of the reflex hammer or tuning fork.

Complex Sensory Functions

STEREOGNOSIS   Stereognosis is the ability to identify common objects, such as a safety pin, button, or coin, by manual palpation of the object with the eyes closed. If language function and subcortical somatosensory pathways are intact, impaired stereognosis (astereognosis) indicates a contralateral abnormality of parietal lobe function, particularly the primary (S1) somatosensory cortex of the postcentral gyrus and its direct connections with the adjacent parietal association cortex of the superior parietal lobule. Astereognosis is often accompanied by agraphesthesia and akinesthesia, but, when seen in isolation, it may be the first sign of parietal lobe dysfunction.

EXTINCTION   Somatosensory extinction refers to a failure to detect the presence of a tactile stimulus on one side when you present two suprathreshold tactile stimuli simultaneously and bilaterally (double simultaneous stimulation, or DSS). For the somatosensory system, the test is most sensitive when the stimuli are applied to homotopic body areas. For this test to be meaningful, there should be no deficits of peripheral, subcortical, or primary (S1) cortical somatosensory function. Do not perform this examination if you have found an elevated threshold to single stimuli on one side. Given otherwise intact somesthetic function, however, unilateral somatosensory extinction is evidence for abnormal function of the association cortex in the contralateral superior parietal lobule and its direct parietal cortical connections. Strictly speaking, the test of somatic DSS is a test of sensory attentional mechanisms and not specifically of somatosensory function. Somatosensory attentional deficits may be accompanied by lateralized attentional deficits in auditory or visual sensory func-

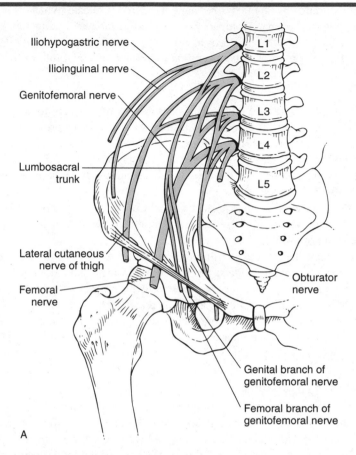

Iliohypogastric nerve

Ilioinguinal nerve

Genitofemoral nerve

Lumbosacral trunk

Lateral cutaneous nerve of thigh

Femoral nerve

L1
L2
L3
L4
L5

Obturator nerve

Genital branch of genitofemoral nerve

Femoral branch of genitofemoral nerve

A

Figure 7-8 *A.* Diagram of the lumbar plexus and its components. *B.* Diagram of the sacral plexus and its components. (Reprinted with permission from DeJong RN: *The Neurologic Examination*, 4th ed. Hagerstown, MD, Harper and Row, 1979.)

tions, particularly if the responsible lesion extends beyond the superior parietal lobule to involve the association cortex near the primary auditory or visual cortex. These deficits are often most evident with lesions that affect the function of the nondominant hemisphere.

DISORDERS OF SENSATION

Sensory Neuropathies

Diseases of sensory nerves cause loss of sensation, often accompanied by positive sensory symptoms (pain, "numbness," paresthesias) within the distribution of a sensory or mixed sensory and motor nerve. The positive symptoms may be caused by spontaneous abnormal discharges originating in diseased nerve fibers, by increases in the excitability

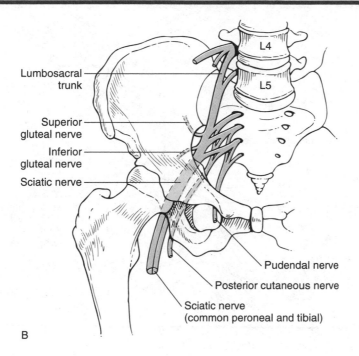

Figure 7-8 *(continued)*

of central cells, or by both processes. Occasionally, especially following traumatic nerve injuries, severe pain, allodynia, and hyperalgesia develop within the distribution of the damaged nerve. These symptoms may be accompanied by local cutaneous signs of abnormally increased or decreased sympathetic nervous system activity affecting the temperature, color, and sweating of the involved limb. Dystrophic changes may be seen, including local osteoporosis and increased or decreased hair growth. The term "reflex sympathetic dystrophy," or "RSD," has been applied to conditions involving some or all of these findings. This term is commonly used but is not favored among practitioners who specialize in pain management, in part because the pathophysiology of these conditions is not understood and because the term suggests a pathophysiologic process that is probably not correct in a large number of cases. Instead, the term "complex regional pain syndrome," or "CRPS," has been suggested for designating those cases in which peripheral nervous system disorders are associated with unusually severe, chronic pain with or without evidence of sympathetic nervous system changes (Stanton-Hicks et al, 1995).

Some neuropathies primarily affect myelinated fibers (acute or chronic inflammatory demyelinating polyneuropathy and some neurotoxic and nutritional neuropathies) and can be initially detected by impaired vibratory or tactile sensation. Neuropathies that damage the finely myelinated or unmyelinated fibers, either primarily or additionally (e.g., diabetes, herpes zoster, amyloidosis, and idiopathic small-fiber neuropathy) are frequently painful and may be detected initially as a thermesthetic deficit and later as a loss of pain and temperature sensitivity.

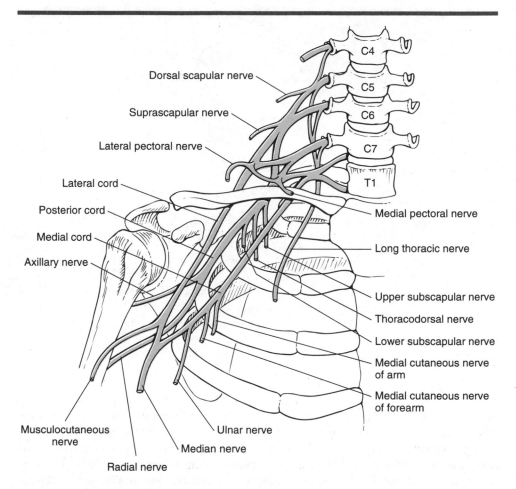

Dorsal scapular nerve

Suprascapular nerve

Lateral pectoral nerve

Lateral cord

Posterior cord

Medial cord

Axillary nerve

C4
C5
C6
C7
T1

Medial pectoral nerve

Long thoracic nerve

Upper subscapular nerve

Thoracodorsal nerve

Lower subscapular nerve

Medial cutaneous nerve of arm

Medial cutaneous nerve of forearm

Musculocutaneous nerve

Ulnar nerve

Median nerve

Radial nerve

Figure 7-9   Diagram of the brachial plexus and its components in relation to anatomic structures of the shoulder and upper chest. (Reprinted with permission from DeJong RN: *The Neurologic Examination*, 4th ed. Hagerstown, MD, Harper and Row, 1979, p 572.)

Radiculopathies

Disorders affecting the sensory function of nerve roots cause symptoms similar to those involving peripheral nerves except that the positive symptoms, especially pain, are within the dermatomal distribution of the involved root and often project into the distributions of adjacent dermatomes. Mechanical irritation of the fifth lumbar root, for example, may produce pain that radiates into both the lateral (first sacral) and dorsal fifth lumbar aspects of the foot. The pain of radiculopathy results, in part, from mechanical stimulation of the dural root sleeve, which is innervated by unmyelinated fibers. CRPS (see above) may be seen as a result of radiculopathy.

The most common radiculopathies are caused by mechanical trauma from osteophytes, bony spurs, and protruding intervertebral discs associated with degenerative changes in the spine and supporting spinal muscles. Infections [herpes zoster, bacterial meningitis, acquired immune deficiency syndrome (AIDS), syphilis] and neoplasms (neurofibromata, meningiomas, malignant lymphomas, and metastatic neoplasms) are prominent considerations in the differential diagnosis of radiculopathies. Sensory loss is likely to involve both myelinated and unmyelinated fiber function. In interpreting the examination, the examiner must keep in mind the functional overlap of dermatomes.

Plexopathies

Lesions affecting the brachial, lumbar, or sacral plexuses cause sensory loss and positive symptoms in somatic distributions that typically overlap peripheral nerve and dermatomal innervation patterns. CRPS may be present in some cases. The sensory findings following lesions involving the lumbar or sacral plexuses are most often within the distribution of one or more of the nerves emanating from the plexus (Fig. 7-8). In the case of the *lumbar plexus*, this includes the genitofemoral, iliohypogastric, ilioinguinal, lateral femoral cutaneous, femoral, genitofemoral, and obturator nerves in the approximate order of lesions involving the upper, middle, and lower portions of the plexus. Lesions affecting the *sacral plexus* are most likely to produce sensory abnormalities within the distribution of the sciatic and, occasionally, pudendal nerves. The *brachial plexus* is affected by disease and injury more often than either the lumbar or sacral plexuses. The location of the sensory abnormality following brachial plexus injury varies systematically with the location of the injury (Fig. 7-9). Often the sensory findings are much less prominent than the weakness because of the overlap of radicular and peripheral nerve innervations. Following lesions of the upper or middle trunk, sensory loss may be found in the lateral upper arm, forearm, and hand. Sensory loss in the distribution of the median nerve accompanies involvement of the lateral cord. Lesions of the lower trunk or medial cord may produce sensory abnormalities throughout the medial aspect of the upper limb, including the territories of the ulnar and median nerves. Sensory loss in radial and axillary nerve distributions follows lesions involving the posterior cord of the brachial plexus.

　Trauma and tumor are the major causes of plexus injury. The brachial plexus is vulnerable to mechanical injuries because of its position between the clavicle and the blood vessels and muscles of the upper limb and cervical spine. This anatomic location can lead to compression of portions of the brachial plexus following displaced clavicular fractures or hypertrophy of the anterior scalene muscle in the presence of a cervical rib (scalenus syndrome). Pain and paresthesias in the distribution of the involved portions of the plexus are common positive sensory symptoms. Partial or complete avulsion of the brachial plexus is a common sequel of motorcycle accidents and frequently leads to chronic pain within the denervated region. This denervation pain syndrome probably results from a combination of afferent discharges from injured and regenerating nerve fibers and increased excitability of central neurons. Pain is also a prominent symptom in the syndrome of brachial plexus neuritis or neuralgia, which presents with the sudden or subacute onset of pain and weakness within the distribution of one or more components of the plexus. The sensory symptoms often precede the onset of weakness. The cause of this condition is unknown, but viral and immune etiologies have been suggested. Recovery is variable, ranging from complete in the case of mild involvement to severe, permanent disability when the plexus is more extensively involved.

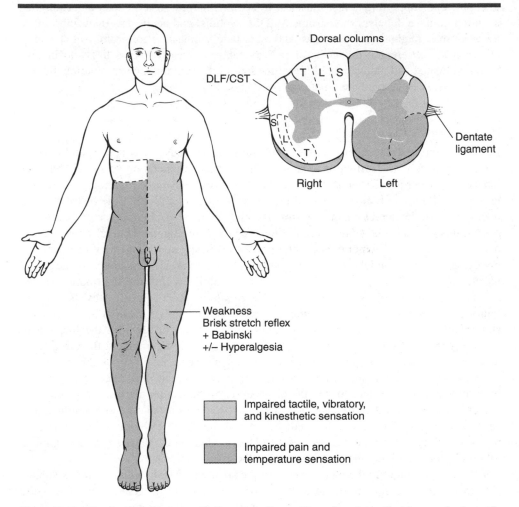

Figure 7-10 Figurine showing sensory findings in the Brown-Séquard syndrome. In this example, the tactile and vibratory sensory deficits begin at the T7–T8 level. The pain and temperature deficit begins at a more caudal level because some spinothalamic fibers ascend ipsilaterally for two or more segments before decussation.

Spinal Cord Lesions

Two major sensory findings are often found with spinal cord lesions: (1) a segmental demarcation of sensory abnormality (sensory level); and (2) a selective involvement of sensory modalities such as pain and temperature or vibratory and tactile sensations (dissociated sensory loss). The sensory symptoms of spinal cord disease reflect the segmental and sensory organization within this structure. Disorders affecting the dorsal (posterior) half of the spinal cord may cause a sensation of "numbness" accompanied by tactile paresthesias below a dermatomal or segmental level. Similarly, lesions involving the ventral spinal cord may cause a selective loss of pain or temperature sensation within the same distribution, at times accompanied by intermittent or nearly continuous pain. Lesions affecting spinothalamic transmission may lead to chronic pain within the area of sensory impairment (central pain) (Casey, 1991). Investigate the location of the sensory deficit by applying repetitive stimuli of equal intensity within the presumed involved region, then move the stimulation toward the normal area. Look for a sensory level by testing the patient's front and back on both sides. Test both dorsal/dorsolateral funicular (tactile and vibratory) and spinothalamic (pain and temperature) functions. Vibratory and moving tactile stimuli are convenient and specific stimuli for testing dorsal spinal cord function. Test kinesthetic sensation even though it is difficult to identify a sensory level with this stimulus. Examine spinothalamic functions with a pin or with hot and cold water in glass tubes. Keep in mind the laminar organization of these afferent pathways and the possibility that disease may affect only part of the ascending fibers. For example, an intramedullary tumor or syrinx at the thoracic level could impair conduction within the *medial* (thoracic) fibers of the spinothalamic tract while leaving the most *lateral* (sacral) fibers intact. This could result in the phenomenon known as "sacral sparing," in which pain and temperature sensations are impaired at the thoracic and lumbar levels but spared in the sacral dermatomes. A similar effect, producing selective tactile sensory deficits, can occur with a lesion affecting transmission within the *lateral* dorsal columns because the segmental lamination within the dorsal columns mirrors that of the spinothalamic tract.

Trauma, tumor, and infectious diseases can affect the spinal cord at any level. There are a few conditions, however, that cause characteristic abnormalities of spinal sensory function. Demyelinating diseases can impair transmission along the major dorsal and/or ventrolateral ascending pathways without directly affecting the spinal gray matter. If most of one side of the spinal cord is involved, for example, the patient may have an ipsilateral loss of tactile and vibratory sensation and a contralateral loss of pain and temperature below the segmental level of involvement. Because of the dorsolateral location of the corticospinal tract, this crossed sensory dissociation is often accompanied by evidence for upper motor neuron involvement on the side of the tactile and vibratory deficit, in which case it is referred to (somewhat incorrectly) as the Brown-Séquard syndrome (Fig. 7-10). Involvement of descending sensory modulating fibers in the dorsolateral funiculus may cause an ipsilateral hyperalgesia. In contrast, an intramedullary tumor or syrinx of the spinal cord may damage the spinal gray matter and the crossing spinothalamic fibers in the anterior spinal commissure, thus producing a selective and profound loss of pain and temperature sensation within a few spinal segments without affecting ascending transmission from other segmental levels. Deep pain may be differentially affected. Infarctions of the spinal cord can produce selective and dissociated sensory losses because of the anatomy of the spinal cord blood supply. Thus, occlusion of the anterior spinal artery can result in a selective, usually bilateral, loss of pain and temperature sensations while infarctions within the territory of the dorsal or radicular spinal arteries, although much less frequent, cause ipsilateral impairment of tactile, vibratory, and kinesthetic sensations. Tumors, particularly neurofibromas, often cause a segmental and radicular sensory deficit (pain and/or tactile) at the level of the tumor accompanied by an impairment of contralateral pain and temperature and/or ipsilateral tactile and vibratory sensation below that level because of compression of the long ascending pathways by the tumor.

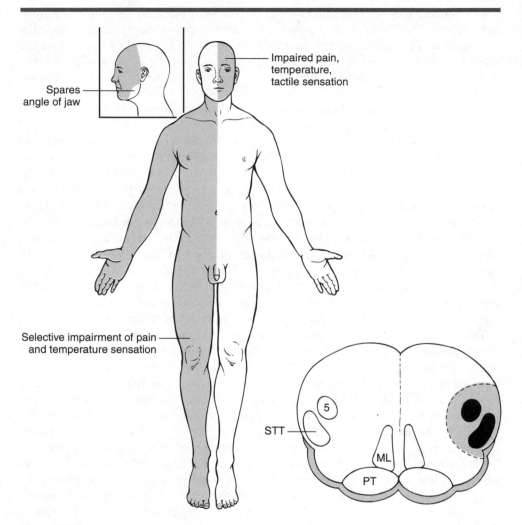

Figure 7-11 Figurine showing a "harlequin" pattern of sensory loss from a lateral medullary lesion. (ML = medial lemniscus; STT = spinothalamic tract; 5 = nucleus and tract of trigeminal nerve; PT = pyramidal tract.) The facial sensory deficit spares angle of the jaw.

Brainstem Lesions

The sensory symptoms accompanying lesions of the brainstem often resemble those found with spinal cord disease, including a dissociated sensory loss because of selective impairment of spinothalamic tract or medial lemniscal function. These pathways remain anatomically separate throughout the medulla, lower pons, and midpons, with the spinothalamic tract occupying a position distinctly lateral to that of the medial lemniscus. Consequently, lesions affecting the lateral medulla or pons are associated with a contralateral loss of pain and temperature in the body, caudal to the distribution of the trigeminal nerve, while tactile and vibratory sensations are spared. As with spinal cord lesions, spinothalamic damage may lead to a chronic pain syndrome within the area of sensory impairment (central pain) (Casey, 1991). Medial lesions, in contrast, cause the opposite pattern of sensory dissociation in which tactile and vibratory sensations are impaired while pain and thermesthesia are preserved. Because the right and left medial lemnisci are close together at these brainstem levels, bilateral tactile and vibratory deficits can occur. At more rostral brainstem levels, medial lemniscal and spinothalamic fibers come into close proximity and occupy a lateral position. Consequently, lateral midbrain lesions may cause a contralateral loss of all somatosensory modalities so that, with respect to sensory abnormality, they are clinically indistinguishable from thalamic or large hemispheric lesions. Because of the persisting segmental lamination of these sensory pathways, brainstem lesions can produce segmental levels of sensory loss, but this is uncommon when compared with spinal cord disease.

Involvement of cranial nerve function is a key characteristic of brainstem lesions. This has important localizing value, especially when considered in conjunction with the pattern of sensory loss. Thus, medial lesions that produce contralateral tactile and vibratory deficits may be associated with ipsilateral impairment of hypoglossal nerve function when the medulla is involved and an ipsilateral sixth nerve palsy when the lower pons is affected. In contrast, lateral lesions at these levels will affect pain and temperature in the contralateral body while impairing ipsilateral ninth and tenth nerve (medulla) or seventh nerve (pons) functions. At both medullary and pontine levels, lateral lesions can cause a "harlequin" pattern of sensory loss because damage to the fifth (trigeminal) sensory nucleus results in an ipsilateral loss of facial sensation while injury of the nearby spinothalamic tract causes a hypoalgesia and thermanesthesia of the contralateral body (Fig. 7-11). Lateral medullary or rostral cervical spinal cord lesions may spare facial tactile sensation and produce a selective, ipsilateral loss of facial pain and temperature sensation because of the preferential distribution of nociceptive afferents to the descending tract and nucleus of the fifth nerve.

Infarctions within the distribution of the vertebral and basilar arteries are the most common causes of brainstem lesions that selectively affect the medial or lateral brainstem, a result of the blood supply to the brainstem being organized into medial penetrating and lateral circumferential branches of the basilar artery at each level of the brainstem. Demyelinating diseases impair conduction along the major afferent pathways, either selectively or together. Sensory impairment may be an early sign of brainstem dysfunction caused by benign or malignant neoplasms within the posterior fossa—and it may be an important sign of medullary involvement in the Arnold-Chiari malformation (type 1).

Thalamic Lesions

Positive sensory symptoms, including intense paresthesias, dysesthesia, and less often pain, frequently accompany lesions in or near the ventral posterior thalamus. These symptoms may persist in the form of a chronic central pain syndrome, sometimes with severe tactile allodynia or hyperalgesia (syndrome thalamique of Dejerine and Roussy) (Casey, 1991), or they may resolve into a feeling of constant "numbness" with intermittent paresthesias. Because of the somatotopic organization within the somatosensory thalamus, the symptoms may be confined to all or part of one contralateral limb or, if the lesion is medial, the contralateral face. More often, however, the symptoms involve most of the contralateral face and body. Examination reveals sensory deficits within and typically beyond the symptomatic area. Because of the extensive convergence of spinothalamic and medial lemniscal inputs onto thalamic neurons, more than one sensory function is usually affected. Thus, pain (including deep pain), thermal, tactile, vibratory, and kinesthetic sensations may be impaired in any combination. The severity of the deficit ranges from a mild to severe elevation of detection threshold; complete anesthesia and analgesia is rare. Usually, the intensity of the impairment precludes testing highly integrated sensory functions such as cutaneous direction sense or sensory extinction.

Vascular lesions, specifically those compromising blood flow within the thalamogeniculate branches of the posterior cerebral artery, are the most frequent causes of selective damage to the ventral posterior thalamus. The thalamus has a very rich blood supply, making it susceptible to the development of abscesses and hematogenous metastases from malignant neoplasms. Demyelinating diseases may affect thalamocortical radiations through the posterior limb of the internal capsule or the lemniscal and spinothalamic inputs to the thalamus, but do not involve the thalamus directly.

Cortical Lesions

PRIMARY SOMATOSENSORY CORTEX   Although paresthesias and sensations of "numbness" can occur, the sensory symptoms from lesions selectively affecting the S1 somatosensory cortex are rarely as pronounced as those with thalamic involvement. Rather, the patient often perceives no sensory abnormality but complains of inability to perform fine or delicate manipulations that depend heavily on tactile information. Central pain syndromes may occur days or months following the lesion. Sensory symptoms may involve all or any part of the contralateral body, but are especially likely to affect the hand and face because of the extensive cortical representation of these cutaneous surfaces. An uncommon, but unique, feature of somatosensory cortical lesions is the development of *somatosensory seizures*, either as simple partial seizures or as an aura for secondary generalized seizures. The progression of the seizure often reflects the somatotopic organization of the cortex, with paresthetic sensations proceeding, for example, from the face and hand to the trunk and leg, or vice versa.

The examination may reveal a mild to moderate elevation of sensory thresholds, but this is usually less severe than the threshold elevations found following thalamic lesions. Pain and innocuous temperature detection thresholds may be slightly elevated. In contrast with thalamic lesions, vibratory sensation is rarely affected. The most profound deficits are found in discriminative functions such as identifying the direction of tactile movement, discriminating two points, and detecting the direction of movement about the interphalangeal joints (kinesthesia). If language functions are intact, tactile discriminative deficits are best examined by testing graphesthesia or stereognosis. Lesions that involve the somatosensory parietal association areas adjacent to the postcentral gyrus cause impaired attention to contralateral somatic stimuli or even to contralateral body parts. If the threshold for the detection of single stimuli is approximately equal bilaterally, an attentional deficit may be revealed by testing double simultaneous stimulation.

Infarctions within the distribution of the middle cerebral artery and its branches are a common cause of somatosensory cortical deficits. Sometimes, as in thalamic lesions, large areas of the contralateral body are involved. However, small lesions may cause localized sensory deficits that are difficult to distinguish from peripheral lesions of roots or nerves. Unless the history or semiology provides a localizing clue, the examiner may have to rely on the character of the sensory deficit, which involves a specific loss of tactile or kinesthetic discrimination rather than a global elevation of all somatosensory thresholds. Like the thalamus, the rich blood supply of the cortex renders it susceptible to embolic phenomena that include abscesses and malignant neoplasms. The overlying dura provides a site for the development of meningiomas and subdural hematomas.

INSULA AND SECONDARY SOMATOSENSORY CORTEX Lesions exclusively affecting the perisylvian somatosensory cortex may cause no symptoms because tactile and discriminative functions can be maintained by the intact S1 cortex of the postcentral gyrus. In some cases, tumors or infarctions involving this region have caused marked loss of pain (Bassetti et al, 1993), associated in some with a central pain syndrome (Casey, 1991) and paroxysms of painful dysesthesias suggesting a focal somatosensory seizure. In one case, quantitative sensory testing revealed marked elevation of pain and temperature threshold, which was relieved following removal of a benign tumor (Greenspan and Winfield, 1992). The basis for these observations may be involvement of thalamocortical projections from nociceptive specific (NS) neurons in the ventral posterior thalamus.

Psychogenic Sensory Abnormalities

Normal individuals vary widely in the degree to which they recognize or attend to sensory symptoms. Psychologic influences, mediated in part by supraspinal and suprabulbar descending sensory control pathways, can greatly magnify the perceived intensity and significance of clinically insignificant somatic sensations—or they can markedly attenuate clinically important symptoms. These psychologic factors, which include normal degrees of anxiety or indifference, should be explored during the mental status assessment and must be considered when interpreting the history of the patient's sensory abnormality. Your knowledge of the normal and pathologic physiology of the nervous system should help you recognize the sensory symptoms of neurologic disease and differentiate these from symptoms that are unlikely to be caused by organic abnormalities. Nevertheless, hubris is a characteristic that the careful clinician must avoid because diseases can present a wide range of symptoms and signs that reveal the limitations of our knowledge.

Normal individuals vary widely in their ability to detect differences among somatic stimuli and in their susceptibility to the acknowledgment of differences that may be suggested by the examiner. Indifference, hostility, anxiety, attentional distractions, and drugs may each contribute to the patient's inability to give reliable responses during the sensory examination, even when the somatosensory system is normal. These variables are added to the unavoidable variation in the intensity of stimuli applied manually by the examiner. To some extent, the variables in the clinical sensory examination can be minimized by reassuring communications with the patient, careful and unambiguous instructions, and by recognizing normal regional variations in somatic sensitivity. Your interpretation of the sensory examination, and your assessment of its validity and reliability, depends on your consideration of all these variables.

Even when all of the above factors have been considered, you will find some patients for whom the sensory examination may be considered reliable but invalid as an indicator of somatosensory function. For example, the patient may consistently indicate that one limb is hypesthetic or hyperalgesic in the absence of any other signs of neurologic abnormality. The region of the sensory abnormality may be unclear, or it may be delimited by anatomic borders rather than peripheral or central patterns of innervation. You may be unable to account for this abnormality based on known neurologic anatomy and physiology. In cases like this, a few noninvasive imaging or neurophysiologic studies should resolve the issue as to whether there has been an unusual presentation of neurologic disease. If organic disease has not been identified, it is usually wise to arrange for a subsequent examination. Often, this course of action is sufficient and the patient is adequately reassured. However, sensory symptoms and signs of psychogenic etiology are sometimes more severe and intractable—and may indicate the presence of a serious psychiatric abnormality. In such cases, it is important to gain the patient's trust and cooperation before referral to a mental health worker or psychiatrist. A short period of mild pharmacotherapy and physical therapy often achieves this goal and leads the patient toward an appropriate psychotherapeutic environment.

REFERENCES

Bassetti C, Bogousslavsky J, Regli F: Sensory syndromes in parietal stroke. *Neurol* 43:1942–1949, 1993.

Bonica JJ: *The Management of Pain*, 2d ed. Philadelphia, Lea and Febiger, 1990.

Casey KL (ed): *Pain and Central Nervous System Disease:The Central Pain Syndromes*. New York, Raven Press, 1991.

Darian-Smith I: Thermal sensibility, in Darian-Smith I (ed): *Handbook of Physiology. Section 1: The Nervous System*. Bethesda, American Physiological Society, 1984, pp. 879–914.

Davidoff RA: The dorsal columns. *Neurol* 39:1377–1385, 1989.

Dyck PJ, Zimmerman I, Gillen DA, et al: Cool, warm, and heat-pain detection thresholds: Testing methods and inferences about anatomic distribution of receptors. *Neurol* 43:1500–1508, 1993.

Fields HL: *Pain*. New York, McGraw-Hill, 1987.

Greenspan JD, Winfield JA: Reversible pain and tactile deficits associated with a cerebral tumor compressing the posterior insula and parietal operculum. *Pain* 50:29–39, 1992.

Haines DE (ed): *Fundamental Neuroscience*. New York, Churchill Livingstone, 1997, Chaps. 16–18.

Kandel ER, Schwartz JH, Jessel TM (eds): *Principles of Neuroscience*, 3d ed. New York, Elsevier, 1991, Chaps. 23–27.

Makous JC, Vierck CJ Jr: Physiological changes during recovery from a primate dorsal column lesion. *Somatosens Mot Res* 11:183–192, 1994.

Matthews PBC: Where does Sherrington's "muscular sense" originate? Muscles, joints, corollary discharges? *Ann Rev Neurosci* 5:189–218, 1982.

Mense S: Nociception from skeletal muscle in relation to clinical muscle pain. *Pain* 54:241–289, 1993.

Patten J: *Neurological Differential Diagnosis*, 2d ed. London, Springer, 1995, Chaps. 8, 11, 13, 14, 16, and 17.

Perl ER: Pain and nociception, in Darian-Smith I (ed): *Handbook of Physiology. Section 1: The Nervous System.* Bethesda, American Physiological Society, 1984, pp. 915–975.

Purves D, Augustine GJ, Fitzpatrick D, et al (eds): *Neuroscience.* Sunderland, MA, Sinauer, 1997, Chaps. 8 and 9.

Ross ED, Kirkpatrick JB, Lastimosa ACB: Position and vibration sensations: Functions of the dorsal spinocerebellar tracts? *Ann Neurol* 5:171–176, 1979.

Stanton-Hicks M, Janig W, Hassenbusch S, et al: Reflex sympathetic dystrophy: Changing concepts and taxonomy. *Pain* 63:127–133, 1995.

Vierck CJ Jr: Tactile movement detection and discrimination following dorsal column lesions in monkeys. *Exp Brain Res* 20:33, 1974.

Wall PD, Melzack R (eds): *Textbook of Pain*, 2d ed. Edinburgh, Churchill-Livingstone, 1995.

Willis WD, Coggeshall RE: *Sensory Mechanisms of the Spinal Cord.* New York, Plenum, 1978.

Willis WD: *The Pain System: The Neural Basis of Nociceptive Transmission in the Mammalian Nervous System.* Basel, Karger, 1985.

JOEL C. MORGENLANDER

THE AUTONOMIC NERVOUS SYSTEM

Patients frequently seek assistance from physicians for complaints referable to disturbances of the cranial nerve, motor, and sensory systems but infrequently complain of dysfunctions of the autonomic nervous system (ANS). Unless physicians specifically inquire about these functions, major disorders can go undetected. Consequently, systematic inquiry about cardiovascular, urinary, sexual, and bowel function is an essential part of a full neurologic evaluation. Clinicians who make these inquiries often are surprised to learn the frequency of disturbances in these functions, particularly in older patients. These patients often assume that their impotence and incontinence, for example, result from normal aging. The ANS can be tested at the bedside only to a limited degree; hence, an accurate and complete history is the key to the detection of autonomic dysfunction. Disorders of autonomic function occur commonly in many neurologic disorders, including neurodegenerative diseases (e.g., Parkinson disease, Alzheimer disease, and multiple system atrophy), spinal cord disorders, and the peripheral neuropathies that involve autonomic fibers, such as diabetic neuropathy.

ANS dysfunction from disorders of the central or peripheral nervous system may add greatly to the morbidity and mortality of these disorders. Autonomic disorders can be divided into primary autonomic failure and secondary disorders. These disorders may be acute or chronic. Primary autonomic disorders are chronic, whereas secondary disorders may be acute or chronic. The primary disorders include pure autonomic failure, autonomic failure as part of multiple-system atrophy, and autonomic failure with Parkinson disease. Secondary autonomic disorders can occur as part of cerebral, brainstem, spinal, and peripheral nervous system lesions. Centrally and peripherally acting medications and toxins may alter ANS functioning.

ANATOMIC CONNECTIONS AND PHARMACOLOGIC FUNCTIONS

The ANS is a division of the nervous system that innervates smooth muscle, cardiac muscle, and the glands of the body. The ANS functions principally on a subconscious level, regulating end organ activity reflexively. Although organs innervated by the ANS,

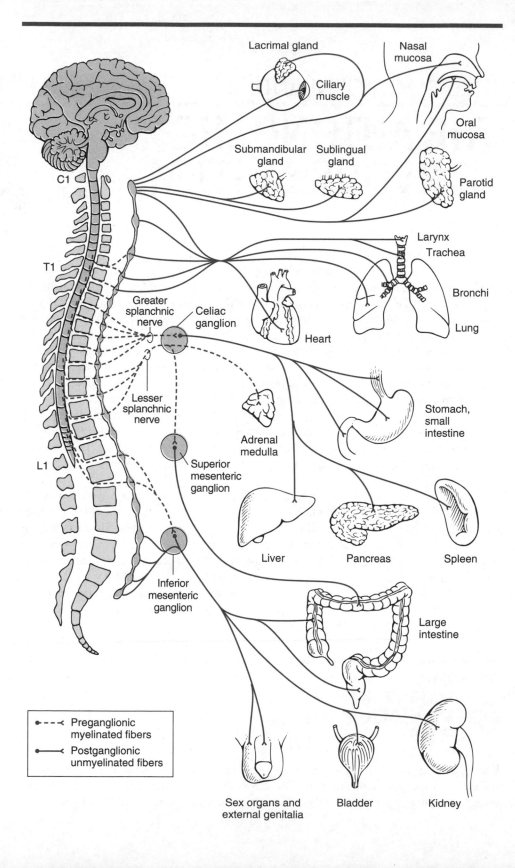

Lacrimal gland

Nasal mucosa

Ciliary muscle

Oral mucosa

Submandibular gland

Sublingual gland

Parotid gland

C1

T1

Larynx

Trachea

Greater splanchnic nerve

Celiac ganglion

Bronchi

Lung

Heart

Lesser splanchnic nerve

Stomach, small intestine

Adrenal medulla

L1

Superior mesenteric ganglion

Liver

Pancreas

Spleen

Inferior mesenteric ganglion

Large intestine

•---< Preganglionic myelinated fibers

•—< Postganglionic unmyelinated fibers

Sex organs and external genitalia

Bladder

Kidney

TABLE 8-1. Autonomic Nervous System Divisions

	Sympathetic	Parasympathetic
General location	Thoracolumbar	Craniosacral
Specific location	Intermediolateral and medial gray T1–L2	Cranial nerves III, VII, IX, X and sacral segments S2–S4
Pathway characteristics	Short preganglionic fibers Long postganglionic fibers	Long preganglionic fibers Short postganglionic fibers
Principal neurotransmitter	Norepinephrine (except sweat glands)	Acetylcholine

such as the heart and the intestines, can perform many functions without input from the ANS, input from the ANS strongly influences these organs, and rapid responses can be mediated via the ANS. Visceral motor neurons influence the organs in response to visceral and somatic inputs in addition to central signaling from the brainstem and hypothalamus. The ANS reaches its effector organ through two neuron circuits. Preganglionic (primary) neurons lie in the brainstem (cranial nerve nuclei III, VII, IX, and X) and the spinal cord (intermediolateral and intermediomedial cell columns). The postganglionic (secondary) neurons are located in peripheral ganglia and innervate end organs.

The ANS has two components: sympathetic and parasympathetic (Table 8-1), each of which is differentiated by its site of origin as well as the transmitters it releases. Many organs receive dual innervation, and the two divisions have opposing effects. In the sympathetic system, preganglionic fibers are usually short, while postganglionic fibers are long; the converse is true of the parasympathetic system. The ratio of preganglionic to postganglionic neurons in the sympathetic division is large; hence, rapid and extreme changes in sympathetic outflow are possible during periods of stress and exercise. The ratio of preganglionic to postganglionic neurons in the parasympathetic division is small, on the order of 1:15 or 1:20, and thus responses to stimulation are focal and controlled. Preganglionic neurons in both divisions utilize the neurotransmitter acetylcholine.

Sympathetic efferent first-order neurons arise in the intermediolateral and intermediomedial cell columns from the T1 to L2 levels of the spinal cord (Fig. 8-1). Myelinated preganglionic fibers exit in the ventral roots to form the white rami communicantes of the thoracic and lumbar nerves (Fig. 8-2). There are 14 white rami on each side, one for each spinal segment. White rami reach the sympathetic trunk and proceed by (1) forming synapses with the paired chain ganglia of the sympathetic trunk, (2) moving rostrally in the sympathetic trunk, (3) moving caudally in the sympathetic trunk, or (4) passing through the sympathetic chain to form synapses with collateral ganglia (celiac or mesenteric). Thus, cervical and lumbosacral ganglia receive from white rami fibers that have

Figure 8-1 The sympathetic division of the autonomic nervous system.

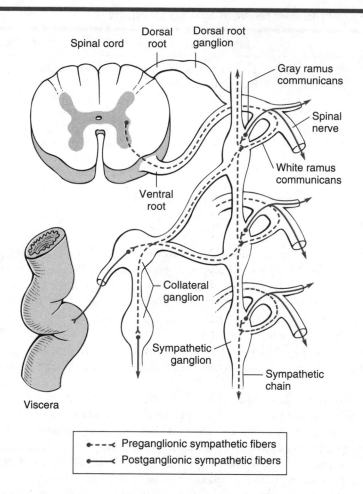

Figure 8-2   Sympathetic division innervation of viscera through the sympathetic and collateral ganglia.

traveled up or down the sympathetic chain. Unmyelinated postganglionic fibers form the gray rami communicantes and travel with spinal nerves or proceed directly to target organs. There are 31 gray rami on each side of the body, corresponding to each spinal nerve or dermatomal level. Norepinephrine is the primary postganglionic neurotransmitter, except in the sweat glands, where the primary neurotransmitter is acetylcholine. The adrenal medulla has only preganglionic innervation. Multiple cerebral nuclei, most importantly the nucleus tractus solitarius, receive afferent information from visceral, skin, and muscle receptors and contribute feedback to the sympathetic system.

    The first four to five thoracic segments form the cervical portion of the sympathetic trunk. The cervical ganglia include the superior cervical, middle cervical, and cervicothoracic (stellate) ganglia. The superior cervical ganglia give rise to the carotid plexus. Fibers from the carotid plexus travel with the carotid arteries, giving rise to the sympathetic innervation of the head. The neck and arms receive sympathetic innervation from

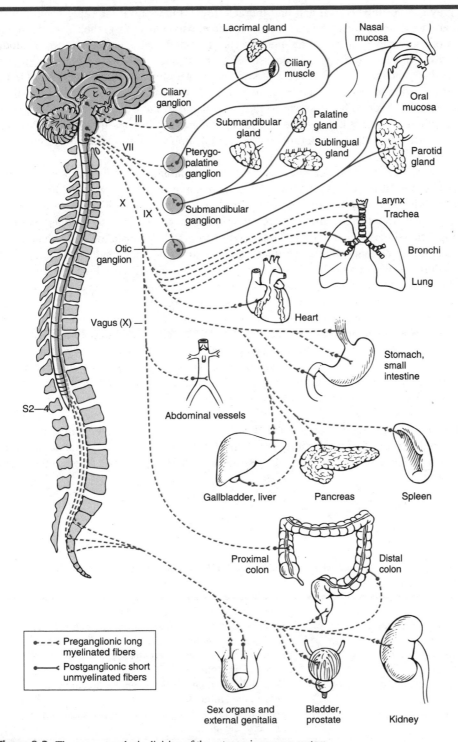

Figure 8-3 The parasympathetic division of the autonomic nervous system.

the gray rami of the cervical and first thoracic roots. Fibers from the same ganglia form the cardiac nerves, which give rise to the cardiac plexus. Fibers from the cervical and upper thoracic ganglia innervate the thoracic viscera. Splanchnic nerves arise from middle and lower thoracic and upper lumbar levels. The greater, lesser, and least splanchnic nerves carry mainly preganglionic fibers to the prevertebral ganglia, which include the celiac, superior mesenteric, and aorticorenal ganglia. Postganglionic fibers from these three ganglia travel with the artery of the same name to their target organ. The lumbar splanchnic nerves carry fibers to the inferior mesenteric and hypogastric ganglia. Postganglionic fibers from these ganglia follow the arterial supply to lower abdominal and pelvic organs.

Parasympathetic first-order neurons have two components: cranial and sacral (Fig. 8-3). The cranial component arises from cranial nerve nuclei III, VII, IX, and X. The Edinger-Westphal nucleus sends preganglionic fibers with the third nerve to the ciliary ganglion and from there to the eye. The superior salivatory nucleus sends fibers with the seventh cranial nerve via the nervus intermedius to the pterygopalatine and submandibular ganglia, which innervate the lacrimal, palatine, submandibular, and sublingual glands. The inferior salivatory nucleus sends fibers to the otic ganglion, which innervates the parotid gland. The dorsal motor nucleus and the nucleus ambiguus send fibers with the tenth cranial nerve to multiple organs in the chest and abdomen.

The sacral component of the parasympathetic system arises from the intermediate gray column of sacral spinal cord segments S2–S4. The preganglionic fibers travel as pelvic nerves destined for the large intestine and urogenital system via the hypogastric plexus. The primary postganglionic neurotransmitter of the parasympathetic system is acetylcholine. Afferent fibers that influence the parasympathetic system travel through cranial nerves II, IX, and X, including those in the baroreflex arc, and through sensory fibers of the sacral roots.

In addition to the regions mentioned above, many areas of the brain communicate with both sympathetic and parasympathetic systems. Further information is available in several excellent review articles and textbooks (Bannister and Mathias, 1992; Low, 1993; Mathias, 1996).

TABLE 8-2. Core Questions to Ask Patients Concerning Autonomic Dysfunction

Pupil	Blurred vision or drooping of eyelids
Cardiovascular	Light-headedness, dizziness, or passing out; palpitations
Sweating	Excessive or diminished; skin temperature regulation
Urinary function	Frequency, urgency, or incontinence; recurrent urinary tract infection
Sexual dysfunction	Difficulty initiating or maintaining an erection; ejaculation difficulties
Gastrointestinal	Dysphagia, abdominal pain, diarrhea, constipation, or fecal incontinence

CLINICAL EXAMINATION OF THE AUTONOMIC NERVOUS SYSTEM

Pupil

Loss of function of the sympathetic innervation of the pupil leads to a Horner syndrome, which consists of anhidrosis on the ipsilateral side of the face, ptosis, a small pupil, and enophthalmos. These changes may be asymptomatic, but some patients complain of visual blurring, especially at night (Table 8-2). Patients usually do not notice anhidrosis and generally cannot provide information about it. The degree of ptosis present usually is not sufficient to obstruct the pupil, and so patients notice it only as a cosmetic problem. Elevation of the lower lid is also present. Subtle lag of pupil dilation in the affected eye may help confirm the diagnosis.

In examining patients with very dark brown eyes, evaluate the pupils carefully because asymmetry may be less apparent than it is in people with light irises. Ask patients with asymmetric pupils about their use of eyedrops, as people often omit mentioning these medications in the history. Patients with congenital Horner syndrome may have an iris that has never become pigmented because of lack of sympathetic innervation.

The finding of a Horner syndrome indicates a lesion of the sympathetic nervous system that can occur within or outside the central nervous system. Dissection of the carotid artery can cause the disorder from involvement of the sympathetic fibers that accompany the artery. Dissection of the vertebral artery causes the disorder through ischemic injury to the brainstem. Lesions of the cervical cord or lower brachial plexus can cause the disorder. The detection of a new Horner syndrome with no other abnormalities should trigger a search for a tumor in the apex of the lung. Sympathetic involvement in the cavernous sinus or a retro-orbital location can be detected by means of the accompanying cranial nerve symptoms and signs. Horner syndrome frequently accompanies retro-orbital headache, particularly cluster headache, but also occurs in other facial pain syndromes.

Chapter 4 reviewed the methods of pharmacologic testing of patients with Horner syndrome to confirm the diagnosis and localize the lesion to the first- and second- versus third-order neuron. Careful examination of the pupil with a bright flashlight in a darkened room usually suffices to confirm the diagnosis in the office or at the bedside.

The parasympathetic fibers innervating the pupil arise in the Edinger-Westphal nucleus in the midbrain and project ipsilaterally to the orbit via the third nerve. Patients with parasympathetic dysfunction to the eye have a dilated pupil and may complain of blurred vision, especially in bright light or during accommodation. If the motor fibers of the third nerve also are involved, strabismus usually results and the patient complains of visual blurring or double vision. In patients with acute severe headache and a unilaterally dilated pupil, a posterior communicating aneurysm compressing the third nerve should be considered. Transtentorial herniation should be suspected in a patient with altered mental status, hemiparesis, and a dilated pupil. As was mentioned in Chap. 4, Adie's tonic pupil consists of a unilaterally large pupil that is poorly reactive to light. Patients with this disorder also may complain of blurred vision, and usually they have areflexia. The means of pharmacologic testing for Adie's tonic pupil is presented in Chap 4. A large pupil can result from ocular trauma and the use of eyedrops such as atropine.

Cardiovascular

Disorders of blood pressure regulation can lead to a variety of symptoms, including dizziness, light-headedness, loss of consciousness, headache, palpitations, numbness, tingling, and weakness. The factors that contribute to blood pressure regulation include reflexes (venoarterial, arterial, cardiopulmonary), humoral systems (circulating catecholamines, renin-angiotensin, atrial natriuretic factors), and blood volume. Changes in the reflex systems usually lead to rapid alteration of blood pressure. The most common cardiovascular symptoms of autonomic dysfunction result from orthostatic hypotension. Orthostatic hypotension is extremely common and has significant consequences but can be overlooked unless it is specifically tested for.

Information from baroreceptors in the aortic arch proceeds through afferents in the ninth cranial nerve and in the carotid sinus through the tenth cranial nerve to the medulla to control blood pressure and heart rate. Efferent information from the parasympathetic nuclei in the medulla is routed through the vagus nerve and influences cardiac rate and rhythm, causing bradycardia when active. A sign of parasympathetic dysfunction is resting tachycardia. This is frequently a prominent and early feature of diabetic autonomic neuropathy. The parasympathetic system can cause vasodilation in the periphery, resulting in lowered blood pressure.

Blood flow and blood pressure can be modulated by many influences, including reflexes in peripheral veins, vessels in visceral organs and muscles, and stretch receptors in the lungs and cardiac chambers. With standing, the reflex action compensates for the gravitational pooling of blood by increasing heart rate and vascular resistance. The sympathetic system increases the heart rate and the speed of cardiac conduction and causes peripheral vasoconstriction.

Measurement of orthostatic blood pressure is a key part of the neurologic examination, especially in symptomatic patients. Take the blood pressure and measure the pulse at least 2 min after the patient has lain down. Repeat the measurements 2 min after the patient has stood up. A decline of blood pressure of at least 20 mmHg systolic and 10 mmHg diastolic provides evidence of postural hypotension. When postural hypotension results from autonomic insufficiency, the increase in heart rate is inappropriately low for the fall in blood pressure.

If a patient has orthostatic hypotension, one can localize the lesion to one of the limbs of the baroreceptor reflex arc to help in the differential diagnosis (Fig. 8-4) (Brazer, 1985). As an initial test, measurement with an electrocardiogram of R-R interval variation with paced respiration can confirm a lesion in the baroreceptor reflex arc. Tell the patient to breathe deeply at a rate of 6 times per minute and give the patient 1 to 2 min to get used to regular deep breathing. Normally the heart rate decreases on expiration and increases on inspiration. Heart rate variability decreases with age. In a subject younger than 65 years, a difference in heart rate of less than 10 beats per minute between inspiration and expiration is usually abnormal. Monitor the R-R interval with a standard rhythm strip. Calculate the ratio of maximal and minimal R-R intervals during expiration and inspiration (E to I ratio). If R-R interval testing is normal, the parasympathetic efferent

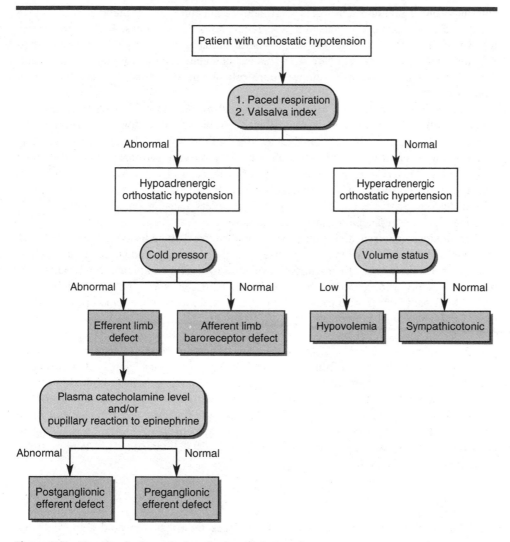

Figure 8-4 Algorithm for the evaluation of orthostatic hypotension.

fibers of the baroreflex arc are intact, suggesting orthostatic hypotension from hypovolemia or sympathicotonic orthostatic hypotension.

The Valsalva maneuver can be used to confirm a lesion in the baroreceptor reflex arc. Instruct the patient to blow into a tube, maintaining a column of mercury at 40 mm for 15 s. Four phases—two during strain and two after release—occur in response to the Valsalva maneuver. Initially, as a result of the increase in intrathoracic pressure, systolic and diastolic blood pressure increase with a fall in heart rate. Subsequently, the blood pressure falls and the heart rate increases because of decreased venous return. A period of continued blood pressure fall occurs with tachycardia followed by blood pressure overshoot and bradycardia. The Valsalva ratio is the ratio of the largest R-R interval after release of pressure to the shortest interval before release. Normally this is greater than 1.2, and abnormal values are below 1.1. This test can be unreliable for many reasons, and the Valsalva maneuver can be studied more reliably in an autonomic nervous system laboratory.

If you detect a baroreceptor lesion, you can perform a cold pressor test to assess the function of the efferent limb. Place the patient's hand in ice water for 1 min. If the blood pressure increases more than 15 mmHg, the efferent limb is intact. If you detect an abnormality of the efferent limb, you can localize the lesion to pre- or postganglionic neurons by looking for denervation hypersensitivity. For instance, 1 or 2 drops of 1:1000 epinephrine applied to the surface of the eye leads to pupillary dilatation in patients with postganglionic lesions. In patients with generalized disorders causing postganglionic lesions, baseline plasma norepinephrine levels may be low.

Carotid sinus hypersensitivity, an uncommon disorder, can be tested at the bedside. Be cautious in using this test and do not use it in patients with known cerebral vascular disease or a carotid bruit. Keep atropine available to treat symptomatic bradycardia immediately. Apply compression to the carotid sinus while measuring pulse and blood pressure. Abnormal findings are a pause of more than 3 s, a symptomatic blood pressure drop of 30 mmHg, and an asymptomatic drop of 50 mmHg.

A test that some clinicians use consists of having the patient sustain hand grip for 30 percent of maximal for 5 min. This causes a rise in blood pressure (diastolic greater than 15 mmHg) and in heart rate from withdrawal of vagal input and increased sympathetic activity. Precise localization of this reflex is uncertain, making this test limited in utility.

Determination of orthostatic blood pressure usually suffices for the evaluation of cardiovascular dysfunction in disorders of the autonomic nervous system. Several more detailed tests of cardiovascular function are performed by neurologists specializing in autonomic nervous system function and by cardiologists (Bannister and Mathias, 1992; Low, 1993; Mathias, 1996).

Sweating

Autonomic dysfunction causing vasomotor changes may result in cold skin, and ultimately, trophic changes may occur. Then the skin may feel dry and warm and appear shiny. Patients with a generalized decrease in sweating may complain of flushing or heat intolerance. Occasionally patients note the absence of sweating on a hot day, with fever, or after a hot bath.

Focal injury of the spinal cord or the peripheral sympathetic nerves can cause localized hyperhidrosis. Many systemic disorders cause generalized hyperhidrosis. Cholinergic responses cause generalized sweating. Piloerection is sympathetically mediated.

A clinical approach to detecting sweating abnormalities using the thermoregulatory sweat test (TST) is to elevate body temperature with a heat lamp and look for localized sweating abnormalities. Sprinkled powdered iodinated corn starch highlights sweating by turning blue. Additional tests of sweat function, such as the sympathetic skin response and the quantitative pseudomotor axon reflex test (QSART), can be useful and usually are performed in autonomic function laboratories.

Urinary Function

Patients with urinary system dysfunction may complain of urgency, frequency, a weak stream, or a sensation of incomplete voiding. Recurrent urinary tract infections are clues to poor emptying.

Sympathetic fibers via the inferior mesentery ganglia innervate the detrusor, aiding in relaxation (Fig. 8-5). Parasympathetic fibers from the sacral cord combine with pelvic nerves to form the pelvic plexus and visceral plexus, which then innervate the detrusor and urethra. Parasympathetic stimulation causes detrusor contraction and bladder emptying. Pudendal motor fibers from the sacral plexus innervate the external urethral sphincter. Urinary continence requires both sensory feedback from the bladder to the sacral spinal cord and feedback from the pontine nuclei and the dorsal medial frontal lobe. Lower motor neuron lesions from disease of the sacral spinal cord (conus medullaris), cauda equina, or peripheral nerves to the bladder cause an atonic or flaccid bladder with a large postvoid residual and overflow incontinence. Upper motor neuron lesions such as spinal cord diseases cause a hyperreflexic bladder with detrusor dyssynergia. Postvoid residuals may not be high, but incomplete emptying occurs. Determination of a postvoid residual is an important test in patients with bladder dysfunction; demonstration of an elevated postvoid residual may lead to a trial of medical therapy or chronic intermittent catheterization, both of which decrease the long-term morbidity from bladder dysfunction. Urologic studies such as cystometry are useful in documenting the specific type of bladder dysfunction and are often helpful in guiding therapy.

Sexual Function

Sexual dysfunction may be the earliest manifestation of autonomic insufficiency but is usually the least frequently volunteered symptom. Males have difficulty initiating or maintaining an erection. There may be an abnormal volume of ejaculate, or retrograde ejaculation may occur, and this can be painful and may result in milky urine. Rarely, women complain of decreased vaginal lubrication. Sexual dysfunction is complex and can result from neurologic, psychologic, pharmacologic, and vascular factors. Nocturnal erections are absent in patients with neurogenic impotence.

The central and peripheral pathways responsible for the sexual response are complex (Rushton, 1996). Sympathetic fibers from the T11–L2 level reach the inferior mesenteric or superior hypogastric plexus to innervate erectile tissue, smooth muscle in the prostate, seminal vesicles, vagina and uterus, and blood vessels in reproductive organs. Parasympathetic fibers from S2–S4 travel through the inferior hypogastric plexus to innervate the same structures. The parasympathetic system functions principally in achieving erection and the sympathetic system in performing ejaculation, although striated muscle adds the rhythmic contraction needed for ejaculation. Diagnostic studies of the cause of impotence are usually the province of urologists or endocrinologists who specialize in sexual dysfunction.

Gastrointestinal Dysfunction

The types of symptoms of gastrointestinal autonomic dysfunction usually are referable to the area of dysfunction. Upper digestive tract symptoms include dysphagia, reflux, nau-

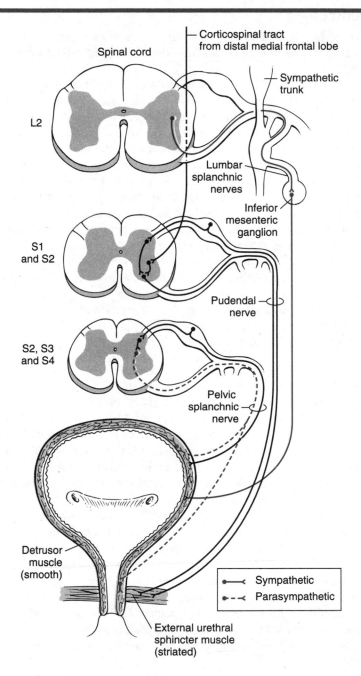

Figure 8-5 Peripheral innervation of the urinary bladder.

sea, vomiting, and upper abdominal pain. Lower digestive tract symptoms include abdominal pain, constipation, and diarrhea (sometimes alternating).

Sympathetic innervation inhibits peristalsis and, when interrupted, can cause excessive contractility or lack of coordination. Sympathetic innervation causes contraction of the upper and lower esophageal, ileocecal, and anal sphincters. The parasympathetic system stimulates peristalsis and mediates sensory feedback through the vagus nerve. The external anal sphincter is solely under somatic motor control (S2–S4). The intrinsic enteric system of nerve fibers controls the rate of peristalsis through both sympathetic and parasympathetic systems.

When taking a history of incontinence of bowel or bladder, you need to differentiate between lack of sensory warning, loss of sphincteric control, and, most frequently, difficulty in getting to the bathroom in time to maintain continence. Examination of anal sphincter tone is an important bedside test in patients with fecal incontinence, but it primarily evaluates the striated muscle of the external sphincter. When patients give a history of bowel or bladder incontinence, clues from the history and physical examination often help in localization. Conus medullaris lesions often cause a combination of upper and lower motor neuron signs that affect the lower extremities (i.e., absent reflexes but extensor plantar reflexes). Cauda equina lesions cause multilevel lumbosacral radiculopathy. Both types of lesions result in perianal numbness. Spinal cord lesions that interrupt ascending sensory pathways cause a decrease or total loss of sensation below the level of the lesion, although sensation in the dermatomes innervated by the sacral roots can be spared owing to lamination of ascending sensory fibers in the spinal cord. Cerebral lesions that produce incontinence may be accompanied by cognitive or other focal neurologic signs.

SUMMARY

In daily practice, patients seldom complain of symptoms referable to the autonomic nervous system; hence, physicians need to focus the history and examination on this system when there are indications that it may be affected. The indictions are when (1) the history suggests primary autonomic failure, (2) the history suggests secondary autonomic failure and documentation of autonomic dysfunction may help narrow the differential diagnosis of the primary disorder, (3) the history or physical examination suggests localized autonomic dysfunction that helps with localization of the underlying disorder and narrowing of the differential diagnosis, and (4) the patient is taking medications that may compromise ANS function. The history should include an inquiry about cardiovascular, the-rmoregulatory, gastrointestinal, urinary, and sexual function. The physical examination should focus on the pupils and the cardiovascular system. Formal laboratory testing can be helpful.

SUGGESTED READINGS

Bannister R, Mathias CJ: *Autonomic Failure: A Textbook of Clinical Disorders of the Autonomic Nervous System*, 3d ed. Oxford, UK, Oxford University Press, 1992.

Brazer SR: The bedside evaluation of orthostatic hypotension. *N Car Med J* 46:213, 1985.

Low PA: *Clinical Autonomic Disorders: Evaluation and Management.* Boston, Little, Brown, 1993.

Mathias CJ: Disorders of the autonomic nervous system, in Bradley WG, Daroff RB, Fenichel GM, Marsden CD (eds.): *Neurology in Clinical Practice,* 2d ed. Boston, Butterworth-Heinemann, 1996, pp 1953–1981.

Rushton DN: Sexual and sphincter dysfunction, in Bradley WG, Daroff RB, Fenichel GM, Marsden CD (eds.): *Neurology in Clinical Practice*, 2d ed. Boston, Butterworth-Heinemann, 1996, pp 407–420.

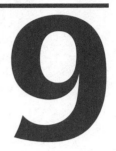

MICHAEL V. JOHNSTON / GARY W. GOLDSTEIN / BRUCE K. SHAPIRO

CHAPTER 9

INFANT AND CHILD NERVOUS SYSTEM

The developing nervous system of infants and young children presents the clinician with continuous changes in behavioral repertoire as well as in neurologic signs and reflexes. These developmental patterns make it challenging to distinguish normal from abnormal signs and also can make it difficult to elicit a child's attention or cooperation for testing. This chapter presents an approach to examining children and an overview of the development of their motor, language, and social skills. The chapter concludes with 10 problem-focused summaries that present scenarios that often are encountered in pediatric neurology practice. Earlier chapters have described the neurologic history and examination in detail, and the information provided here is either unique to infants and children or especially important in this age group.

APPROACH TO NEUROLOGIC EVALUATION IN CHILDREN

Begin the neurologic evaluation of an infant or young child with a quiet, relaxed conversation with the parent or caretaker about the history in the child's presence. Do not have the child undressed and put into a gown to await the physician; this is counterproductive to a good neurologic evaluation. A period of introduction gives the child a chance to relax and gain confidence that you mean no harm and often gives you a chance to observe some of the child's development and behavior. If the child has not brought toys or books to the visit, provide some in the office or waiting room for the child to bring into the examining room. As the inquiry about the chief complaint and history begins, toddlers and young children often sit on the carpeted floor playing with toys, and the appropriateness of this play sometimes provides valuable information. With hospitalized children, pause a few minutes before beginning the examination, since a more aggressive approach often leads to tears and resistance. For most infants and toddlers, begin the examination while the child is comfortably seated in the caretaker's lap with most of the child's clothing still on. A great deal of information can be gathered from observation alone, such as the child's posture, strength, and symmetry of movements. The formal examination is typically opportunistic, eliciting information that is least traumatic to obtain first and later proceeding to more stressful issues, such as the retinal examination. Generally, it is best to accomplish the parts of the examination that require cooperation before the child is manipulated. It usually is possible to manipulate the feet and legs to elicit tone and strength without causing distress while the child is comfortable. These procedures are described in more detail below, but first it is useful to learn more about the child's problems and developmental milestones so you can plan and focus the examination.

SPECIAL FEATURES OF PEDIATRIC HISTORY TAKING

The Chief Complaint and Current Illness

In addition to complaints such as loss of consciousness and headache, which occur frequently in both adults and children, certain complaints are particularly common in pediatrics. They include developmental delay, hypotonia or hypertonia in infancy, head growth that is too great (macrocephaly) or too little (microcephaly), school failure or learning disability, hyperactivity, trouble with hearing or eyesight, and an unusual appearance that suggests a genetic syndrome. In addition to understanding how to evaluate these complaints, you need to ascertain how they emerged. Generally, the current illness fits one of four different patterns (Lyon, Adams, and Kolodny, 1996). One pattern occurs in relatively *static* disorders, in which the disorder emerges as a delay in the acquisition of skills from an early age. For example, many types of mental retardation become apparent first as a lag in developmental milestones that is fairly consistent throughout infancy and childhood up to adolescence. At each age, mental age as a percentage of chronologic age remains fairly stable. In contrast, a *degenerative* pattern is seen when development progresses normally but then stops and previously acquired skills are progressively lost. A variation of the degenerative pattern occurs in children who begin with a maturational delay typical of a static disorder but then reach a plateau, failing to progress or actually beginning to deteriorate. A *metabolic* or *intermittent* pattern of illness is seen in children who have a sudden decline in neurologic abilities and who then either regain their developmental progression with no permanent disability or progress, but at a slower rate than expected and/or with some permanent disability. The metabolic pattern of disorders often includes a stuttering or remitting-relapsing course but also may include illnesses with only one episode. In clinical practice, these patterns all occur fairly frequently and the distinction between them is often challenging. Textbook distinctions between static and degenerative disorders often are blurred in clinical practice, making it important to inquire carefully about the child's developmental progress before the current illness, progress since the illness, and any evidence of a recurring or cyclic pattern.

History of Developmental Milestones

The child's neurodevelopmental achievements provide an essential context for evaluating the child's neurologic complaints, and you should get an impression about them at the outset, when you inquire about the current illness and past medical history. Information about development often permits you to determine how deeply you need to search for historic risk factors in the past history, such as disorders of pregnancy and events in the neonatal period. The neurodevelopmental history itself often can be abbreviated if caretakers report that development was entirely normal. Nevertheless, you should ask some pointed questions about each of the four major realms of development: language, fine motor, gross motor, and personal and social adaptation. For example, with a 1-year-old you should ask about the ability to stand independently, say a word or two besides "mama, dada," hold an object with the thumb and index finger alone (pincer grasp), and assist with dressing. If the child can accomplish all these tasks, you usually can move on to the rest of the history, taking time independently to check the parents' answers during the physical examination. Truly normal development provides a different, simpler context for certain common disorders. For example, a brief first seizure in a child with entirely normal neurodevelopmental milestones suggests a different approach to the patient than does a seizure in a child with marked developmental delay or a regression in development.

If you suspect that the child's development is delayed, ask about all four realms of development with the intention of directly evaluating development during the examination. The reason for taking a detailed developmental history is twofold: It gives parents an opportunity to give their "expert" knowledge about the child, and it provides information that you may not able to elicit from the child during the examination. It is not unusual for infants or children to stop speaking completely during the examination. Often parents will elicit certain behaviors during the history by saying, "See, she does this," when it would take you many attempts to coax the same behavior from the child. Parents are often unhappy with evaluations that do not give them an adequate opportunity to show the child's strengths and focus excessively on "tests." If a serious look at developmental milestones is warranted, for example, to determine whether development has reached a plateau or deteriorated, have the parents bring in "baby books," photographs, or videotapes, since they may not recall the child's milestones accurately.

After years of examining children, clinicians learn most of the key neurodevelopmental milestones and become able to form reasonably accurate estimates of developmental levels. Nevertheless, many still find it useful to refer to the types of timetable charts included in this section, especially those for the development of language.

GENERAL FEATURES OF DEVELOPMENT

From "Head to Toe"

While the details of development are important, several general features help tie them together. For example, infant development proceeds from head to toe. One of the first developmental events that often can be appreciated in full-term newborns is the ability to fixate on a large red ring or develop optokinetic nystagmus when large stripes are moved across the field of view. These events represent some of the first evidence of visual-parietal cortical function in humans. The centrally located special senses of smell, sight, and hearing all get an early start, and facial motor acts lag just a bit behind: Smiling appropriately at the mother occurs at about 4 to 6 weeks of age, and a delay in this milestone is generally noteworthy. The ability to open the hands and grasp a rattle (4 months) and the ability to transfer it to the opposite side (5 months) occur before activities more distant from the brain. Standing, holding on to the furniture, standing alone, and walking come only at the end of the first year.

Development Occurs in Stable Sequences

Motor, language, and social development occur in sequences that are generally very stable. (Capute and Accardo, 1996). Gross motor development is the major focus between 6 and 18 months as the child moves from static sitting to independent walking. Walking represents the functional threshold for gross motor function and occurs at about 1 year. Gross motor milestones are easy to observe and usually are recalled accurately but are not strongly related to cognition. Fine motor abilities are less easy to observe than are gross motor abilities, do not lend themselves to historic reporting after the attainment of unilateral reach, and must be elicited after that time. Fine motor function begins with a diminution of fisting and progresses to the mature pincer grasp and voluntary release. Shortly after 1 year of age, the cognitive requirements of the tasks usually confound the measurement of fine motor abilities. The dynamic tripod used to support a pen is the functional threshold

TABLE 9-1. Motor Development Milestones in the First Year

Age	Gross Motor	Fine Motor
Newborn	Clears face (prone)	
2 months	Chin up (prone)	
3 months	Supports on forearms (prone)	Hands unfisted
4 months	Supports on extended arms (prone)	Brings hands to midline
	Rolls prone to supine	
5 months	Rolls supine to prone	Transfers objects
	Sits with arm support	
6 months	Sits without arm support	Reaches unilaterally
		Whole hand grasp
7 months	Locomotion in prone (creeps)	
8 months	Locomotion in quadruped (crawls)	
	Comes to sitting	
	Pulls to stand	
9 months	Cruises	
11 months	Walks (one hand held)	Pincer grasp
12 months	Walks (independently)	Voluntary release

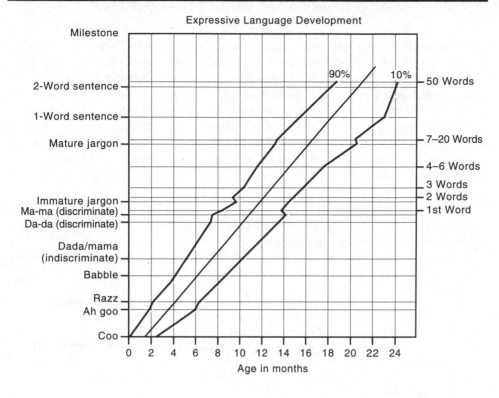

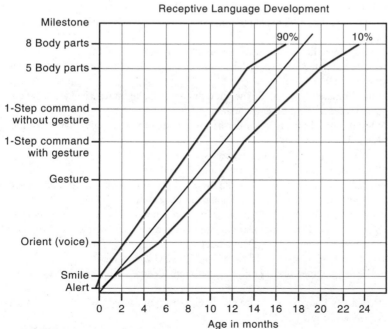

Figure 9-1 Ages at which normal children acquire expressive and receptive language milestones. (Reprinted with permission from Capute AJ et al: Clinical linguistic and auditory milestones scales: prediction of cognition in infancy. *Dev Med & Child Neurol* 28:762–771, 1986.)

for fine motor function and occurs at approximately age 30 months. Motor milestones are listed in Table 9-1. A disproportionate delay in gross and fine motor milestones usually occurs in association with upper motor neuron signs in children with cerebral palsy.

Language milestones are the most predictive of later cognitive function and generally can be reported by parents in a nearly concurrent fashion (Capute et al, 1986). Although most professionals do not focus on language development before a child can produce words, distinct milestones are present from birth onward. A set of sample questions that can be used to gather information about language development up to age 2 years is shown in Table 9-2, and language development milestones are listed in Table 9-3 and Fig. 9-1.

TABLE 9-2. Sample Questions for Parental Reporting of Linguistic and Auditory Milestones

Alert: When did the infant recognize presence of sound by blinking, starting, or moving any part of the body?

Social smile (communicative smile): When did the infant smile at you when you talked to him or her or stroked his or her face? When could you get him or her to smile?

Coo: When did the infant produce long vowel sounds in a musical fashion?

Orient to voice: When you enter a room and the baby does not see you at first, does she or he turn immediately to the correct side when you speak to him or her, or does she or he search for you, sometimes looking first in the right direction and sometimes not?

Ah-goo: When did the baby first say "ah-goo"?

Razz: When did the baby first give you the "raspberry"?

Babble: When did the infant first babble (demonstrate repetitive strings of vowel/consonant combinations)?

Gesture language: When did the infant wave bye-bye or play pat-a-cake?

Mama/dada (indiscriminately): When did the child first say "dada" or "mama" but without reference to the mother or father?

Mama/dada (discriminately): When did the child first refer to the father as "dada"? When did the child first refer to the mother as "mama"?

First word: When did the child say his or her first word other than "dada," "mama," or family names? Name it.

Second word: When did the child have two words? Name them.

Third word: When did the child have three words? Name them.

One-step command without gesture: When did the child first follow simple commands such as "give me—" or "bring me—" not accompanied by a gesture?

Four to six words: When did the child have a four- to six-word vocabulary? Name them.

Immature jargon: When did the child begin to jargon—to run unintelligible words together in an attempt to make a "sentence"? (Demonstrate)

Seven to 20 words: When did the child have a 7- to 20-word vocabulary?

Mature jargon: When did the child's jargon begin to include intelligible words? (Demonstrate)

Body parts: How many body parts can the child point to when named? Which ones? When could she or he point to five? Eight?

Two-word phrases: When did the child start to put two words together in a phrase? (Not a sentence, frequently both nouns).

50 words: When did the child have a 50-word vocabulary?

Two-word sentences: When did the child put a noun and a verb together in a sentence?

TABLE 9-3. Expressive and Receptive Language Milestones (CLAMS) for Ages 2 Weeks to 36 Months

Age (months)	Expressive Language Milestones	Receptive Language Milestones
0.5		Alert
1.5	Coo	Smiles
4.0	Ah-goo	Orients to voice
4.5	Razzing	
5.0		Orients to bell I
6.5	Babbles	
7.0		Orients to bell II
7.5	Dada/mama, nonspecific	
9.0		Understands "no"
		Gestures
		Orients to bell III
11.0	Dada/mama, specific	Follows one-step command with gesture
11.5	First word	
12.0	Immature jargon	
12.5	Second word	
13.0	Third word	
14.0		Follows one-step command without gesture
15.0	4–6 words	
16.5	Mature jargon	Recognizes five body parts
17.0	7–20 words	
18.0		Points to one picture
		Recognizes eight body parts
19.0	Two-word combinations	
20.5	Two-word sentences	
21.0	50 words	Points to two pictures
24.0	3 pronouns, indiscriminately	
30.0	3 pronouns, discriminately	
36.0	250 words	
	Three-word sentences	
	Gives age, sex, name	
	Repeats three digits	

Language delay is found in children with mental retardation, hearing loss, central communication disorders, and autism. Language can be divided into receptive and expressive components. Hearing impairment is a common cause of both types of problems. Isolated expressive language or speech disorders can be delays without lasting developmental consequences.

Social adaptive or personal milestones include independent skills in self-feeding, dressing, bathing, and toileting as well as in interactive "social skills" (Table 9-4). Sequences of development in this area reflect the coupling of motor, cognitive, and language abilities

TABLE 9-4.   Personal Social Development

Age	Feeding	Dressing	Toileting and Grooming
6 months	Chewing		
9 months	Hold own bottle Finger feeds		
12 months		Assists Pushes arm through sleeve if started Pulls off socks	
15 months	Drinks from cup (unassisted)		
18 months	Feeds self with spoon		Indicates need to toilet
24 months		Pulls up pants Takes off shoes	Toilets for bowel movements
30 months	Feeds self with fork		Toilets for urination Washes hands
36 months		Puts on socks Unlaces shoes Unbuttons	
4–5 years		Buttons	Wipes self after bowel movement Brushes teeth
5–6 years	Uses knife for spreading	Ties shoes	
6+ years	Uses knife for cutting		Combs hair

and their application to a "real-world" context. Delays in this area often occur in children with generalized developmental delay and mental retardation, children with disorders of fine motor function, children with cerebral palsy, and sometimes in children with syndromes that feature defects in social skills, such as autism and fragile-X syndrome.

Speed of Psychosocial Development Predicts Final Destination

The rate at which normal children acquire new skills has been measured for years in many populations and forms the basis of a number of tests of infant development, such as the Cattell Test of Infant Development and the Bayley Scales of Infant Development (Capute and Accardo, 1996). The principle underlying all these tests is that if a child is delayed, the rate at which the child accomplishes these tasks provides a general estimate of the child's eventual level of mature achievement. This is not as true in normal children, for their rate of milestone acquisition does not predict later achievement very strongly. For example, if a child's developmental milestones at ages 1 year, 2 years, and 3 years are appropriate for a 6-month-old, 1-year-old, and 1.5-year-old, the child is very likely to reach an adult IQ in the range of 50 and a "mental age" of 8 years. This principle applies to children in whom developmental milestones are delayed in all realms (language, fine motor, gross motor, social-adaptive), not to children lacking a few skills that could result from specific neurologic disorders. Some children who appear to be slow in development may prove to be "late bloomers," but these children usually have uneven development with some exceptional skills and some retarded skills, not a global delay in all realms.

Some Milestones Are More Important Than Others

The developmental milestones included here generally are considered meaningful because they occur fairly uniformly at about the same time and in the same sequence in most children. Failure to acquire them or a delay usually indicates a problem, although it is prudent not to rely on only one or two alone. Many skills that children acquire are variable in onset and have little diagnostic importance. A summary list of major developmental expectations is given in Table 9-5.

TABLE 9-5. Developmental Expectations by Age

Failure to achieve age-appropriate expectations is the
most common presentation of developmental disabilities.

Age	Expectation	Typical Questions
Newborn	Physiologic stability Functioning organs Normal morphology	
3–6 months	Interaction with environment	Does he or she see? Does she or he hear? Does he or she respond differently to his or her mother (soothing, eye opening, cooing)? Periodicity
6–18 months	Motor achievement	Fine and gross motor delays
18–36 months	Language achievement	Delayed language milestones Achievement of milestones
30+ months	Play Fine motor Behavior	Attention Preacademic skills (drawing, coloring, cutting) Dressing
72 months	Academic achievement	Reading achievement Atttention and behavior

History of Pregnancy, Labor, Delivery, Neonatal Period

Obtain and record information about the pregnancy, labor, delivery, and neonatal period in the history of all pediatric patients. The information you need to obtain about the pregnancy includes its length and any problems, including bleeding; infections, including sexually transmitted diseases; and a history of maternal smoking and drug ingestion, both therapeutic and drugs of abuse. Ask about other medical disorders in the mother, including thyroid disease, toxemia, and gestational diabetes. Ask the patient's mother about other siblings and previous pregnancies, including spontaneous or elective abortions. Obtain and record the child's birth weight, presentation, mode of delivery and estimated gestational age based on menstrual history and a standardized examination, Apgar scores, neonatal complications, and length of hospital stay. If the pregnancy or neonatal period was complicated, obtain the actual records, since the parents' memory may be inexact as a result of the stress of the events. If the pregnancy was complicated, a considerable amount of data may be available, including fetal ultrasounds and biophysical profiles. Interpret cautiously parents' recollections about events in the neonatal period and their link to the child's current problems until the entire case record and evaluation become available. For example, infants with cerebral palsy from an intrauterine disturbance of brain development often display signs in the neonatal period at term, such as cyanosis and transiently low Apgar scores, that can falsely suggest a perinatal brain insult.

Other Past Medical History

Elicit other elements of the past medical history as is done in the examination of adults with neurologic disorders, including hospitalizations, major illnesses, injuries, and operations. Children are more vulnerable to abuse than are adults, and this is often repetitive. Consider child abuse, especially in infants with subdural hematomas or unexplained skull fractures or other injuries. Children with mental retardation and behavior disorders frequently are victims of sexual abuse and injury. If appropriate, ask about prescribed drugs and allergies to drugs or other substances, including alcohol and drugs of abuse. Inquire about immunizations and infectious diseases, including the timing of diphtheria-pertussis-tetanus (DPT) injections and measles vaccination and the timing and type of polio vaccination. A history of travel or origin outside the United States requires detailed questions about disorders such as malaria, tuberculosis, and cysticercosis that have important neurologic complications.

Review of Systems

In the review of systems proceed as you would in an adult but keep in mind that many neurologic disorders in children and treatment of these disorders have associated systemic complications and that many systemic disorders have neurologic manifestations. For example, patients with neurocutaneous disorders and epilepsy have prominent skin abnormalities, and children with ataxia-telangiectasia or acquired immune deficiency syndrome (AIDS) commonly have disorders associated with an immune deficiency. Ask about eyesight and hearing. Hearing disorders are common causes of language delay even when parents believe the child's hearing is normal. Disorders of swallowing and gastroesophageal reflux are common in children with chronic neurologic disorders and in infants lead to regurgitation, bad breath, pain, irritability, and occasionally apnea. Respiratory obstruction and sleep apnea occur frequently in children with neurologic disorders and can contribute to increased intracranial pressure. Signs of depression may indicate that a psychiatric disorder is contributing to a learning disability. Signs of thyroid dysfunction occur fairly frequently in children with Down syndrome. Children with spinal cord disorders often have serious secondary problems with skin breakdown and urinary tract infection. The ketogenic diet used to treat certain children with refractory seizure disorders commonly is associated with renal calculi.

Family History

Many genetic disorders that cause neurologic disease in children are still being described and reported. Hence, it is essential that you take a careful family history. We have encountered numerous children with disorders assumed to be sporadic who later turned out to have a genetic and/or metabolic disorder. Childhood migraine and learning disabilities are two striking examples of this. Cognitive problems giving rise to school failure and attention deficit and/or hyperactivity disorders often affect relatives in multiple generations. Children who once were thought to have extrapyramidal or dyskinetic cerebral palsy have been diagnosed with glutaricaciduria type I or mitochondrial disorders. Children with neonatal strokes may have clotting disorders secondary to homocystinuria or protein C or protein S deficiency with a family occurrence of venous thrombosis.

Social History

In obtaining the social history, take into consideration the vulnerability of children to neurologic disorders from abuse and infectious diseases. In certain urban centers, the risk for lead poisoning is directly related to poverty and substandard, poorly maintained housing.

NEUROLOGIC PHYSICAL EXAMINATION IN INFANTS AND CHILDREN

Neonates and Infants

Begin the examination of neonates and infants with observation of level of alertness and resting posture. Newborns spend a considerable amount of time sleeping but generally can be aroused easily with tactile stimulation or gentle movement of the extremities. Even in sleep, an infant's extremities are held in flexion, and extension of the limbs with external rotation of the hips (the "frog leg" position) may be a sign of hypotonia and muscle weakness. When you hold an infant upright and gently rock the head from side to side, the child's eyes generally will be open. Failure to respond with eye opening to a few minutes of stimulation may indicate a depressed level of consciousness. At this time, evaluate the appearance of the infant's face and head as well as that of the rest of the body and note dysmorphic features. Certain facial appearances may suggest specific types of neuro-

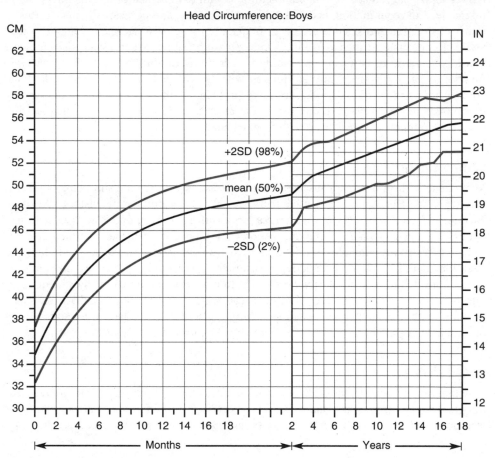

Figure 9-2 Head circumference growth for normal boys. (Reprinted with permission from Nellhaus G: Composite international and interracial graphs. *Pediatrics* 41:106, 1968.)

logic disorders; for example, a narrow face with an oval open mouth may suggest a congenital myopathy. Midfacial anomalies commonly occur in children with fetal alcohol syndrome and holoprosencephaly. Palpate the anterior fontanelle, measure the head circumference, and insert it on the head chart to determine growth percentile (Figs. 9-2 and 9-3). Bulging and firmness of the fontanelle may indicate elevated intracranial pressure, especially if pulsations are absent.

Serial plotting of the head circumference over time can give important diagnostic information. A large head that continues to grow along the same percentile line may indicate normal growth, while head circumferences that cross percentiles can reflect abnormalities such as hydrocephalus and neoplasms. A decline in head growth reflected in a fall in percentiles also can indicate a disruption of brain growth, for example, from a degenerative disease or infection. Measurements above or below 2 standard deviations (SD) from the mean (macrocephaly or microcephaly) can be associated with genetic disorders such as neurofibromatosis (macrocephaly) and holoprosencephaly (microcephaly). Never-

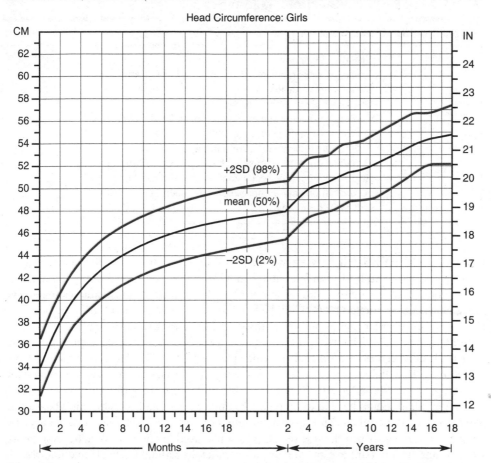

Head Circumference: Girls

Figure 9-3 Head circumference growth for normal girls. (Reprinted with permission from Nellhaus G: Composite international and interracial graphs. *Pediatrics* 41:106, 1968.)

theless, individuals who are otherwise normal also may demonstrate growth outside 2 SD. In some cases, large or small head size is familial, and sometimes you will find it useful to measure and plot the parents' head circumferences.

Look for abnormal postures such as opisthotonus and torticollis, which may be obvious or subtle. Persistent neck and shoulder retraction in premature infants can be a sign of later neurodevelopment dysfunction or developmental delay. Arthrogryposis or fixed deformities of the hands or feet may indicate disorders, such as neuromuscular diseases, that lead to decreased fetal movement. Similarly, easily dislocated hips may indicate a congenital neuromotor disease. Observe the infant for other signs of illness, such as respiratory distress, that may be associated with lung, heart, or neuromuscular disease and cutaneous signs of infection or genetic disorders such as tuberous sclerosis. Examine the skin completely to detect cutaneous signs that may be hidden, such as the small white spots of tuberous sclerosis.

TABLE 9-6. Earliest Visuomotor Milestones

Age, months	Milestone
1	Visually alerts, orients
	Visually fixates momentarily on face and/or red ring
	Moves eyes vertically
	Displays little to no head movement
2	Coordinates eye movements with limited head movements
	Follows past midline through 180° arc
	Follows in prone but not across midline
3	Coordinates eye movement with complete head turning
	Begins coupling eye-head coordination with eye-hand
	coordination and/or upper extremity function
	Follows red ring in a circle

CRANIAL NERVES Shortly after birth, a full-term infant can fix momentarily on a red ring or a face, and by 1 month an infant should be able to follow the ring horizontally for a short distance to either side (Table 9-6). Even in a newborn, oculovestibular eye movements can be elicited by rocking the head from side to side, and this is the best way to look for extraocular muscle palsies at this age. Pupillary responses may be sluggish at birth but should be symmetric. Unilateral pupillary constriction can be seen with a sympathetic lesion secondary to a high brachial plexus injury. This asymmetry is best observed in a dimly lighted room. Most babies have bluish irises at birth, but a sympathetic lesion may cause the affected iris to remain blue after the other one turns brown. At 6 weeks the infant should be able to fix on the examiner's eyes and possibly imitate a smile, and by 3 months the infant can follow a red ring throughout 180 degrees horizontally (see Table 9-6). A cloth strip with wide red stripes can be used to elicit optokinetic nystagmus, which along with pursuit eye movements tests parietal-occipital cortical function. Developmental disorders may cause oculomotor apraxia, a disturbance of eye coordination requiring that the child move the head to move the eyes. A crude visual field examination generally can be performed at 3 to 4 months by distracting the infant with a toy in central vision and bringing another bright moving object in from the side. The infant's eyes generally will dart quickly to the peripheral object, indicating the child's perception of it. Funduscopic examination is important in infants because of numerous congenital infections and genetic disorders that produce retinopathies, but it generally is left to the end of the examination. Some of the important disorders that can be detected at the bedside with funduscopy include retinitis of rubella or cytomegalovirus (CMV), the retinal pits in girls with Aicardi syndrome, and the retinal hemorrhages of shaken baby syndrome or subarachnoid hemorrhage. Trigeminal and facial nerve function can be tested as they are in older individuals, although the corneal reflex is inconsistent until a few months of age. The development of a social smile at 6 weeks of age is an important milestone that requires the participation of cortical visual function as well as the facial musculature. Hearing is difficult to test reliably in infants, but alerting to a loud noise or bell is generally present by 1 month, and an infant orients to voice at about 4 months. If you or the parents are concerned about hearing, you should order a specialized audiologic test. Premature or otherwise "high-risk" infants generally have routine hearing screens in the nursery. Glossopharyngeal or vagus nerve dysfunction may be suspected if the infant has difficulty swallowing, but otherwise do not examine the gag reflex or you may cause discomfort or vomiting. Stridor may be a sign of vagus nerve dysfunction in infants with posterior fossa disorders such as Arnold-Chiari malformation, which is commonly seen in association with meningomyelocele. Observe the size and movement of the tongue to detect hypoglossal dysfunction. Prominent atrophy and fasciculations of the tongue can be seen in babies with motor neuron or Werdnig-Hoffmann disease.

POSTURES, STRENGTH, AND PRIMITIVE REFLEXES   To assess strength in the neck muscles, lift a supine infant's arms or shoulders a few inches upward and look for head lag. Newborns and infants up to 4 weeks of age generally have considerable head lag when being pulled into the sitting position. By 3 months the infant stiffens the neck as the shoulders are lifted. Abnormal stiffness in the neck or back muscles can be

Primitive Reflex: Tonic Labyrinthine Reflex

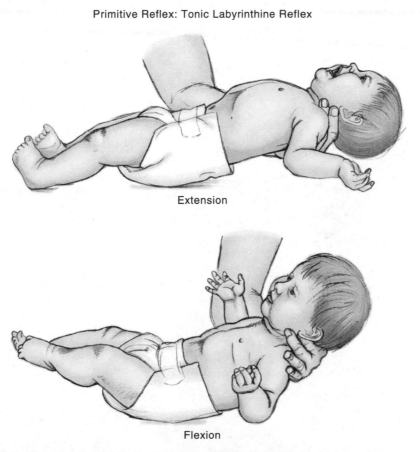

Extension

Flexion

Figure 9-4   The tonic labyrinthine reflex is elicited by flexing and extending the neck.

pathologic in the first few weeks of life. In newborns, lifting the shoulders quickly usually elicits the Moro reflex of flexion of the arms. This reflex also can be elicited by holding the shoulders and head several inches above the examining surface and gently but quickly letting the head fall back 1 or 2 in. The response should become fatigued after a couple of trials, and persistence may indicate a state of heightened excitability such as that seen in Tay-Sachs disease patients. An asymmetric Moro response can be seen in central or peripheral nerve or brachial plexus lesions such as those in Erb palsy, while a weak response in a newborn may indicate a depressed level of consciousness. The Moro response usually is hard to elicit by 6 months of age in normal infants. Three other primitive reflexes mediated at a brainstem level usually can be elicited during the first 4 to 5 months: the tonic labyrinthine response, the asymmetric tonic neck reflex, and the positive supporting reflex. As illustrated in Fig. 9-4, flexion of the neck evokes the tonic labyrinthine response, which includes mild symmetric flexion of the arms and legs. Turning the head to either side elicits the asymmetric tonic neck, which generally is associated with extension of the arm and leg ipsilateral to the face (Fig. 9-5). This reflex is prominent at 3 to 4 months of age, and infants at this age often assume this posture spontaneously. Both the

Primitive Reflex: Asymmetric Tonic Neck Reflex

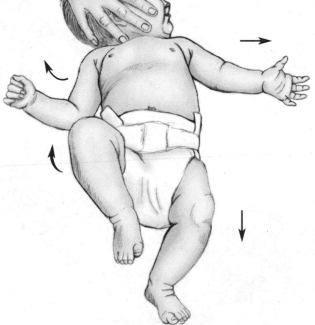

Figure 9-5 The asymmetric tonic neck reflex is elicited by turning the head to one side. This causes the "fencing posture" in which the infant extends the arm and leg on the side to which the head is turned.

Primitive Reflex: Positive Supporting Reflex

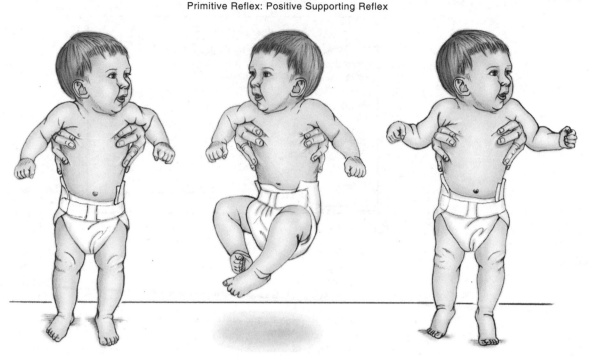

Figure 9-6   The positive supporting reflex is elicited when the child's feet touch a firm surface. Antigravity muscles in the legs and trunk contract and support the child's weight while the examiner provides balance.

asymmetric tonic neck reflex and the tonic labyrinthine reflex probably represent stereotyped reflexive responses to sensory inputs from the eighth cranial nerve and proprioceptive fibers from cervical muscles. The positive supporting reflex can be used to evaluate leg function in infants (Fig. 9-6). As is shown in Fig. 9-7, the prominence of primitive reflexes diminishes progressively up to about age 6 months as the normally flexed posture of the newborn extremities becomes extended and volitional movements of the hands, fingers, and legs emerge. In normal young infants, these reflexes are typically variable and fatigue with repetition. Persistence of these primitive reflexes into the second half of the first year may indicate congenital motor disorders such as cerebral palsy, especially if they are very stereotyped and repetitive after multiple repetitions. You can evaluate resistance to passive manipulation of the limbs ("tone") by passive flexion and extension, keeping the neck in a neutral position because the primitive reflexes powerfully influence muscle stretch responses. A full-term newborn holds the arms and legs in a flexed position, and the examiner typically grasps the hands, forearms, or feet and extends the limbs momentarily, letting them fall back to their flexed position. The postures of the extremities vary with gestational age, and small premature infants typically lie with extremities extended and have reduced resistance to passive manipulation in flexor groups compared with term infants. Most nurseries routinely rate extremity "tone" and joint flexibility as part of a standardized score (e.g., Dubowitz score) to estimate gestational age. Evaluate rigidity, characterized by increased resistance to passive manipulation in flexors and ex-

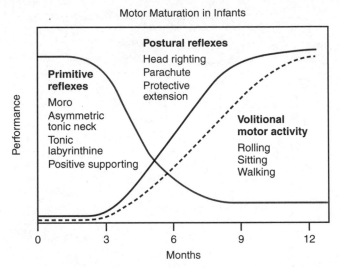

Figure 9-7   The infant's motor repertoire progresses in the first year from primitive reflex-driven activities, to adaptive postural reflexes to volitional activities such as sitting and walking. Persistence of reflex-driven activity in the latter part of the first year suggests a defect in cortical motor control.

tensors throughout the range of movement, and spasticity, characterized by a velocity-dependent increase in resistance as in the examination of older individuals. Examination of resistance to passive manipulation in the hips is important because spasticity in the lower extremities (e.g., in spastic diplegia) commonly increases tonic contraction adductor groups in the thighs, pulling the femurs upward and out of the hip joint.

It is important to assess muscle strength as well as resistance to passive manipulation in a sick neonate, but this cannot be done in the same detail as in an adult. Newborns with true weakness generally show signs of a long-standing disorder in utero such as high arched palate, dislocated hips, breech presentation, arthrogryposis, or a bell-shaped chest as seen in type I Werdnig-Hoffmann disease, myotubular myopathy, or myotonic dystrophy. Acute weakness in infants typically leads to hypotonia (decreased resistance to passive manipulation of the limbs along with decreased movement and respiratory difficulty) as seen in infantile botulism. True muscle weakness suggests peripheral neuromuscular disease, while hypotonia alone suggests a central nervous system (CNS) origin. In young infants, a prominent head lag and a weak Moro may be seen in both central hypotonia and neuromuscular weakness, but the other signs help localize the site responsible for the weakness.

EMERGING FINE AND GROSS MOTOR SKILLS   During the latter part of the first 6 months of life, as the dominance of stereotyped brainstem reflexes such as the Moro and asymmetric tonic neck subside, cortical control of the limbs emerges, manifested as opening of the fists and flexion of the elbows, grasping at objects such as rattles, and finally transfer of objects from one hand to the other at 5 months (Figs. 9-8 through 9-10). This is a more informative set of motor functions than trunk rolling, which may emerge at 3 to 4 months, because rolling depends primarily on axial spinal musculature and to a lesser extent on crossed corticospinal pathways. Hand and arm movements in the first 6

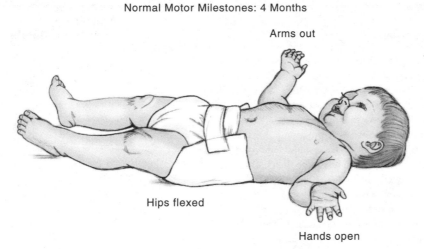

Figure 9-8   The normal 4-month-old has lost some of the flexed posture of the newborn and has begun to extend the arms and hands.

months may have a choreoathetoid quality that normally fades as mature hand control is obtained. The hand and finger sequence of development continues through the rest of the first year with acquisition of the ability to grasp objects with the thumb and several fingers and finally the mature "pincer" thumb and index finger grasp at age 11 months. You can evaluate this sequence by observation or by giving the infant a small, harmless object such as a raisin to grasp. This also serves as a test of visual acuity. The infant is ambidextrous at this point, as handedness generally is not developed until 18 months. At 11 months, the "parachute" response also emerges, which is a thrusting movement of the forearms when you hold the infant's body facedown over the examination table. By evaluating the pincer grasp and the parachute response at 11 months, you may detect hemiparesis resulting from cerebral lesions. By this time the infant usually can come to a sitting position and sit unsupported with a reasonable ability to prevent falling backward or to one side. In evaluating fine motor as well as visuospatial development, you should use standardized items from the Cattell Scale of Infant Development (Capute and Accardo, 1996) (Table 9-7).

DEEP TENDON REFLEXES AND THE BABINSKI   The deep tendon reflexes in the extremities can be elicited as in adults with practice and some modification of technique. The biceps reflex is usually elicitable, but the triceps, brachioradialis, and deltoid reflexes may be challenging. Reflexes at the knees and ankles generally can be evoked and may be very active in a normal newborn, with 3 to 4 beats of clonus not unusual before 6 months of age. If the reflexes are asymmetric, check the position of the head and neck because of their influence on spinal cord reflexes. The Babinski response is usually active up to 1 year of age and then fades by about 18 months (Table 9-8). The reflex is generally well developed with extension of the great toe and complete fanning of the other toes and can be elicited over a wide area of the skin of the foot. Development of spasticity can cause tightening of the Achilles tendons (heel cords), which may actually diminish the ankle reflexes. Reflexes such as the jaw jerk and signs of frontal lobe dys-

TABLE 9-7.   Age of Attainment of CAT Milestones

Milestone	Mean Age of Attainment, Months
Visually fixates momentarily on red ring	1
Lifts chin off table in prone	1
Visually follows ring horizontally and vertically	2
Lifts chest off table in prone	2
Visually follows ring in a cricle	3
Supports on forearms in prone	3
Blinks in response to hand rapidly approaching eyes	3
Unclenches hands at rest more than half the time	4
Manipulates fingers	4
Supports on wrists in prone	4
Pulls down ring	5
Transfers object from one hand to the other	5
Regards pellet	5
Obtains cube	6
Lifts cube	6
Reaches for objects with thumb and forefinger sliding across table surface	6
Attempts pellet	7
Pulls out peg	7
Inspects ring	7
Pulls ring by string	8
Secures pellet	8
Inspects bell	8
Performs three-finger scissor grasp	9
Rings bell	9
Looks for toy dropped over edge	9
Combines cube and cup	10
Uncovers bell	10
Fingers pegboard	10
Displays mature overhand pincer movement	11
Looks for cube hidden under cup	11
Releases one cube in cup	12
Marks with crayon	12
Reaches for toy around intervening glass pane	14
Pushes peg in and out	14
Solves pellet-bottle with demonstration	14
Solves pellet-bottle spontaneously	16
Puts round block in formboard	16
Scribbles in imitation	16
Puts 10 cubes in cup	18
Solves round hole in reverse formboard	18
Spontaneously scribbles with crayon	18
Completes pegboard spontaneously	18
Obtains object with stick	21
Solves square in formboard	21
Builds tower of three cubes	21

TABLE 9-7. Age of Attainment of CAT Milestones (*Continued*)

Milestone	Mean Age of Attainment, Months
Attempts to fold paper	24
Builds train of four cubes	24
Imitates stroke with pencil	24
Completes formboard	24
Makes horizontal and vertical strokes with pencil	30
Solves three-hole formboard rotated 180 degrees	30
Folds paper with definite crease	30
Builds train of four blocks with fifth block as smokestack in imitation	30
Builds bridge of three cubes	36
Draws circle	36
Names one color	36
Draws a person with head plus one other body part	36

function in older children and adults, including the suck, root, and palmomental, are well developed in newborns and fade over the first year.

CEREBELLAR FUNCTION AND SENSATION Classical signs of cerebellar dysfunction are difficult to elicit even at 1 year of age, possibly because the nervous system adapts differently to cerebellar dysfunction present from early in development compared with dysfunction acquired after a period of normal development. Delay in sitting and walking is the most common sign of chronic cerebellar disorders in young infants, and appendicular tremor is less common. Acute cerebellar hemorrhage occurs occasionally in newborns and typically presents with apnea, a diminished level of consciousness, and signs of cranial nerve dysfunction. In infants with basal ganglia injury, dyskinetic rather than choreoathetoid movements may appear when mature finger control should be emerging. The sensory examination in infants is difficult, and only the most severe losses generally can be detected. Infants with hemiparesis should be evaluated for nociceptive and touch sensation because a combined sensory and motor loss has a much worse prognosis than does motor loss alone for effective use of the extremities. The level of a disorder of the spinal cord can generally be determined by moving a sterile pin up the abdomen and thorax and looking for the site that evokes discomfort. Spinal cord disorders are common in patients with traumatic or congenital disorders such as spina bifida. These infants typically have prominent vasomotor instability in the skin below the lesion and a patulous anus. The anal wink reflex may be preserved if a segment of cord remains functional below the level of the lesion. It usually is easy to palpate a full bladder in an infant, and bladder emptying usually can be elicited by stroking the lower abdominal skin over the bladder, the Crede maneuver.

Older Infants and Toddlers

You can change the strategy of your examination in children toward the middle of the second year as infants begin to stand, take steps, and run. Unless they are ill, children at this age usually are in constant motion in the examination situation and often are unwill-

Motor Milestones: 4 Months

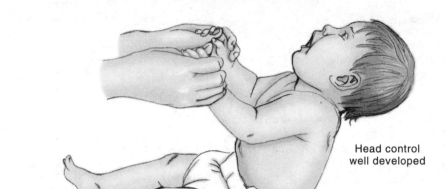

Head control
well developed

A

4 Months

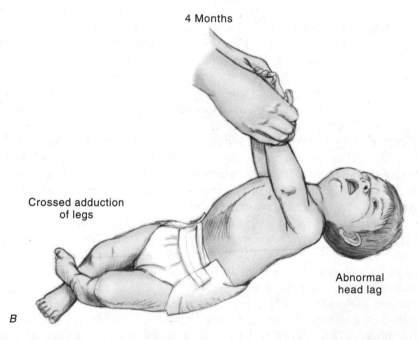

Crossed adduction
of legs

Abnormal
head lag

B

Figure 9-9   A. The normal 4-month-old infant has good head control when brought to a sitting position. B. Head lag is abnormal at four months, and strong crossed adduction of the legs is a sign of possible spasticity.

Normal Motor Milestones

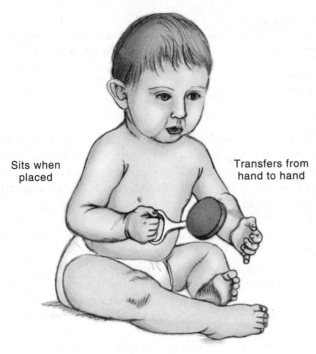

Sits when
placed

Transfers from
hand to hand

A   6 months

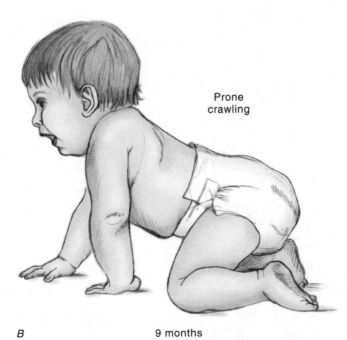

Prone
crawling

B   9 months

Figure 9-10   A. The 6-month-
old can usually sit when placed
and is beginning to transfer objects from one hand to the other.
B. The 9-month-old infant is usually beginning to crawl.

TABLE 9-8. Appearance and Disappearance of Reflexes

Reflex	Appearance	Disappearance, months
Moro	Newborn	6
Babinski	Newborn	18

ing to sit on an examination table. Children from 18 months to 3 years of age are usually reluctant to cooperate with strangers, especially those in white coats. The child's constant motor activities give you an opportunity to gather information about fine and gross motor abilities from simple observation as the child plays with toys, runs down the hallway, and interacts with the caretaker. Children at this age gain language abilities quickly, going from "mama, dada" at 11 months to approximately 50 words with 2-word sentences at 2 years of age (see Tables 9-3 and 9-7). One examination is usually sufficient to evaluate language, and the caretaker's history can be important and helpful.

By 18 months to 2 years of age, most congenital motor disorders can be assessed on examination. Signs of spasticity are usually apparent by 4 to 6 months, consisting of either hemiparesis or spastic diplegia with spasticity in the lower extremities greater than the arms (Fig. 9-11). A child with a hemiparesis usually has established strong handed-

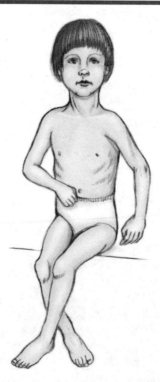

Figure 9-11   A typical pose assumed by a child with the spastic diplegia form of cerebral palsy. High tone in the hip adductors produces scissoring which impedes walking.

ness on the opposite side by then, while a child with spastic diplegia is usually not walking and has persistent Babinski signs with spasticity or passive manipulation of the limbs, tight heel cords, brisk deep tendon reflexes, and tight adduction of the legs at the hips. Children with basal ganglia disorders from injury or metabolic diseases usually manifest choreoathetosis, rigidity, and delay in fine and gross motor milestones by this time. In contrast to spastic diplegia caused by damage to periventricular white matter, the motor disability from basal ganglia disorders affects the upper extremities more than the lower. In children with traumatic lesions, some of the abnormalities of motor function seen in the toddler may diminish as the child grows older, probably as a result of reorganization of the developing brain.

Neurologic disorders that begin in older infants and toddlers usually cause dysfunction similar to that in older children and adults. For example, acute cerebellar ataxia following viral infection or medication causes truncal ataxia; cerebellar hemisphere tumors lead to ipsilateral limb kinetic tremors; and cranial nerve dysfunction presents signs similar to those in adults. Nevertheless, spinal cord disorders are difficult to detect because they often require a reliable sensory examination.

School-Age Children (Ages 4 to 12 Years)

As children approach the time for preschool and elementary school, the traditional neurologic examination becomes feasible, although you need to make allowances for the child's short attention span and potential fearfulness in the examination setting. The neurologic symptoms at this age are similar to those in adults, for example, headache, seizures, and other changes in consciousness and muscular weakness. In the infant and young toddler motor and immature language development are dominant features, but in the school-age child cognitive development occurs rapidly and many disorders of attention and intellect begin to emerge. You are likely to be asked to evaluate disorders in children of this age that are more obvious to school personnel than to parents. Some of these "school problems," attention problems, and reading and learning disorders become apparent at this age in part because parents may not have the critical skills to pick them up at home and in part because the more complex intellectual demands made on the child in school uncovers the deficits. While most adults are accustomed to a stable set of reading, writing, and reasoning skills, a school-age child is required to make quantum jumps each year, and many of the abilities required have not been "tested" in the past. These problems reach the neurologist more frequently currently than in the past because of accumulating evidence that they have an organic brain-based cause and because school achievement is viewed as more important for economic survival than it was in the past.

The neurologic evaluation of childhood disorders of attention and learning includes a standard physical and neurologic examination as well as a battery of tests that generally are not used by neurologists in evaluating adults (Rapin, 1995). The history and examination are focused on potential neurologic and genetic disorders that may underlie these conditions. Genetic neurologic disorders can range from the relatively common, such as fragile-X syndrome and neurofibromatosis, to the rare, such as adrenoleukodystrophy and metachromatic leukodystrophy. The neurologic examination should include an evaluation of coordination and balance as well as fine motor skills.

Developing Mental Abilities

Performance in school is a major task for children between 4 and 12 years of age. Early difficulties in school are often related to failure to attain basic skills in language, behavioral, or motor functions. Later-onset difficulties frequently stem from a child's inability to meet the demands of the classroom. School performance requires the successful integration of behavioral, language, and motor abilities. Poor written expression may result from disturbances of motor function, language skills, or organization of thought. Social interaction is primarily verbal. Language competence is a major determinant of school success, and delayed language development is the key to the diagnosis of mental retardation. Language disorders that are present at school entry usually predict poor reading abilities. Quantification of language abilities is easier to achieve before age 3 than afterward. Preschoolers should be able to use mature syntax, tell stories, master sequenced language tasks (counting, alphabet, days of the week, telephone number), and summarize. Early in elementary school the language focus shifts from oral to print, and children learn to assign sounds to symbols and to decode words. Third-grade children begin to use inferential thinking, and reading comprehension is a major focus. Children with pragmatic language disorders may present with social difficulties because of their poor conversational skills. Toward the end of elementary school, children move from page reading to chapter reading, tell jokes, and use inferential thinking to interpret proverbs.

Children with disordered receptive language may have difficulty following spoken directions, long response latencies ("zone out"), poor short-term auditory memory and/or processing (manifested by frequent use of "huh?"), and difficulties with humor. Disordered language expression may be marked by a disinhibited or tangential speaking style; frequent use of "umm," "uhh," or "like"; and single-word or reduced responses to open-ended questions. Older children may show difficulty in maintaining social banter and interacting in the gymnasium or cafeteria, where the language demands are high and the structure is more variable.

Attentional Disorders

Attention is the behavioral attribute most commonly linked to school performance. There are many aspects of attention, including initiating, sustaining, inhibiting, and shifting, but sustained attention is a major focus. Attention must be interpreted within the context of age, cognition, and functional ability. Most parents whose children have a disorder report that their child has poor attention in only certain situations and may do well in playing video games or watching television. Perseveration is a common symptom and is manifested verbally by repetitive asking of questions or by difficulty with transitions. Distractibility, hyperactivity, disorganization, and social immaturity frequently accompany inattention, and you need to judge them by comparison to age-matched peers. Distractibility may be manifested by inability to complete tasks or by focusing on minor extraneous stimuli.

You may not observe hyperactivity in the office setting, and this disorder may not be fully appreciated at home, but only in the classroom. In younger children hyperactivity is usually motoric, but as the child ages, verbal or cognitive hyperactivity becomes more prominent. Hyperactivity can be measured by direct observation or recording, performance on a standard task, interview, or with behavioral checklists. Many clinicians use behavioral checklists because they are easy to use, but you need to be cautious in interpreting them because they rely strongly on the impressions of the reporter.

Children with primary attentional dysfunction must be distinguished from those who lack ability to perform academic tasks. Disordered attention is seen in attention deficit hyperactivity disorder, mental retardation, Tourette syndrome, mixed receptive-expressive language disorders, specific learning disability, hearing loss, anxiety disorder, and mood disorders (depression and bipolar disorder). It is uncommon for seizure disorders to present as isolated attentional disorder. Disorders of mood, irritability, and anxiety usually do not cause isolated attention deficit hyperactivity disorder.

Motor Function Complaints

Motor dysfunction in school-age children can present not only with signs of gross motor dysfunction such as hemiparesis or ataxia but also with problems in speech articulation, dressing, putting on shoes, handwriting and copying, and making adventitious movements while sitting or standing quietly. Complaints occurring later in school include difficulty with note taking, incomplete assignments, and avoidance of writing. Caretakers also may complain about hypotonia, dyscoordination, or asymmetric function as a child begins to participate in organized sports in elementary school. These symptoms should be evaluated carefully because they have the potential to cause major disabilities and often reflect ongoing neurologic disorders. You need to distinguish between delays in the maturation of abilities, for example, learning to copy carefully or learning to ride a bicycle, from neurologic disorders that require remediation.

You should obtain information in the history not only about language, behavioral, and motor function but also about displays of emotion, socialization, and play. Ask specifically about grades, current performance (academic and behavioral), past performance, academic assistance required, and homework accomplishments. Homework is an important area of inquiry because it reveals information about how well the child is able to perform classwork, organize ideas, and interact with the parents. Nonperformance of homework is a common source of conflict between parent and child.

Neurologic Examination of School-Age Children

The techniques of neurologic examination, including mental status testing, can be used in children as they grow older, but you need to observe a child carefully before making demands. You should look for mild dysmorphisms, abnormalities of skin pigmentation, and asymmetry of growth. Some childhood disorders, such as tuberous sclerosis, neurofibromatosis, and ataxia-telangiectasia, may manifest skin or conjunctival signs only after age 6.

When you talk with the child, you can assess articulation, richness of responses to open-ended questions, use of fillers ("umm," etc.), following directions, telling jokes, and using figurative language. You should assess the resistance to passive manipulation of the limbs and in particular compare the resistance at the shoulders and the hips. Proximal instability because of weakness and hypotonia of shoulder muscles may be misinterpreted as intention tremor. Children above the age of 5 years generally can participate reliably in assessment of position sense, graphesthesia, or stereognosis. Children can distinguish their left from their right sides by age 5 and the examiner's left and right sides by age 7. You can assess reading with a graded word list such as the Wide Range Achievement Test-3. Formal psychologic evaluation is generally required to assess adequately the cognitive abilities of school-age children.

Subtle ("Soft") Signs of Neurologic Disorders

Many authors have identified a relationship between childhood disorders of attention, memory, and learning and disturbances of motor control. Some of these disturbances, such as overflow of movements from one hand to the other (synkinesia) or clumsy rapid alternating movements, have been called subtle signs or "soft" signs because they are not necessarily considered abnormal and may suggest a maturational delay rather than a definite pathology. Nevertheless, these motor signs can reflect disruption of a "neurologic core" that is located at the interface in the brain where motor control is adjacent to cognitive control (Denckla and Roeltgen, 1992). These signs can be assessed semiquantitatively with protocols such as the Revised Neurological Examination for Subtle Signs, which includes age-standardized norms, speed, and skill in activities including tandem walking, hopping, finger to nose testing, overflow movements, and finger tapping (Denckla, 1985). Slowness, imprecision, loss of rhythm, and overflow of movements identified by these tests are strongly associated with disorders of attention and behavior but not with dyslexia (Denckla and Rudel, 1978; Denckla et al, 1985). Some of these disorders, such as overflow movements, may reflect inability of the nervous system to direct a discrete movement (such as pointing a finger) while suppressing closely associated movements. A similar defect in motor inhibition and control may be involved in attention deficit and/or hyperactivity syndrome. In contrast to these motor signs, sensory findings such as defective graphesthesia and finger agnosia have an uncertain association with neurodevelopmental abnormalities in children.

Evaluation of subtle neurologic signs can be especially helpful in the diagnosis of problems with handwriting. Observation of the child's pencil grasp provides important information, since deviations from the normal mature grasp are associated with motor disorders (Deuel, 1995). Handwriting speed can be measured with the Ayres Handwriting Speed Test. Children with handwriting problems often have choreiform movements or slowness of finger sequencing (sequential tapping of each finger against the thumb). Choreiform movements that disrupt writing often appear as lapses in postural stability when the child stands with the eyes closed and the arms held out. Slow finger sequencing correlates with poor or dyspraxic illegible handwriting (Berninger and Rutberg, 1992). At times the finding of abnormal motor control associated with poor handwriting may lead to a recommendation for occupational therapy or for a school program that de-emphasizes handwriting, possibly using a computer keyboard.

INTEGRATING DATA FROM THE NEUROLOGIC HISTORY AND EXAMINATION

You need to use information gathered from the history and examination to generate hypotheses to be evaluated using additional tests or a period of observation. The stage of development greatly influences the manifestations of neurologic disorders in infants and children, making it difficult to provide a specific diagnosis on the first visit. For example, mental retardation from a gene defect may present in infancy as a motor delay, and only with time does it become apparent that all areas of development are delayed. Autism often presents as a period of language regression in a relatively normal toddler who then begins to regress socially. Many undifferentiated disorders in infants or young children become clear as more specific disabilities develop in older children. For this reason, it is important to put the findings from the history and examination in the context of the child's total developmental profile. Table 9-9 shows how disorders can be placed in subgroups, using undifferentiated data from young children to generate diagnostic hypotheses for future evaluation.

CLINICAL VIGNETTES OF NEUROLOGIC HISTORY AND EXAMINATION IN PEDIATRIC NEUROLOGIC DISORDERS

Eight-Year-Old Boy with Difficulty in School

The parents of an 8-year-old boy referred him for consultation because of academic underachievement. He was then in the second grade at school and had difficulty staying in his seat, interacting with other children, and completing classroom assignments. He had

TABLE 9-9. Dissociation of Development
Contrasting rates of development within individual streams show patterns that permit early diagnosis

	Gross Motor	Fine Motor/ Problem Solving	Language	Personal and Social
Cerebral palsy	Decreased	Decreased	Normal	Decreased
Mental retardation	Normal	Decreased	Decreased	Decreased
Communication disorder	Normal	Normal	Decreased	Normal
Autism	Normal	Normal	Decreased	Decreased

been an A student previously, but recently he had become a C student and was beginning to voice concerns about his abilities and was experiencing low self-esteem.

PAST MEDICAL HISTORY   His mother had a normal pregnancy, he has been healthy, and he takes no medications.

DEVELOPMENTAL HISTORY   He walked at 11 months, initially as a toe walker, and flatfooted after about a month. He ran as soon as he walked. He had difficulty learning to ride a bicycle and was successful only at 7 years of age. He developed handedness at 4 years, initially left and then right. He learned to tie his shoes at age 7. He was slow in buttoning, experiencing difficulty in the sequencing of movements needed, but eventually became successful. Language development was precocious, and he was speaking in sentences by 20 months of age. He knew colors and the alphabet by age 3. His articulation has been clear. When he was a preschooler, his parents at times found it difficult to comprehend his stories. He frequently left out facts or started in the middle of the story and worked outward. He does not summarize well and intrudes himself into conversations.

He has had a high level of motor activity. His mother reports that she was "black and blue" from his kicking in utero. He destroyed his crib by standing against the rail and rocking and has been "on the go" constantly. His attentional skills have been variable. He could sit down and watch television or play Nintendo for 2 hours at a time; however, he had difficulty staying in his seat in the classroom. He frequently asked questions that were not related to the topic at hand. From the beginning of school his teachers noticed that his activity level was high. He did not fight or have adverse interactions with other children. At home he had difficulty settling down for sleep but did not wake up during the night. He was enuretic three nights per week.

FAMILY HISTORY   His father failed third grade because of poor handwriting and hyperactivity. He did well subsequently and developed his own business. He was known to have substantial drive. The patient's mother had no school-related problems.

PHYSICAL EXAMINATION   Growth was normal. Head circumference was at the fiftieth percentile. He was active and fidgety and stood while performing tasks with paper and pencil. His affect seemed normal. Mild facial asymmetry was noted, but the cranial nerves were otherwise normal. Resistance to passive manipulation was decreased in the shoulders. His elbows could be brought together behind his back and crossed. Hamstring range was normal to mildly decreased in the legs. Deep tendon reflexes were symmetric. When walking, he had mild postural disturbances on the right with toe walking and heel walking. He displayed choreoathetoid movements in the hands on standing with the arms extended and the eyes closed. He had a poor pencil grasp, symmetric synkinesis on finger apposition, and excessive use of proximal musculature with rapid alternating movements. Sensory examination was normal. Handwriting speed was slow, and he missed several words in the paragraph he was copying. He was decoding words at an appropriate level for his grade.

IMPRESSION   Based on the history from parents and teachers, he appeared to have a learning disorder with difficulty with writing and reading as well as attention deficit with hyperactivity disorder (ADHD). His father may have shared this diagnosis. Evidence of a disorder of motor coordination was consistent with the ADHD working diagnosis. He was referred for psychologic testing, and the WISC-III revealed a bright average intellect without significant scatter. On the Woodcock-Johnson Psycho-Educational Battery, he was in the low average range on reading comprehension and in the average range in decoding. He scored 2 SD from the mean on a scale for ADHD, and his written language skills were 2 SD below his IQ scores.

One-Year-Old Infant Who Did Not Sit or Stand

The infant was a 1-year-old boy whose parents were concerned because he did not sit or stand holding on to furniture. His legs seemed stiff, and it was sometimes difficult for the mother to diaper him because the thighs were held together much of the time. Otherwise, the child had been well.

Past medical history indicated that the child had been generally well with no medications or allergies. He had never been hospitalized, and immunizations were up to date. Pregnancy lasted 39 weeks, and the infant was delivered uneventfully after a 9-h labor. In the nursery, the baby was slow to begin breast-feeding and had jaundice with a bilirubin to 12 mg/dL. He stayed in the nursery for 4 days before going home.

Developmental history indicated that his language and social milestones were normal. He smiled appropriately at 4 weeks of age and progressed normally through cooing and babbling to the point of saying "mama" and "dada" appropriately at this time. He transferred a rattle from one hand to the other at 7 months and began to roll from front to back at 5 months. He did not sit when placed and was not able to come to standing, although he did stand momentarily on his toes when held by his hands. His parents felt there has been no progression; the child simply failed to gain the expected motor skills.

FAMILY HISTORY   Both parents were healthy except that the mother had Graves disease 3 years prior to this pregnancy and was treated with thyroidectomy and thyroid replacement medications. There were no other children in the family.

NEUROLOGIC EXAMINATION   The infant was happy and playful in mother's lap, and height, weight, and head circumference were in the thirtieth percentile. General physical examination was normal for age, as were cranial nerves. Resistance to passive manipulation was normal in the shoulders but increased in the hips, and the thighs were held together tightly. The child could pick up a raisin with a pincer grasp using the thumb and the first two fingers. Resistance to passive manipulation in the legs was increased in the knee extensors, and the heel cords were tight with the ankles plantarflexed. Deep tendon reflexes were increased 3+ in both arms at the biceps, and there was some spread from the brachioradialis reflex to the biceps. In the legs, reflexes were 4+ at the knees and ankles, with clonus at the ankles. The patellar reflex spread to the thigh adductors on the opposite side. The plantar responses were extensor bilaterally. Sensation was intact. The back was straight without scoliosis. Sensation was intact in all four extremities. The child had no tremor or obvious ataxia of the extremities.

IMPRESSION   Examination revealed spasticity confined to the lower extremities with tight hip adductors and increased reflexes with abnormal spread, a good explanation for the inability to sit or stand alone. Function of the hands appeared mildly impaired with a "two-fingered" pincer grasp rather than the "fine" index finger–thumb expected at 11 months, and historically the baby was a few weeks late to transfer objects between hands. Language and social skills were appropriate for age. The conclusion was that the child had the cerebral palsy syndrome with spastic diplegia resulting from involvement of white matter motor fibers serving the legs more than the arms. Magnetic resonance imaging (MRI) scan of the brain confirmed the clinical impression, showing moderate enlargement of the lateral ventricles with a symmetric high T2 signal along the edge of the ventricles indicating periventricular encephalomalacia (PVL). Generally associated with premature birth, spastic diplegia also occurs in infants born at term whose white matter was injured prior to 32 weeks of gestation. In this case, the mother's thyroid disorder may be linked to white matter injury (Kuban and Leviton, 1994).

Infant with Developmental Delay and Hypotonia

The parents of a 7-month-old girl asked for an evaluation of motor delay and floppiness that seemed to be getting worse. The child would not bear weight on the legs, had difficulty feeding from a bottle, and had lost some body weight.

Past medical history indicated that the child was born in breech presentation at term and had no neonatal problems. The child received no medications and had no allergies, and the immunizations were up to date. The child went home from the nursery at 2 days of age and seemed normal.

Developmental history revealed that the child made consonant sounds such as "dada" but did not say any real words. The child smiled appropriately at 5 weeks and was awake, alert, and interactive. She could sit if propped but could not come to a sitting position alone. She did not put weight on her legs, and they usually dangled when she was held by the shoulders. Generally, the baby felt "floppy" compared to the mother's previous child.

Family history was negative for any neurologic diseases.

EXAMINATION   The infant made good eye contact when sitting on the mother's lap, smiled, followed the examiner around the room, and laughed at times. Height, weight, and head circumference were at the fiftieth percentile. Cranial nerve examination showed normal eye movements and pupillary reactions. Facial nerve function and hearing seemed normal. There was a gag response, but the tongue seemed smaller than normal and had "wormlike" movements under the surface. The baby was hypotonic, and there was a slight head lag when she was picked up. She slipped through the examiner's hands when picked up at the chest, but she was able to move the arms and shoulders actively. The legs were weak, and she could not lift them off the examining table when lying down. She lay supine with legs extended and externally rotated at the hips. Muscle mass appeared normal in the arms and legs. Reflexes were 1+ at the biceps but absent in the legs. Plantar responses were flexor. Sensation was intact to pinprick. She had no ataxia of the limbs.

IMPRESSION   The infant was hypotonic as reported by the parents but was also clearly weak, especially in the legs, suggesting a peripheral neuromuscular disorder. Absence of reflexes in the legs suggested either a neuropathy or a motor neuron disorder, but the atrophy of the tongue with fasciculations strongly suggested a motor neuron disorder, possibly Werdnig-Hoffmann disease. The breech presentation at birth was consistent with an early-onset neuromuscular disorder that interfered with the fetus's ability to assume the vertex position. An electromyogram (EMG) and muscle biopsy confirmed the diagnosis of Werdnig-Hoffmann motor neuron disease type II.

Two-Year-Old with Loss of Consciousness

A 2-year-old boy was seen with a history of loss of consciousness that occurred twice, once a few days before examination and another a month earlier. Both episodes were similar. The onset was with the child crying out as if in pain, screaming for a few seconds, and then appearing to be continuing to scream but without sound. His face was initially bright red but then turned white, and he fell to the ground. He lay there for about 30 s and then began jerking movements in his arms and legs for just a few seconds. He regained consciousness after about 5 min and seemed sleepy. He seemed exhausted after the spell and took a long nap later in the afternoon. After that he appeared normal again.

Past medical history indicated that he had been in good health. Gestation and delivery were normal, and he had no operations or hospitalizations. Immunizations were up to date, and he took no medicines and had no allergies. An electrocardiogram (ECG) when he was taken to an emergency room was normal.

Developmental history revealed that he walked at 12 months and could run several steps. He transferred objects between hands at 5 months and could help his caretaker undress him. He had used a fine pincer grasp since 11 months of age. He had a vocabulary of about 50 words.

Family history revealed that he had two brothers who were healthy. His father was given phenobarbital as an infant for about a year, but he does not know why.

PHYSICAL EXAMINATION   General physical examination was entirely normal. His skin was clear, and eyesight and hearing were normal. The cranial nerves, muscle strength, muscle bulk, coordination, and resistance to passive manipulation of the limbs were normal. No signs of ataxia were found. The deep tendon reflexes were normal in amplitude and symmetric, and the plantar responses were flexor. The gait was normal, and he ran appropriately for a 2-year-old. Sensation was intact.

IMPRESSION   The patient's history of loss of consciousness at this age could be consistent with breath-holding spells, a seizure disorder, ingestion of a toxin, hypoglycemia, episodic vertigo, or ataxia. The history of screaming turning to paleness and loss of consciousness at this age strongly suggested breath-holding spells followed by a short period of myoclonus secondary to the syncope. The father's history could indicate that he had the same disorder, which sometimes occurs. The normal ECG suggested that the disorder is not one of the familial prolonged QTc syndromes predisposing to ventricular fibrillation. Ingestion of a toxin, intoxication by an inherited metabolic disease, and hypoglycemia were unlikely because of the nature of the spell and because of its repetition. Children with episodic ataxia or vertigo generally are awake and distressed by their condition, and they often vomit. This patient exhibited a classic pediatric neurologic syndrome that can be evaluated by using the history and physical alone without further neurodiagnositc testing.

Coma with Seizures in a 5-Year-Old Girl

A 5-year-old girl was evaluated after an episode of seizures with coma lasting 5 days. She experienced symptoms of flu with vomiting several days before the onset of the present illness and then developed repetitive tonic convulsive movements with loss of consciousness and no response to deep pain. She was treated with anticonvulsants and intravenous fluids and gradually woke up on the fifth day. She continued in her normal state for 6 months. In the hospital, the laboratory testing was normal, including blood glucose, electrolytes, amino acids, and blood ammonia. Liver enzymes were mildly elevated.

Past medical history indicated that she was born weighing 8 lb and had a normal neonatal course. In infancy, she tended to vomit easily, and several episodes of vomiting required oral rehydration. She had never been hospitalized and took no medications. The parents reported that she did not feel well if she slept too late in the morning, and she felt better after eating breakfast. Immunizations were up to date, and she had no allergies or food aversions.

Developmental history revealed that she had normal early language, motor, and social milestones. At 3 or 4 years of age, she appeared to fatigue easily and did not want to run very long.

Family history indicated that a brother had died of a similar illness about a year before. After several days of coma he developed a cardiac arrhythmia and could not be resuscitated. The mother and father, who are not related, had no medical history. They had only two children.

NEUROLOGIC EXAMINATION The patient was a pleasant, friendly girl with no dysmorphic features. Height and head circumference were at the thirtieth percentile, and weight was at the sixtieth percentile. General examination was normal, including the skin and heart. Mental status was normal with no disturbances of memory, speech, language, or reasoning. Motor activity was normal, and affect was appropriate. Cranial nerves and fundi, muscle strength, resistance to passive manipulation, and deep tendon reflexes were normal. There were no pathologic reflexes. Muscle bulk seemed reduced, but no fasciculations were seen. There was no ataxia, and gait was normal. Sensation was normal.

IMPRESSION The episodes of seizures with protracted coma in both siblings suggested an inherited metabolic disorder. The signs are similar to sporadic episodes of "Reye syndrome" after a viral illness, except that Reye syndrome is associated with elevated ammonia levels. The history suggested that the patient had had previous, milder episodes of illness associated with vomiting as an infant. The history of the patient limiting her physical exertion and feeling better after eating in the morning and her examination suggested that her ratio of adipose to muscle tissue might be elevated. The history suggested that the disorder represented an inborn error of metabolism, a disorder of energy metabolism such as glucose or fatty acid metabolism, or a mitochondrial disease. During a fast, she had very little rise in ketone bodies when free fatty acids rose and glucose fell modestly, suggesting a defect in fatty acid oxidation. This type of disorder also would be compatible with the brother's history of cardiac arrest since fatty acids are a source of energy for the myocardium.

Movement Disorder in an 8-Year-Old Child

An 8-year-old girl was seen for worsening of a movement disorder. She had been unable to walk since 15 months of age when she became ill during an episode of gastroenteritis. At that time she became obtunded and had random, rapid choreiform movements of her arms and head. She recovered over the next week but was unable to make any sounds and was hypotonic. Over the next several months, movements improved in the arms and legs and she regained the ability to sit but not walk. She had been given the diagnosis of choreoathetoid cerebral palsy. Recently she had developed some pain and stiffness in the legs.

Past medical history except for the preceding illness was unremarkable. Immunizations were up to date, she took no medicines, and she had no allergies. She weighed 8 lb at birth, which was uneventful. She had other childhood illnesses but no more episodes of encephalopathy.

Developmental history indicated that she had normal developmental milestones before 15 months of age. At 1 year of age, she was able to say "mama" and "dada" appropriately, could pick up a raisin with the thumb and forefinger of either hand, and was interactive socially. She also could pull to stand along furniture and was taking several steps without assistance.

Family history revealed that the parents had two other normal children. There was no history of a previous illness.

NEUROLOGIC EXAMINATION   The patient was a thin, alert girl with head circumference and height in the fiftieth percentile and weight in the tenth percentile. She seemed appropriately interactive but did not speak or make sounds. She was able to use a communication device to respond appropriately to questions, and her responses suggested that she was normally intelligent. Cranial nerves were all normal with the exception of difficulty opening and closing her mouth and protruding her tongue. Passive movement of the extremities revealed increased resistance that was even throughout the range of motion with no spastic quality. The arms and legs were held extended outward in fixed postures that changed from time to time. She appeared to have normal strength, but her movements were limited by hypertonicity. When the neck was flexed, the stiffening of the arms in extension worsened, whereas with extension of the neck the arms flexed at the elbows. Deep tendon reflexes were symmetrically increased to 3+, but the reflexes depended on her limb postures, which could be changed by the position of her neck.

Babinski signs were present bilaterally. She had awkward fine motor movements and some athetoid movements of the fingers. She was unable to write. There was no evidence of ataxia, and sensation appeared to be intact.

IMPRESSION   The history indicated that she suffered a brain injury at 15 months of age. Before that time her developmental milestones were normal. This is not consistent with choreoathetoid cerebral palsy, which is a congenital disorder that delays motor milestones in the first year. The examination indicated that the hypertonicity represents rigidity and the fixed postures indicate dystonia, two findings that point to a disorder of the basal ganglia. The variability in resistance to passive manipulation of the limbs over time and the persistence of the symmetric tonic neck responses are typical of infantile extrapyramidal disorders, and lack of speech production is also commonly seen in these disorders. Pain may be produced by muscle spasm itself or by disorders of joints produced by muscle stiffness and maintenance of the extremities in unusual positions. The sudden onset of injury to the basal ganglia in an otherwise normal child at 15 months during an acute illness most likely resulted from an infectious and/or inflammatory or genetic metabolic disorder. Mitochondrial disorders and other disorders of energy metabolism are particularly likely to injure the basal ganglia in infants. In this case, urine sent for organic acid determination indicated high levels of glutaric acid and metabolites, consistent with glutaricaciduria type I from a deficiency of the mitochondrial enzyme glutaryl-CoA dehydrogenase. The history and examination led to the correct diagnosis because the history was incompatible with the diagnosis she carried of "cerebral palsy," and the examination revealed basal ganglia dysfunction, which frequently is due to inborn errors of metabolism in infants. This history and examination findings prompted metabolic testing.

Seizures in a 3-Month-Old Infant

A 3-month-old infant girl was seen for episodes that appeared to be seizures beginning 10 days previously. The episodes consisted of repetitive flexing movements of the arms and legs with flexing of the neck that occurred about every 2 s and appeared in clusters of 50 to 100. The spells often occurred when the infant was waking up in the morning and after naps. At other times she was free of spells, but she seemed less interested in her surroundings than she had been before they began.

Past medical history indicated that she was born after a term gestation with no problems and that the delivery was uneventful. She was a poor feeder for the first 2 weeks, requiring the mother to change to a formula from breast-feeding, but otherwise she seemed normal to her mother. The infant was the mother's first child. She had one set of immunizations, including DPT. Otherwise she had no illnesses or operations. She did not appear to have any allergies and took no medications.

Developmental history revealed that she smiled frequently at 8 weeks, but her mother was uncertain whether the response was related to interactions with her or to other stimuli. At the time of examination, she was making cooing sounds and could open her hands.

Family history indicated no history of epilepsy in the family. The parents were both healthy and worked as schoolteachers.

NEUROLOGIC EXAMINATION The infant was well nourished and had no dysmorphic features. The height and weight were in the fiftieth percentile, and the head was in the twenty-fifth percentile. The skin, including the lower back, showed no depigmented or hyperpigmented spots. General physical examination was normal with no hepatosplenomegaly. Eye examination revealed small abnormalities in the retina that looked like "pits." Both optic discs were slightly pale. The baby was not able to fix and follow a mirror and a red ring. The rest of the cranial nerves were normal. The baby could open the hands but did not take a rattle in either hand. Resistance to passive manipulation was reduced, and when the baby was picked up at the shoulders, the head lagged back about 30° before coming up with the body. Deep tendon reflexes were symmetric and 2+, and the plantars were extensor. Sensation was intact.

IMPRESSION The parents brought a videotape of the episodes that confirmed the impression from the history that the infant was having infantile spasms. Infantile spasms have a strong association with genetic and metabolic disorders such as tuberous sclerosis and disturbances of brain development such as migrational disorders and porencephaly. The developmental history indicated delayed development, since smiling in an appropriate social context should occur by age 6 weeks. The examination indicated reduced resistance to passive manipulation. Head lag, which should disappear by 3 months, remained present, and visual function was impaired. The findings, including the retinal abnormality and the female sex, suggest the diagnosis of Aicardi syndrome. This syndrome consists of agenesis of the corpus callosum and brain parenchymal malformations in addition to abnormalities of the spinal lamina. The outcome is uniformly poor. An MRI of the brain confirmed this diagnosis. Signs of tuberous sclerosis (TS) manifested by small depigmented spots on the back were not found. The MRI also would have been useful to rule out TS, since brain tubers are often seen in infants at a time when the characteristic facial adenoma sebaceum and depigmented "ashleaf" spots have not yet developed.

Developmental Regression in a 6-Month-Old Infant

A 6-month-old infant boy was evaluated for slowed development over the previous 6 weeks. The baby seemed normal after a term gestation and weighed 9 lb. He took avidly to the breast and had been a good feeder. He smiled appropriately at his mother at 5 weeks of age, and she was sure that he fixed and followed her around the room when he was 3 months of age. Over the previous few weeks he did not seem to be making visual contact with her as much as before, and he generally seemed less interested in his environment. She also noticed recently that he seemed "jumpy" around noises such as the telephone ringing.

Past medical history revealed no medical illnesses and no surgery. He took no medications and had no allergies. Immunizations were up to date.

Developmental history indicated that until recently his motor and language social skills were normal. He had been babbling and saying "dada." He could grasp a rattle and begin to transfer it from one hand to the other at age 5 months. He could roll from front to back. He was a very pleasant, interactive baby until the previous few weeks.

Family history revealed that the parents were unrelated with no previous history of neurologic diseases in the family. The parents emigrated from Russia to the United States 4 months before the birth of this baby, and this is the first child for each parent.

NEUROLOGIC EXAMINATION   The patient was an awake, well-developed, well-nourished baby with growth parameters that included head circumference at the fortieth percentile. Skin and general physical examination, including liver and spleen, were normal. He reacted to a bright light with eye closure, but seemed inattentive to a large red ring, looking at it only momentarily. Hearing was normal, but a strong startle response occurred with the sound of a bell. Funduscopic examination showed pale discs with a red spot near both maculae. The rest of the cranial nerves were normal. Resistance to passive manipulation of the limbs was mildly reduced, but there was no head lag and the extremities were strong. Deep tendon reflexes were 3+ and symmetric, and the plantars were extensor. He sat well when placed and transferred large objects from hand to hand but did not pick up a raisin held in front of him.

IMPRESSION   The neurologic examination confirmed the parents' concern about the baby's visual attentiveness, demonstrating lack of age-approriate ability to fix and follow objects and reach for a small piece of food. The history suggested a degenerative course because the baby acquired abilities that were lost and skill acquisition reached a plateau. Lack of visual attentiveness, red maculae ("cherry-red spot"), and excessive startle pointed to a tentative diagnosis of Tay-Sachs disease resulting from abnormal accumulation of GM_2 gangliosides in the brain secondary to lack of hexosaminidase A. A cherry-red spot, caused by degeneration of retinal ganglion cells surrounding a normal redness of the macula also can be seen in other storage diseases, such as GM_1 gangliosidosis. Later in the course of the disease, the head circumference typically increases because of storage of ganglioside. Prepregnancy screening is available for this autosomal recessive disease, which is particularly common in Ashkenazic Jews from eastern or central Europe, but this family was not able to participate.

Severe Hypotonia in a Newborn

The infant was seen for consultation after a full-term gestation complicated only by moderate polyhydramnios. The infant was born weighing 7 lb in the breech position and was found to have fixed contractures of both feet in a "clubfoot" position. The baby needed bag and mask ventilation for 5 min to start breathing but then breathed normally. In the nursery, he was floppy and had poor sucking, requiring a nasogastric feeding tube.

Past medical history and developmental history were not contributory.

Family history indicated that the mother was 30 years old and had been followed by an ophthalmologist since receiving lens implants for cataracts 3 years previously.

NEUROLOGIC EXAMINATION   The baby was lying supine with the legs extended and the hips rotated outward in a "frog leg" position. The arms were also extended at the baby's sides. The face and head seemed elongated and narrow, and the palate was arched. The funduscopic examination and the cranial nerve examination including the tongue were normal, but the baby had a weak sucking reflex. The extremities showed arthrogryposis of the hands and feet, more severe in the legs than in the arms. When the baby was raised off the bed by the arms, the head flopped back with no neck support. The extremities showed no movement against gravity. Deep tendon reflexes were present at the biceps and knees and were 2+. Plantar stimulation elicited a grasp response bilaterally. Sensation was intact.

IMPRESSION   The baby's examination showed marked hypotonia with evidence of muscle weakness. The contractures of the hands and feet, evidence of muscle weakness, narrow face and high arched palate, and preserved deep tendon reflexes suggested a primary muscle disease. The breech presentation is also consistent with a neuromuscular disorder, while the polyhydramnios could indicate that the baby's poor sucking and swallowing reduced the circulation of amniotic fluid in utero. The mother's history of cataract surgery at a young age sparked the interest of the examiner, who evaluated her and found that she also had a long narrow face with some complaints of arm weakness when combing her hair over the last several years. She demonstrated myotonia in her hands when the thenar eminence was struck with the percussion hammer, and significant proximal muscle weakness was demonstrated on neurologic examination. The examiner also noted early atrophy of the temporalis muscles on her face. The mother's EMG was positive for myotonia, and a diagnosis was made of myotonic dystrophy, an autosomal dominant disorder that often includes cataracts and endocrine disorders. The baby's EMG and nerve conduction studies were normal, and a diagnosis of neonatal congenital myotonic dystrophy was made. Myotonia is seldom found before age 3 years. Sucking problems are particularly prominent in this neonatal neuromuscular disease. Inheritance is virtually always from the mother.

A 7-Year-Old Boy with School Problems and a Seizure

A 7-year-old boy was seen for problems first noticed at school. He had been a precocious reader at home and had no trouble with first-grade work, but several months after starting second grade, the teacher reported to his parents that he seemed uninterested in work in the classroom. He got out of his seat frequently. Previously cooperative, he become hard to discipline. The teacher put him in the front row of the class, but the behavioral problems persisted. At home, his parents noticed that he seemed less alert at breakfast than at other times and seemed to stumble more when running than he had previously. He showed signs of hyperactivity. One week before the visit, he had a generalized seizure while at school.

Past medical history indicated that he was the second child, his birth came after a full-term pregnancy, and he weighed 7 lb at birth. The neonatal period was unremarkable. He had no allergies and was taking no medication. Immunizations were up to date. There were no operations or medical illnesses.

Developmental history revealed that all his language, social, fine motor, and gross motor milestones were appropriate for his age, and he showed an early interest in reading.

Family history indicated that his father had been treated for attention deficit disorder as a child and retained some restlessness. There was no family history of other neurologic disorders. The parents have three children: a girl, this child, and a younger boy, all healthy.

NEUROLOGIC EXAMINATION He was a well-developed, well-nourished boy with appropriate growth measurements and head circumference in the fortieth percentile. Examination of his skin and the general examination were unremarkable. He seemed less mature than his age, frequently breaking into conversations between parents and physician and needing to be reminded to sit down. At times he did not appear to hear what his mother was saying, requiring that she repeat herself. Examination of the fundi was unremarkable. When shown words appropriate for the first grade, he was not able to identify any of them. His cranial nerve examination was normal except for the question about hearing. Muscle bulk and strength seemed normal, but resistance to passive manipulation was increased in the lower extremities. Deep tendon reflexes were hyperactive in the lower extremities, 4+ at the knees, and 3+ at the ankles. The plantar responses were extensor bilaterally. Reflexes in the upper extremities were 2+ and symmetric. His gait was narrow and stiff, his running was awkward, and he tripped several times. Sensation was difficult to test because of poor cooperation.

IMPRESSION This 7-year-old developed problems with attention and reading in the second grade that are relatively common and experienced a brief seizure. His father had exhibited similar behavior in school, and disorders of attention and behavior are frequently inherited. The parents' concern about his stumbling when running was confirmed during the examination, and signs of corticospinal pathology were identified, with a stiff gait, brisk reflexes, and bilateral Babinski responses. These signs in an otherwise normal child support the impression of the parents that the disorder was new and progressive. Although the signs of cortical dysfunction, including loss of ability to read and distractibility, initially drew attention to the child's problem, on examination he had prominent long tract signs that pointed to a disorder of white matter. At this age, two disorders of white matter—X-linked adrenoleukodystrophy (ALD) caused by accumulation of very long chain fatty acids and metachromatic leukodystrophy, a recessively inherited defect in arylsulfatase activity—can cause a combination of cognitive, behavioral, and motor problems that involve the legs predominantly. Suspicion of a vision and hearing problem in this boy suggested the diagnosis of ALD, and seizures occur in 20 percent of these patients. This disorder also typically caused adrenal insufficiency, which is often clinically inapparent at diagnosis. In this patient an MRI of the brain suggested ALD because of the characteristic "butterfly" pattern of posterior occipital lobe dysmyelination and high plasma very long chain fatty acids. Increasingly, both ALD and metachromatic leukodystrophy are being treated with bone marrow transplantation, but the procedure generally is not effective in symptomatic ALD boys. However, the younger boy can now be tested, and bone marrow transplantation can be offered if he has the disease but is presymptomatic.

SUGGESTED READINGS

Berninger VW, Rutberg J: Relationship of finger function to beginning writing: Application to diagnosis of writing disabilities. *Dev Med Child Neurol* 34:198, 1992.

Capute AJ, Accardo PJ: The infant neurodevelopmental assessment: A clinical interpretive manual for CAT-CLAMS in the first two years of life; II. *Curr Probl Pediatr* 26:279, 1996 .

Capute A, Accardo PJ: *Developmental Disabilities in Infancy and Childhood*, 2d ed. Baltimore, Paul H. Brookes, 1996, p 529.

Capute AJ, Palmer FB, Shapiro BK, et al: Primitive reflex profile: A quantitation of primitive reflexes in infancy. *Dev Med Child Neurol* 26:375, 1984.

Capute AJ, Palmer FB, Shapiro BK, et al: Clinical linguistic and auditory milestone scale: Prediction of cognition in infancy. *Dev Med Child Neurol* 28:762, 1986.

Denckla MB: Revised neurological examination for subtle signs. *Psychopharm Bull* 21:773, 1985.

Denckla MB, Roeltgen DP: Disorders of motor function and control, in Rapin I, Segalowitz SS (eds), Boller F, Grafman J (series eds): *Handbook of Neuropsychology*. Vol. 6: *Child Neurology*. Amsterdam, Elsevier, 1992, p. 455.

Denckla MB, Rudel RG: Anomalies of motor development in hyperactive boys. *Ann Neurol* 3:231, 1978.

Denckla MB, Rudel RG, Chapman C, Krieger J: Motor proficiency in dyslexic children with and without attentional disorders. *Arch Neurol* 42: 228, 1985.

Deuel RK: Developmental dysgraphia and motor skills disorders. *J Child Neurol* 19 [Suppl 1]:S6, 1995.

Kuban KCK, Leviton A: Cerebral palsy. *N Eng J Med* 330:188, 1994.

Lyon G, Adams RD, Kolodny EH: *Neurology of Hereditary Metabolic Diseases of Children,* 2nd ed. New York, McGraw-Hill, 1996, p 379.

Rapin I: Physicians' testing of children with developmental disabilities. *J Child Neurol* 10 [Suppl 1]:S11, 1995.

LARRY JUNCK / JAMES W. ALBERS / IVO DRURY

LABORATORY EVALUATION

CHAPTER 10

COMPUTED TOMOGRAPHY

Description

Computed tomography (CT) uses x-rays emitted from a source and confined to a plane oriented perpendicular to the long axis of the body. On the opposite side of the head or body, the fan-shaped beam of x-rays reaches an array of 600 or more detectors, where the x-ray intensity is converted to an electrical signal. The x-ray source and detectors are rotated serially through a range of angles through the head. Data from the detectors in the various projections permit estimation of x-ray attenuation in each picture element (pixel) using a computer algorithm called *filtered back-projection.* x-ray attenuation is closely related to electron density in the tissue, and tissues or substances with a high atomic number such as calcium and metals have the highest density on CT.

CT is often performed before and after intravenous infusion of a contrast agent containing iodine. A local increase in attenuation after contrast infusion is called *contrast enhancement.*

Indications and Findings

CT is best at showing calcific structures, including the skull and calcific abnormalities in the brain, and blood, including subarachnoid blood and epidural, subdural, and cerebral hematomas. It is also very good at showing the ventricles and cerebral spinal fluid (CSF) spaces. With the use of iodinated contrast agents, it is very good at showing brain neoplasms. It is less reliable for showing small abnormalities or subtle changes such as abnormal white matter. It is not nearly as reliable as magnetic resonance imaging (MRI) at showing posterior fossa abnormalities. Its major advantages over MRI include its speed, greater availability, and lesser expense, while a disadvantage (especially in pregnancy) is the small radiation exposure. CT is nearly always the preferred approach to brain imaging in emergency situations, including the acute evaluation of trauma, suspected subarachnoid hemorrhage, and cerebral ischemia (Figs. 10-1 to 10-3). It is also good for evaluating hydrocephalus (Fig. 10-4) and, when necessary, for detecting mass lesions in patients with headaches. CT imaging of the spine is excellent for showing vertebral lesions but of no value for showing the spinal cord or nerve roots.

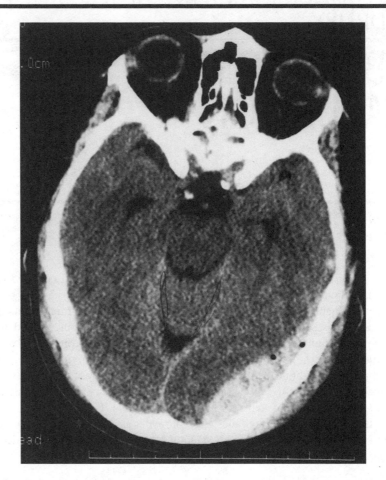

Figure 10-1   CT showing acute epidural hematoma. This 61-year-old woman suffered a head injury due to a fall while ice-skating. In addition to the hematoma, the scan shows air within the hematoma (probably from mastoid air cells) and scalp edema.

Contrast infusion is not needed in most emergency situations. Because of the risk of anaphylaxis from the iodinated contrast agent, contrast infusion should be avoided in patients with known allergy to these agents. In some cases, it may be justifiable to infuse nonionic contrast agents which have a lower risk of allergy, in patients with known allergy to ionic agents or to give contrast agents after antihistamine and steroid premedication starting 24 h prior to the scan. Because of the risk of nephropathy, contrast infusion should be avoided when possible in those patients who are dehydrated, those who are medically unstable, and those with advanced renal disease or diabetes mellitus.

Contrast enhancement usually indicates disruption of the blood-brain barrier with passage of the contrast agent across leaky capillaries. Enhancement is commonly seen in neoplasms, abscesses, and infarcts. Enhancement can also be seen within normal arteries

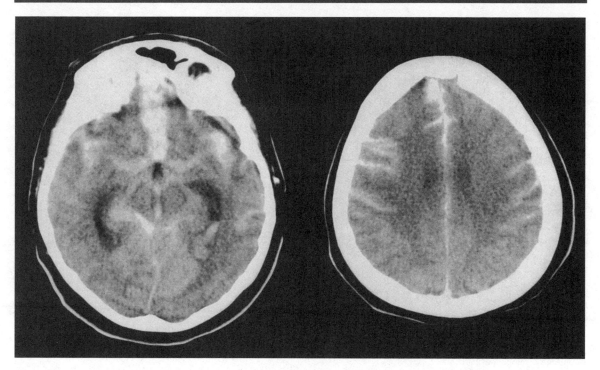

Figure 10-2   CT in subarachnoid hemorrhage. At the base of the brain (*left*), blood can be seen as high attenuation (white) in the interhemispheric fissure, the sylvian fissures, and the cisterns surrounding the midbrain. At the higher brain level (*right*), blood can be seen in the sulci.

and veins, including the circle of Willis and the large venous sinuses, as well as within abnormal vascular structures such as aneurysms and vascular malformations.

MAGNETIC RESONANCE IMAGING

Description

Magnetic resonance imaging (MRI) utilizes a large magnet with a strong magnetic field. MRI relies on the interaction of the spin associated with protons (and, to a lesser extent, neutrons) with this magnetic field. Among the elements present in biologic tissues, many such as ^{12}C, ^{16}O, and ^{40}Ca have an even number of protons resulting in a net spin of zero and no magnetic moment. Nuclei with an odd number of protons such as ^{1}H, ^{19}F, and ^{31}P are *paramagnetic* nuclei with a non-zero spin. In the absence of a magnetic field, the spins are randomly oriented. Such nuclei act like small magnets when placed in a magnetic field and will rotate or *precess* around the direction of the field lines. In addition, a slight excess of nuclei become aligned parallel with the magnetic field, a process called *magnetization*. With MRI, the magnetization is disrupted by radiofrequency (RF) pulses.

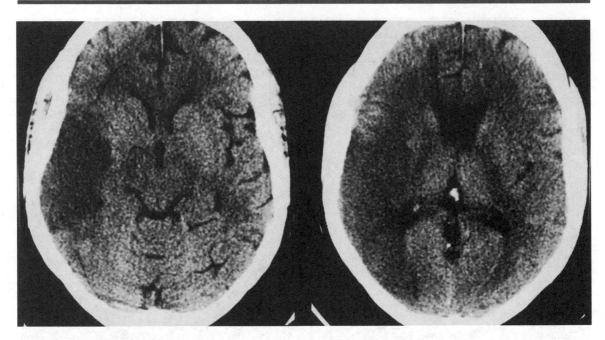

Figure 10-3 CT showing cerebral infarct. The large middle cerebral infarct in this 32-year-old woman occurred as a complication of chronic myelogenous leukemia.

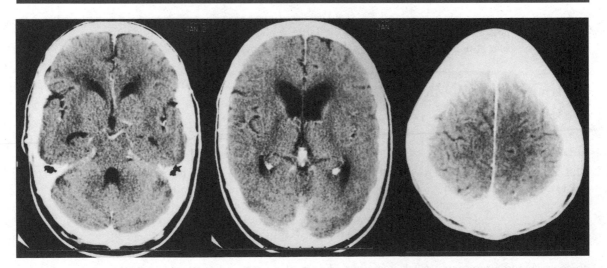

Figure 10-4 CT scan in normal pressure hydrocephalus. This 68-year-old man had a progressive gait disturbance and fatigue 2 years after treatment for cryptococcal meningitis. The scans show enlarged lateral ventricles (including dilated temporal horns) and third ventricle. Attenuation is decreased in the periventricular region. The sulci near the vertex are not enlarged, indicating the absence of generalized brain atrophy. His symptoms improved after ventriculoperitoneal shunting.

The interaction of the RF pulses with nuclei depends on the local magnetic field, and a gradient purposely introduced in the magnetic field results in localized sensitivity to the pulses. After each pulse, the nuclei return toward their previous alignment on a time scale of ~1 s or less (*relaxation*), emitting RF signals proportional to their initial degree of alignment. Detection of these radio waves provides information about the density and local magnetic field characteristics of these nuclei and serves as the physical basis for MRI. Variations in the applied RF pulses and in the time at which the system "listens" for RF responses result in a variety of types of images. The images most commonly obtained emphasize the physical parameters T1 and T2, as well as the proton density. Just as CT is often performed with contrast agents containing iodine, MRI is generally performed with contrast agents containing the paramagnetic substance gadolinium. Gadolinium rarely causes side effects, and except in rare patients known to have gadolinium allergy and in pregnant patients, gadolinium is nearly always used with MRI.

Some patients experience claustrophobia that interferes with completion of MRI. Diazepam 10 mg, taken orally ~30 min prior to the scan, usually permits successful completion in adult patients who do not have contraindications to this medication.

Indications and Findings

MRI can be used for brain imaging for nearly any clinical indication, but because it costs more than CT, it is best reserved for situations in which it has advantages over CT. It is clearly superior for evaluating patients with epilepsy; suspected multiple sclerosis and other white matter diseases; cerebral vasculitis; vascular malformations; small, deep infarcts; and lesions of any type in the brainstem and cerebellum. It demonstrates some large infarcts and tumors better than CT, but CT is often adequate in these situations. MRI may be preferred in patients who, due to allergy, cannot receive iodine-based contrast agents with CT. Although not conclusively proved safe in pregnancy, MRI may be preferred to CT when imaging is necessary during pregnancy because of the lack of known effects on the fetus.

Most contraindications to MRI are related to the possibility of movement of ferromagnetic objects in the strong magnetic field (e.g., aneurysm clips or metallic foreign bodies in the eye) or of current induction in metallic implants (e.g., pacemakers and pacing wires left in place after cardiac surgery). The common types of MRI images are depicted in Figs. 10-5, 10-6, and 10-7 and described in Table 10-1. T1-weighted images are useful for showing overall brain anatomy and for evaluation of CSF spaces; they are most useful for demonstrating hydrocephalus, atrophy, cysts, and malformations. *Gadolinium enhancement* on T1-weighted images is most commonly seen in lesions with blood-brain barrier breakdown such as neoplasms, abscesses, meningeal inflammation, infarcts, and relatively acute plaques of multiple sclerosis. Enhancement is also useful for demonstrating vascular structures such as aneurysms and vascular malformations. T2-weighted images are sensitive to edema and to subtle changes in tissue characteristics. T2-weighted images are best for distinguishing parenchymal lesions from surrounding brain (e.g., multiple sclerosis plaques, small infarcts, and edema). FLAIR images are similar to T2-weighted images, but the signal from CSF is suppressed, leaving CSF dark. FLAIR is the best sequence for demonstrating disease adjacent to CSF spaces (e.g., in the periventricular region) and is excellent for showing parenchymal lesions anywhere in the brain. Proton

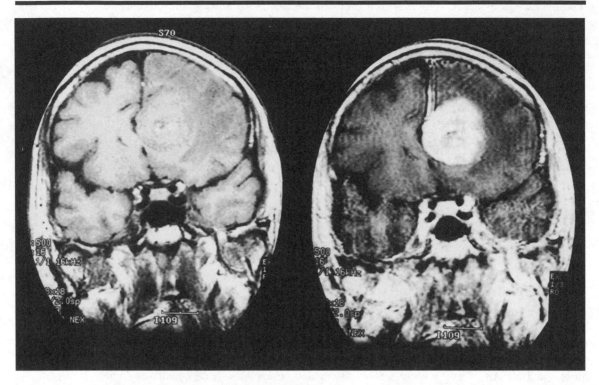

Figure 10-5   T1-weighted coronal MRI showing glioblastoma multiforme. The image without gadolinium (*left*) shows mass effect, effacement of sulci, midline shift, heterogeneous abnormal signal in the mass, and homogeneous low signal adjacent to the mass. The increased brightness in the tumor after gadolinium (*right*) is due to the passage of gadolinium across abnormal tumor vessels that lack the normal blood-brain barrier.

density images are useful for showing water distribution because free protons (hydrogen nuclei) are present in higher density in water than in other molecules. Proton density images, like T2-weighted and FLAIR images, are good for demonstrating lesions in brain parenchyma, but they are also excellent for gray-white differentiation. Blood is visualized less well with MRI than with CT, but usually parenchymal hemorrhage can be identified.

TABLE 10-1.   Features of Different Types of MRI Images

	T1-Weighted	T2-Weighted	Proton Density	FLAIR
Normal gray matter	Dark	Bright	Bright	Gray
Normal white matter	Bright	Dark	Dark	Gray
CSF	Very dark	Very bright	Gray	Very dark
Features best demonstrated	Anatomy	Parenchymal lesions, white matter disease	Gray-white differentiation	Parenchymal lesions

The imaging characteristics of intracerebral blood depend on its age and are summarized in Table 10-2.

SPECIAL APPROACHES USING MAGNETIC RESONANCE

Magnetic Resonance Angiography

Magnetic resonance angiography (MRA) is most commonly performed using the time-of-flight approach. With this method, the brain signal is suppressed by a rapid succession of slice-selective RF pulses causing nuclei within the slice to lose their spin alignment and hence generate little signal. Inflowing blood, in contrast, is not affected by the pulses and generates a strong signal, creating bright images of flowing blood. Another approach, direct perfusion-sensitive T1 contrast, can also generate angiographic images.

MRA provides excellent visualization of large vessels and effectively shows thrombosis, embolism, stenosis, and dissection of large vessels in the neck or head. It is also good for showing aneurysms and arteriovenous and venous malformations. It has not yet

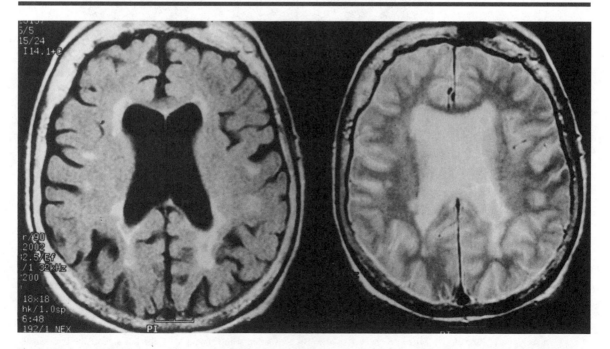

Figure 10-6   MRI in multiple sclerosis. The FLAIR image (*left*) and T2-weighted image (*right*) both show extensive periventricular signal abnormality. The periventricular lesions are more obvious in the FLAIR image because the CSF is dark whereas the lesions are bright.

TABLE 10-2.   Imaging Features of Intraparenchymal Blood on MRI

Stage	Time	Biochemical Form	T1	T2
Hyperacute	Minutes to hours	Oxyhemoglobin	Dark	Bright
Acute	Hours	Deoxyhemoglobin	Dark	Dark
Acute	Days	Methemoglobin (extracellular)	Bright	Bright
Subacute	Weeks	Transferrin, lactoferrin (extracellular)	Bright	Bright
Chronic	>2 months	Ferritin, hemosiderin (in phagocytes)	Iso	Dark

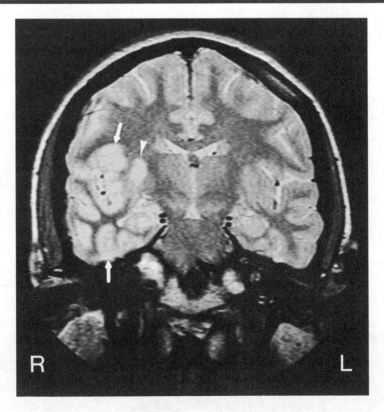

Figure 10-7   MRI in cortical dysplasia. By convention with CT and MRI, the left side of the brain is displayed on the viewer's right. This 33-year-old woman has a long history of choreiform and dystonic movements, predominantly on her left side. Proton density images show abnormally thick cortex (pachygyria) in the right insula and temporal lobe (*arrows*). The right basal ganglia are also abnormal (arrowhead).

COLOR PLATES

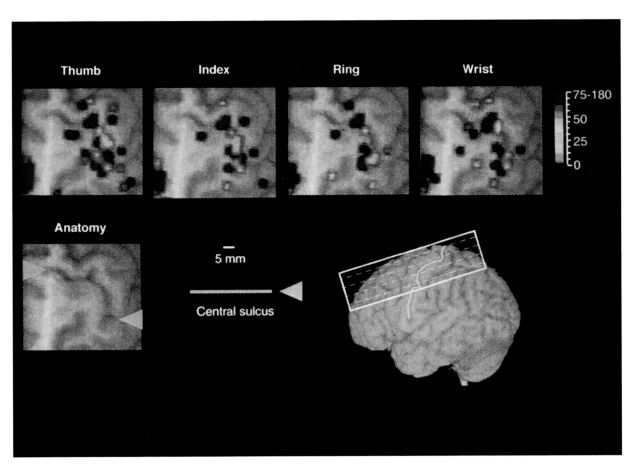

PLATE 1   fMRI study of the hand representation in primary motor cortex. The images show the regions activated by movement of the right thumb, index finger, and ring finger, and by moving the hand at the wrist. Areas shown in color are areas of increased oxygen saturation of hemoglobin due to increased blood flow. The lateral surface of the left hemisphere is toward the right, and anterior is down. Most activations are on the anterior margin of the central sulcus. In contrast to the classical view of the cortical representation of the hand portrayed with the homunculus, these results show a more complex representation with multiple, overlapping regions corresponding to different parts of the hand. (With permission from Jerome N. Sanes. Reprinted from Science 1995; 268:1775–1777. Copyright © 1995, American Association for the Advancement of Science.)

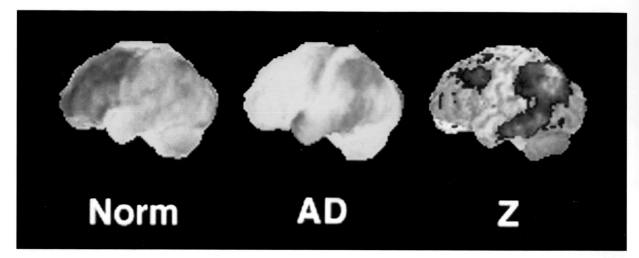

PLATE 2 Alzheimer's disease studied with PET and 18F-fluorodeoxyglucose (FDG) to assess cerebral glucose metabolism. Images are left lateral views emphasizing cerebral cortex. The left image shows mean metabolism in 40 normal elderly subjects, while the center image shows mean metabolism in 39 patients with Alzheimer disease. In the right image, areas that are significantly decreased in Alzheimer disease patients are shown in color as statistical Z scores. The patients with Alzheimer disease have decreased metabolism in the temporal lobe, parietal lobe, and to a lesser extent frontal lobe, sparing primary motor and primary visual cortex. (Images were provided by Satoshi Minoshima.)

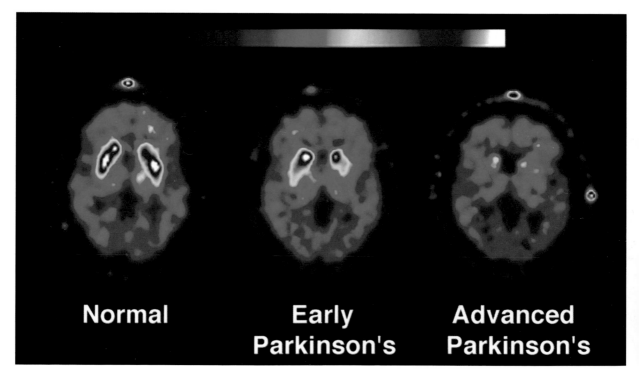

PLATE 3 PET slices obtained using [11C]-dihydrotetrabenazine, a ligand for the transporter that pumps dopamine into presynaptic vesicles. Uptake in the striatum represents dopamine uptake in the nerve terminals of the nigrostriatal projection. The left image shows normal binding in the caudate and putamen in a healthy elderly person. The middle image from a patient with early Parkinson disease shows the typical pattern of asymmetrically reduced binding, while the right image shows markedly reduced binding bilaterally in advanced Parkinson disease. (Images were provided by Kirk Frey.)

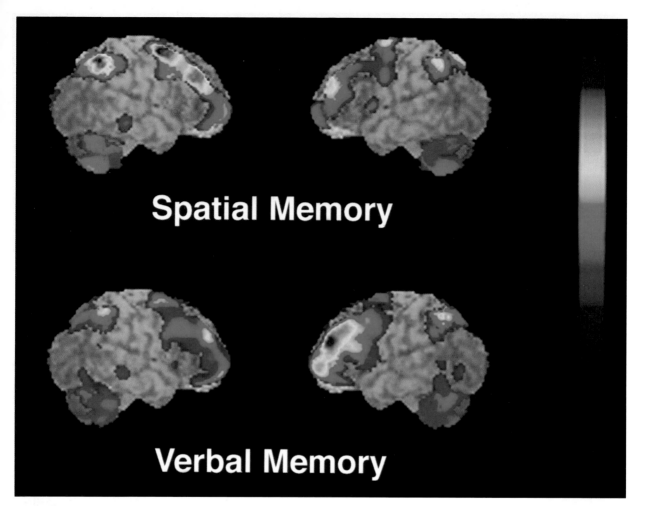

PLATE 4 PET activation studies of working memory. Working memory is defined as memory for short-term storage (seconds) during ongoing mental processes. In both the spatial memory and verbal memory tasks, normal subjects viewed a screen where a letter would appear at varying locations every 3 s. In the spatial memory task, subjects were asked to indicate whenever the location of the letter matched that of the letter presented 9 s earlier, while in the verbal memory task, they were asked to indicate whenever the letter of the alphabet matched that presented 9 s earlier. Scans using [15O]-H2O as a blood flow tracer were performed during the memory tasks, and scans performed during tasks that were similar but did not require memory were subtracted. The PET results are shown in color, overlain on a representation of the brain surface derived from MRI. Differences shown in red and yellow are generally significant. Both tasks activated frontal and parietal cortex, the spatial task predominantly in the right hemisphere and the verbal task predominantly in the left hemisphere. (Images were provided by Robert A Koeppe, John Jonides, and Ed Smith.)

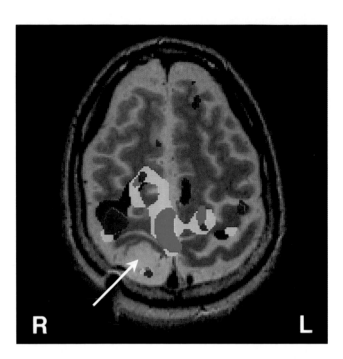

PLATE 5 PET activation scans in a patient with a brain tumor. The colored areas are regions activated during left finger tapping (red) and foot movements (yellow) and during vibratory stimulation of the left hand (blue) and foot (green). The PET images are overlain on an MRI that shows his tumor (arrow), an anaplastic oligoastrocytoma. The most prominent activations are in the primary motor cortex and primary sensory cortex of the right hemisphere. Less prominent activations are seen in the left hemisphere (ipsilateral to the movements and sensory stimuli). Small, colored regions remote from the primary motor and sensory cortex probably represent PET image noise. This image was used to help guide surgical resection of the tumor.

PLATE 6 Ictal SPECT. Scans were performed during a partial seizure and in the interictal state using SPECT and HMPAO, a blood flow tracer. Perfusion in the R temporoparietal region is decreased in the interictal state but is nearly identical to that in the contralateral hemisphere during the seizure. Subtraction images (ictal minus interictal, shown in color in the bottom row) show the areas of cerebral cortex thought to be involved in the seizure.

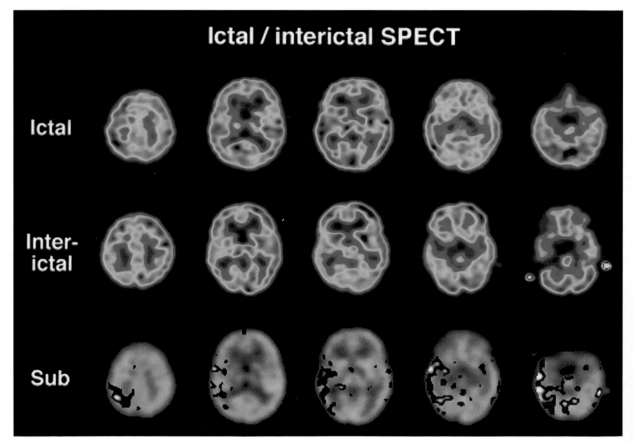

achieved the crisp resolution of catheter angiography, which remains the procedure of choice for evaluating small intracranial branches and for showing the neck of aneurysms.

Functional Magnetic Resonance Imaging

Functional magnetic resonance imaging (fMRI) refers to a variety of techniques that can be expected to come into increasing use in clinical research and potentially into routine clinical management of certain neurologic problems. The most common approach uses the blood oxygen level dependent (BOLD) technique. During a motor, language, or cognitive task or during sensory stimulation, brain regions activated by the task show increased blood flow but little or no change in oxygen metabolism. As a result the capillary and venous oxygen tension *increases* in the brain regions activated, and hemoglobin saturation increases. fMRI demonstrates the local increase in oxyhemoglobin in the activated regions.

fMRI is primarily used in brain mapping research to demonstrate the brain regions involved in various tasks (see Color Plate 1). Early studies focused on regions activated by motor tasks, sensory activation, and language production. Further studies are focusing on localization of different types of memory, complex sensory discrimination, complex aspects of language function, and executive control. Complex activities typically involve a network of widely separated brain regions, and a major goal of activation studies is to determine the function of each region participating in such a network. In patients with various diseases, fMRI studies can assess the function of regions involved by the disease, as well as the effects of plasticity resulting in the shifting of functions to other brain regions. In patients with brain tumors and vascular malformations, fMRI can demonstrate the relationship between the lesion and critical brain regions such as primary motor cortex and primary language areas, and such information can be useful in guiding neurosurgical resections.

Magnetic Resonance Spectroscopy

Magnetic resonance spectroscopy (MRS) takes advantage of the effect of interactions within the same molecule on the spin properties of a paramagnetic nucleus. It is thus closely related to nuclear magnetic resonance techniques used in analytic chemistry. MRS has not yet achieved the exquisite resolution typical of other MR techniques; most MRS analyses are performed on volumes of at least several cubic centimeters, but MRS can also be used to make images of specific chemical moieties in the brain.

The strength of the MRS signal depends on the natural abundance of the paramagnetic nuclide in the brain, as well as the signal intensity per nucleus. ^{31}P can be used to assess the abundance of ATP, ADP, and AMP; phosphocreatine; and pH, measured indirectly by the relative abundance of HPO_4^{2-} and HPO_4^{-}. ^{1}H MRS can be used to assess the abundance of lactate, a marker for regions where glycolysis outpaces oxidative metabolism; *N*-acetylaspartate, present primarily in neurons and axons; glutamate/glutamine; creatine; choline; and myo-inositol, an osmoregulator and a precursor of the inositol phosphate family of intracellular messengers.

MRS has shown promise in studying focal and diffuse brain diseases as well as metabolic diseases of muscle, but its potential role in routine neurologic diagnosis remains to be defined.

POSITRON EMISSION TOMOGRAPHY

Description

Positron emission tomography (PET) utilizes injected radiopharmaceuticals. Most commonly these are trace doses of natural metabolic substrates or drugs that act on the brain. The positron-emitting nuclides available include ^{15}O, ^{11}C, and ^{13}N, and ^{18}F. A wide range of biologically important compounds can be labeled with these nuclides. When a positron-emitting nuclide decays, the positron emitted typically travels 2 to 7 mm before annihilating an electron. The resulting energy is emitted in the form of two gamma rays traveling in opposite directions. Positron tomographs are designed to register an *event* when two gamma rays of the appropriate energy are detected almost simultaneously on opposite sides of the head. The line connecting the two detectors where the gamma rays were detected defines the source of the event. After $\sim 10^6$ events are recorded, a backprojection algorithm similar to that used for x-ray CT is applied, resulting in an image showing the distribution of the positron emitter.

The most common type of PET scan is that for measurement of metabolic rate for glucose using the glucose analog [^{18}F]-fluorodeoxyglucose (see Color Plate 2). Other common variables measured with PET are listed in Table 10-3 and include cerebral blood

TABLE 10-3. Radiopharmaceuticals for PET

Radiopharmaceutical	Pharmacology	Process Measured
[^{15}O]-H$_2$O	Water	Cerebral blood flow
[^{15}O]-O$_2$	Oxygen	Oxygen metabolism
[^{18}F]-Fluorodeoxyglucose	Glucose analog	Glucose metabolism
[^{11}C]-Flumazenil	Benzodiazepine antagonist	GABA/benzodiazepine receptors
[^{11}C]-Fluorodopa	Levodopa analog	Presynaptic dopaminergic sites
[^{11}C]-DTBZ (dihydrotetrabenazine)	Ligand for vesicular monoaminergic transporter	Presynaptic dopaminergic sites
[^{11}C]-Raclopride	D2-receptor antagonist	D2 receptors
[^{11}C]-Diprenorphine [^{11}C]-Cyclofoxy [^{11}C]-Carfentanil	Opiate receptor ligands	Opiate receptor density

flow, oxygen metabolism, presynaptic nerve terminals assessed as sites of neurotransmitter synthesis or reuptake, and neurotransmitter receptors assessed with radiolabeled ligands (see Color Plate 3). With each type of scan, serial images of the distribution of the positron emitter are entered into a mathematical model that depicts the predicted behavior of the radiopharmaceutical, permitting calculation of the important variables. Although with some types of scans the goal is visual analysis of images, more commonly the goal with PET is quantification of aspects of brain function in the relevant brain regions.

PET has yielded a number of important results from activation studies (see Color Plates 4 and 5). Typically $[^{15}O]$-H_2O, a tracer of cerebral blood flow, is injected two or more times during different states of cerebral activity. Often one of these states is a resting state, and the other is a cognitive, motor, or sensory task. Subtraction of the images in the two states permits identification of regions that are more active in one of the states. PET activation scans can be used for the same goals as fMRI, described above. The relative merits of PET and fMRI for activation scans will become clearer over the next few years.

Most applications of PET in neurology are in research, but PET is clinically useful in some situations. Perhaps the most common and best established clinical application is in evaluating patients with partial epilepsy who are candidates for surgical procedures such as temporal lobectomy. The epileptic focus is surrounded by a zone of hypometabolism that can be demonstrated with PET fluorodeoxyglucose scans in 70 to 85 percent of these patients, and this information can be useful in identifying the region to be resected. Fluorodeoxyglucose PET can demonstrate a typical pattern of parietal and temporal hypometabolism in Alzheimer disease (see Color Plate 2). In patients who have received radiation treatment for brain tumors and have a progressive focal abnormality in the brain, fluorodeoxyglucose PET can be useful in distinguishing recurrent tumor, which typically has high metabolism, from radiation necrosis, which has low metabolism. PET can be used to assist in selecting patients with unresectable aneurysms or vascular malformations for carotid ligation. In such patients carotid ligation is associated with approximately 30 percent risk of major stroke. PET with $[^{15}O]$-H_2O during temporary balloon occlusion of the carotid is useful in predicting which patients have adequate collateral flow and should therefore be considered candidates for carotid ligation. Finally, PET activation studies can show the location of important brain regions such as primary motor cortex, and this information can be used by neurosurgeons during surgical resection of brain tumors and vascular malformations (see Color Plate 5).

SINGLE PHOTON EMISSION TOMOGRAPHY

Description

Single photon emission tomography (SPECT), like PET, can be used to demonstrate the distribution of radiopharmaceuticals in the brain. With appropriate selection of radiopharmaceuticals, processes of biologic interest can be evaluated (see Color Plate 6). The radionuclides most commonly used with SPECT are ^{123}Iodine and ^{99m}Technetium. Whereas in PET detection of two gamma rays defines an event recorded by the tomograph, with SPECT, detection of a single gamma ray emitted by the radioactive decay defines an event. Compared with PET, SPECT has the major advantage that the radiopharmaceuticals and tomographs are much less expensive, and SPECT is thus much more widely available. Disadvantages of SPECT compared to PET are that labeling compounds of biologic interest with the available nuclides is more challenging, the longer half-life of the nuclides results in higher radiation exposure, and resolution (ability to show detail) is not as good as that of PET.

Indications and Findings

The most common type of SPECT scans for studying the brain are those used to study cerebral blood flow (see Color Plate 6). SPECT scans of this type can demonstrate regional hypoperfusion in patients with large infarcts; the clinical usefulness of such scans remains a matter for investigation. Promising results have been obtained in patients with partial epilepsy; if a blood flow tracer is injected during a seizure, it can demonstrate increased perfusion of the involved cortex, and this information can be used to evaluate patients for epilepsy surgery. SPECT scans to study neurotransmitter receptor pathways are in an earlier stage than PET scans for this purpose, but promising results have been obtained with ligands for presynaptic cholinergic terminals and for benzodiazepine receptors (Table 10-4).

TABLE 10-4. Radiopharmaceuticals for SPECT

Radiopharmaceutical	Pharmacology	Process Measured
[^{99m}Tc]-HMPAO (hexamethylpropylen-amine oxime, or exametazime) [^{99m}Tc]-ECD (ethyl cysteinate dimer, or bicisate)	Lipid-soluble agents	Cerebral perfusion (approximates cerebral blood flow)
[^{123}I]-β-CIT [2β-carboxymethyoxy-3β-(4-iodophenyl)tropane]	Ligand for dopamine transporter	Presynaptic dopaminergic sites
[^{123}I]-IBVM (iodobenzovesamicol)	Ligand for vesicular acetylcholine transporter	Presynaptic cholinergic sites
[^{123}I]-Iomazenil	Benzodiazepine antagonist	GABA/benzodiazepine receptors

LUMBAR PUNCTURE

Indications and Contraindications

The most common purpose of lumbar puncture (LP) is to obtain CSF for analysis. In many disorders, CSF exam will provide a specific diagnosis, such as some types of meningitis, leptomeningeal carcinoma, and subarachnoid hemorrhage. In other disorders, CSF exam is supportive though not diagnostic of a specific disease, for example, multiple sclerosis, Guillain-Barré syndrome, aseptic meningitis, and central nervous system (CNS) vasculitis. When the diagnosis is unclear and a wide differential diagnosis must be considered, CSF exam can be helpful. LP can be indicated for pressure measurement, for example, when you suspect idiopathic intracranial hypertension (pseudotumor cerebri) or are evaluating chronic hydrocephalus. LP may be performed for a large-volume CSF withdrawal (CSF tap-test) to aid in diagnosing normal pressure hydrocephalus. Finally, LP is performed for intrathecal injections, for example, of the contrast agent for myelography, the radionuclide for isotope cisternography, antibiotics for certain infections, and antineoplastic drugs for leptomeningeal carcinoma.

Contraindications to LP include the presence of a large intracranial mass lesion or obstructive hydrocephalus, because CSF withdrawal can precipitate herniation. When a mass is present, factors associated with increased risk of herniation include substantial midline shift; radiographically evident obstruction of the basal cisterns; middle fossa location, especially with occlusion of the basal cisterns; and posterior fossa location, especially with obstruction of the fourth ventricle. Another contraindication is an intradural or extradural abnormality (most commonly a neoplasm) blocking the spinal canal, because CSF withdrawal can worsen spinal cord compression and cause acute deterioration. Other contraindications include coagulopathy (e.g., platelet counts less than 50,000/mm^3, intravenous heparin, subcutaneous low-molecular-weight heparin) and infection in the lumbar region where the needle is introduced.

Procedure

Obtain informed consent either verbally or in writing, according to institutional practice. Proper positioning of the patient is a key to success. Place the patient in the lateral recumbent position with the hips flexed. The spine should be horizontal, and the plane of the sacrum should be vertical. Bring the lumbar spine into maximal flexion by asking patients to bring their knees to the chest and wrap their arms around their knees. Neck flexion is not necessary. Explore the location for needle introduction by palpating the landmarks. Use interspace L3–L4, L4–L5, or L5–S1. Identify these interspaces by palpating the iliac crests, which are at the level of the L3–L4 interspace. Palpate the spinous processes to establish the midline and, when possible, to identify an entry point between two spinous processes. When you have difficulty performing an LP, especially in obese patients, performing the LP in the seated position may be advantageous because you can identify the midline more easily.

Use sterile technique to put on sterile gloves. Use of a local anesthetic is optional; if used, it should be injected intradermally and subcutaneously using a short needle, but not deeply. Introduce the LP needle, usually 20 or 22 gauge and 3 1/2 in. long. The needle is angled ~20 degrees rostrally. For a small adult, the depth of insertion needed is about half the needle length, but for a very large adult (~250 to 300 lbs., or ~110 to 135 kg), nearly the full length of insertion may be needed. For an even larger person, a longer needle may be needed. Advance the needle to a depth slightly less than that needed. Thereafter, advance the needle in ~5-mm steps, removing the stylet at each step to check for fluid in the hub of the needle. Often, you can feel a "pop" when the needle punctures the dura. If you strike bone, withdraw the needle and select a new angle of approach; you may need to reassess the midline location or aim the needle more rostrally or more caudally. Once you obtain fluid, measure the opening pressure, then collect fluid. Note the presence of blood on the initial fluid obtained, as this observation can help with interpretation of the cell count, as described below.

CSF Analysis

When you suspect subarachnoid hemorrhage, examine the fluid for xanthochromia (yellow or straw coloration). Subarachnoid hemorrhage can be distinguished from a bloody tap with fair reliability by immediate centrifugation. With subarachnoid hemorrhage, some breakdown of red blood cells (RBCs) should leave the supernatant xanthochromic, but with a bloody tap, the supernatant will be clear. Another helpful procedure when you suspect subarachnoid hemorrhage is to count the cells in the first and last tube; with subarachnoid hemorrhage, the two tubes should yield similar RBC counts, but with a bloody tap, you find a declining RBC count. A bloody tap can alter the white blood cell (WBC) and protein results. One simple procedure to correct these values is to reduce the WBC count by $1/mm^3$ and the protein by 1 mg/dL for every 600 RBCs/mm^3. A more accurate procedure is to determine the individual patient's WBC/RBC and protein/RBC ratios from peripheral blood and to use these values to adjust the CSF values.

Examination of cell count, differential, glucose, and protein are nearly always indicated. Do not routinely request other tests such as cultures; use them only in situations where you suspect relevant disease entities.

Normal CSF values are given in Table 10-5. Usually there should be no RBCs, provided the tap was not bloody, and no neutrophilic WBCs. A WBC count as high as 30/mm^3 may be normal within the first month of life. When the serum glucose is elevated (e.g., due to diabetes or IV infusions), measurement of serum glucose helps with the interpretation of the CSF glucose. CSF glucose is usually 0.5 to 0.8 times serum glucose in normoglycemic patients, but glucose values 0.3 to 0.5 times the serum glucose can be expected in hyperglycemic patients. Conversely, CSF glucose is commonly higher than 0.8 times serum in infancy. CSF total protein is normally 24 to 45 mg/dL but may be somewhat higher in normal infants and in normal elderly persons.

Patterns typical of various diseases are also shown in Table 10-5. RBCs are not usually increased in infectious, inflammatory, and neoplastic disorders except herpes simplex encephalitis, where up to 1000 RBCs/mm^3 are commonly present. It is helpful to divide the WBCs into two types, neutrophilic and mononuclear. The early WBC response in viral (aseptic) meningitis may be neutrophilic, but mononuclear cells are likely to predominate

TABLE 10-5. Typical CSF Findings in Normals and in Various Disorders

	RBC (per mm³)	WBC (per mm³)	Differential	Glucose (mg/dL)	Protein (mg/dL)
Normal	0	0–5	All mononuclear	45–80, or 0.5 to 0.8 times serum glucose	15–45, (higher in the elderly)
Bacterial meningitis	0	500–10,000	Mostly neutrophils	0–40	100–500
Cryptococcal meningitis	0	0–800	Mostly lymphocytes	20–80	20–500
Tuberculous meningitis	0	25–100	Mononuclear and neutrophils	20–80	45–200
Viral meningitis	0	5–500	Mostly mononuclear	Usually normal	15–100
Herpes simplex encephalitis	0–1000	5–1000	Mononuclear and neutrophils	Usually normal	15–400
Encephalitis due to other viruses	0	5–1000	Mononuclear	Usually normal	15–100
Subarachnoid hemorrhage	1000–500,000	Elevated in proportion (early) or out of proportion (late) to RBCs	Mononuclear and neutrophils	Usually normal	Elevated in proportion (early) or out of proportion (late) to RBCs
Leptomeningeal metastasis	0	0–1000	Mononuclear	0–80	20–1000
Multiple sclerosis	0	0–50	Mononuclear	Normal	20–100
Guillain-Barré syndrome	0	0–50	Mononuclear	Normal	20–500

within 12 to 24 h. A low glucose is common in bacterial meningitis and leptomeningeal carcinoma. CSF glucose may also be somewhat low in chronic meningitis of various causes, and more rarely it can be low with viral meningitis, viral encephalitis, and subarachnoid hemorrhage. Mild elevations in protein are typical of numerous neurologic disorders. Extreme protein elevations >500 mg/dL occur most commonly with partial or complete blockage of the spinal canal. Clotting of CSF associated with very high protein is known as Froin syndrome.

Helpful tests on CSF include Gram's stain and culture when you suspect bacterial meningitis; fungal smear and culture, acid-fast bacilli smear and culture, and cryptococcal antigen for subacute or chronic meningitis; polymerase chain reaction (PCR) for certain infections, especially herpes simplex; cytology when you suspect leptomeningeal malignancy; and oligoclonal bands and IgG index when you suspect multiple sclerosis or other immune-mediated illnesses. Latex agglutination tests for bacterial antigens are available for *Streptococcus pneumoniae, Haemophilus influenzae, Neisseria meningitidis,* Group D streptococcus, and *E. coli* type K1; because of low sensitivity and specificity, however, these tests are useful only in patients with meningitis in whom previous antibiotic treatment has reduced the likelihood of positive bacterial cultures. A positive reagin test (e.g., Venereal Disease Research Laboratory, or VDRL) on CSF can support the diagnosis of neurosyphilis, but CSF examination for this purpose is indicated only in patients with a positive serum FTA-ABS, as the latter test is highly sensitive and specific for prior syphilis infection.

ELECTROENCEPHALOGRAPHY

Electroencephalography (EEG) is a technique that measures temporal changes in summated postsynaptic potentials from the superficial layers of the cerebral cortex. Currently, EEG is used principally in two major areas of clinical practice, seizure disorders and alterations in mental status. Technicians record EEGs and physicians interpret them. Interpretation is usually performed after completion of the study, but in emergency situations, you should view the EEG on site while it is being recorded. The technician places a series of electrodes in symmetric locations over the scalp and connects them to a specialized recording device. Typically, a routine EEG recording takes 30 min. While the EEG is being recorded, the technologist documents patients' behavioral state (i.e., awake, drowsy, stuporous), asks the patients to perform certain tasks to judge their level of alertness, has them open and close their eyes, and performs activation procedures such as hyperventilation and photic stimulation. The technologist observes the patient closely and indicates on the record any alteration in responsiveness, seizure-like activity, or responses to noxious or auditory stimuli. In certain clinical circumstances, such as status epilepticus, a physician may administer antiepileptic drugs (AEDs) intravenously during the study.

Description of Normal EEG

The appearance of the normal EEG changes from birth through teenage years, then remains relatively unchanged until at least age 80 years. The EEG also changes markedly with the behavioral state of the patient. In interpreting EEG studies, you need to be familiar with changes that may be explained by age and state of consciousness. EEG rhythms are divided into four normal-frequency bands: delta ($<$4 Hz), theta (4 to 7 Hz), alpha (8 to 13 Hz), and beta ($>$13 Hz). The potentials are small; most scalp-derived EEG activity is between 10 and 100 microvolts (μV). In the normal awake adult whose eyes are closed, the most prominent background rhythm consists of sinusoidal 30- to 60-mV, 9- to 10-Hz alpha activity over the parieto-occipital region that attenuates when the eyes are open

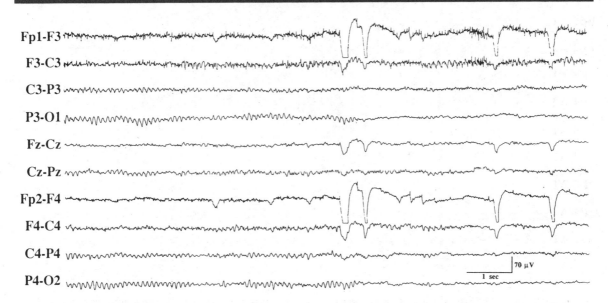

Figure 10-8 Normal EEG. Symmetric, sinusoidal, 10-Hz activity over the parieto-occipital regions which attenuates with eye opening. Recorded from a healthy young adult in relaxed wakefulness.

(Fig. 10-8). A mixture of faster and slower frequencies predominates over the more anterior head regions and is relatively unaffected by eye opening or closure. In younger children, the rhythms are somewhat slower and less organized. In very advanced age (>80 years), there is some slowing of this dominant posterior rhythm and a greater amount of intermittent, more focal slowing.

Hyperventilation provokes physiologic slowing of the background rhythm and further intermittent slowing in many normal subjects. These changes are most pronounced in young children. Intermittent photic stimulation may evoke a repetitive, time-locked occipital rhythm at the frequency or a harmonic of the frequency of the photic stimulus in normal subjects. Drowsiness and sleep result in characteristic changes in the EEG background, including increasing amounts of slower frequencies. There are characteristic EEG features to drowsiness, each stage of nonrapid eye movement (REM) sleep, and REM sleep itself. In many patients with seizures, it is particularly valuable to record the EEG in sleep or after sleep deprivation since abnormal waveforms may be seen more commonly in these recording conditions than in well-rested, awake subjects.

EEG and Epilepsy

Nearly every epileptic syndrome can be categorized as follows: (1) idiopathic (i.e., with no known insult but often occurring on a heredofamilial basis) or symptomatic (i.e., due to some underlying insult); and (2) generalized (i.e., due to a diffuse brain abnormality) or partial (i.e., due to a more local brain abnormality). Patients with idiopathic epilepsies have normal background, while patients with symptomatic epilepsies usually

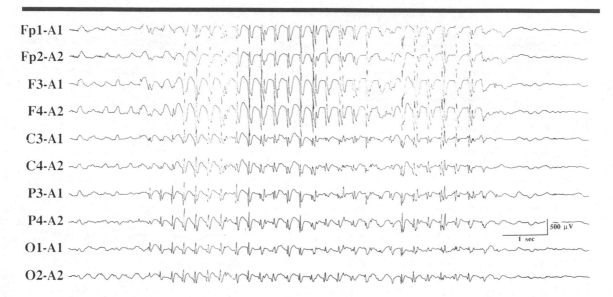

Figure 10-9   Train of 3.5-Hz generalized spike-wave activity with frontal maximum recorded from a teenager with absence seizures.

have an abnormal background. Epileptiform discharges seen in patients with generalized epilepsies are generalized (Fig. 10-9), while those with focal (partial) epilepsies are focal. Analysis of the EEG in the epilepsies begins with an assessment of the background activity. Epileptiform abnormalities on the EEG may be either interictal (i.e., occur in between seizures) or ictal (seen during the course of a clinical seizure). Interictal discharges are spikes, sharp waves, or spike-wave complexes, and their morphology, topography, frequency, appearance, and response to different activation procedures will vary depending

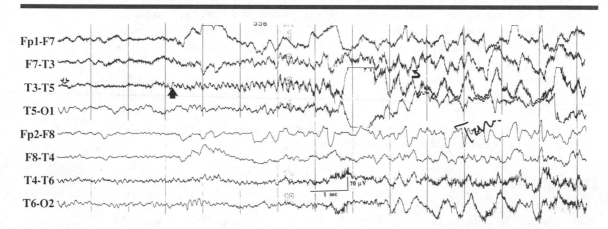

Figure 10-10   Complex partial seizure. The seizure begins with a focal voltage attenuation in the left temporal region (*open arrowhead*) evolving to rhythmic theta activity (*closed arrowhead*) and then bilateral rhythmic delta activity maximal left hemisphere (*curved arrow*). The seizure was associated with oral automatisms and loss of awareness.

on the patient's underlying epileptic syndrome. Ictal EEG discharges are more prolonged than interictal activity and show an evolution in frequency, morphology, and topography during a clinical seizure, especially in the partial epilepsies (Fig. 10-10). EEG recordings may be combined with concurrent video monitoring of behavior in the investigation of patients with epilepsy. This can be accomplished for up to several hours as an outpatient study or over days in an inpatient epilepsy monitoring unit. Video-EEG monitoring is useful in establishing a diagnosis of epilepsy or demonstrating that a patient's spells are nonepileptic in nature. In patients with medically refractory complex partial seizures, video-EEG allows the precise localization that is needed for resective surgery. Approximately 40 percent of patients who undergo epilepsy surgery require additional video-EEG monitoring with intracranial electrodes because the ictal activity is insufficiently localized on scalp electrodes.

EEG recordings are immensely valuable in the care of patients with status epilepticus. An EEG should be obtained as quickly as possible, but treatment of status epilepticus should never be delayed while awaiting an EEG recording. EEG can confirm status epilepticus and exclude the rare patient who has pseudo-status epilepticus. It also monitors the response to treatment given acutely. Occasionally EEG will demonstrate subclinical (electrographic) seizures when overt seizure activity is not apparent, indicating an incomplete response to treatment. A conclusive diagnosis of nonconvulsive status epilepticus may only be made by concurrent EEG recording. Psychogenic causes of unresponsiveness can be determined with certainty by a normal EEG during an episode.

EEG and Other Disorders

EEG abnormalities that are slower than expected for the age and behavioral state of the patient are termed slow-wave abnormalities. These may be generalized or focal, and intermittent or persistent, the latter defined as present for >80 percent of an EEG recording. Slow-wave abnormalities can be seen in patients with epilepsy, but when they occur without other associated abnormalities, they are nonspecific. Focal slow-wave abnormalities imply a local disturbance of cortical and sometimes adjacent subcortical structures in the focal epilepsies, but they also can occur in other conditions such as stroke, brain tumors, severe migraine, or in localized brain injury after head trauma. Generalized intermittent slowing occurs most commonly in diverse encephalopathies. The frequency of the slowing and the percent to which it is present in the EEG correlate with the severity of the encephalopathy. Stuporous patients will show a moderate degree of slowing of background rhythms and brief trains of even slower waveforms intermittently. Stimulation of the patient accelerates the background frequency. Comatose patients show a more marked and persistent degree of slowing that typically does not change with stimulation. Occasionally, comatose patients have EEG findings highly suggestive of a particular etiology. A combination of unreactive delta rhythms with superimposed widespread beta activity should lead to a suspicion of overdose with barbiturates or benzodiazepines. In heavily sedated patients or patients who are paralyzed with neuromuscular blocking agents, EEG recordings are an extremely useful bedside measure of the integrity of brain function. EEG is one of the confirmatory tests that can be useful in establishing a diagnosis of brain death. EEG should be used to confirm brain death only when the patient has met all clinical criteria for the absence of any brain function due to a known and irreversible cause. EEG provides a measure of the function of the neocortex only. It is crucial that the patient's blood pressure and temperature be normal or close to normal at the time the study is performed and that the patient be on no CNS depressant agents.

In patients with well-defined focal brain lesions such as tumors or stroke, there is no indication for the routine use of EEG. A characteristic EEG pattern seen in severe focal encephalitis or other acute focal brain lesions is known as periodic lateralized epileptiform discharges (PLEDs). PLEDs are high-amplitude, regularly recurring sharp waves on a background of marked voltage and frequency attenuation.

The EEG has no particular utility in the investigation of patients with degenerative disorders of the nervous system with one notable exception. Patients with the acute or subacute presentation of a dementing illness should have one or more EEG recordings performed searching for the generalized periodic sharp wave complexes of Creutzfeldt-Jakob disease.

EVOKED POTENTIALS

Evoked potentials are responses produced from different levels of the nervous system with a relatively fixed latency following a stimulus. Responses may be recorded from the nerves, subcortical tracts and nuclei, or cortical segments of a stimulated pathway. In clinical practice the most commonly used potentials are visual, auditory, and somatosensory.

Due to the their low amplitude, adequate characterization of the potentials requires averaging of multiple responses to the stimulus. With averaging, the randomly occurring background EEG signal diminishes while the fixed latency responses of interest persist. The amplitude of the individual evoked response determines the number of responses that must be averaged. With visual evoked responses the occipital cortical responses elicited by an alternating pattern produced on a TV screen may be well seen with as few as 100 stimuli. The much smaller scalp activity generated within the brainstem in response to auditory stimuli requires averaging at least 1000 responses. At least two sets of stimulus trials must be obtained to ensure reproducibility. The peak latency and amplitude of the responses to right- and left-side stimulation need to be compared, irrespective of the stimulus being used. Each laboratory must establish its own normal controls, standardizing the laboratory's particular recording derivations, techniques, and environment. Studies in normal subjects should include both sexes and a wide age range including those over 60 years of age. Significant abnormalities are defined as prolongation of latencies beyond three standard deviations of the control population. Reduction in amplitude of the responses is less useful than prolongation of latency. The level of patient cooperation needed differs among stimulus modalities. With pattern reversal visual stimuli, full patient cooperation and attention is crucial. For brainstem auditory and somatosensory stimuli, the best responses often are obtained while the patient is relaxed, drowsy, or asleep.

Commonly Used
Evoked Potentials

Visual evoked potentials are generated from the occipital cortex and recorded from the mid-occipital region of the scalp. The stimulation is monocular with the patient focusing on the center of a TV screen where an alternating pattern appears. The clinically important response is the P100 wave, a positive peak with a latency of about 100 ms.

Brainstem auditory evoked potentials are generated within various structures in the subcortical auditory pathways. They are elicited with monaural stimulation consisting of repetitive clicks. The clinically useful responses are obtained within the first 10 ms after stimulation. The potentials are recorded at the vertex of the scalp.

Somatosensory evoked potentials are most commonly produced by electrical stimulation of a peripheral nerve, typically the median nerve in the arm or the posterior tibial nerve in the leg. With median nerve stimulation, sequential waveforms that are detected originate in the brachial plexus, dorsal root entry zone, dorsal columns and nucleus cuneatus, medial lemniscus, thalamus, and somatosensory cortex. With lower extremity stimulation, a peripheral nerve potential, caudal spinal cord potential, and somatosensory cortex potential can be recorded.

Use of Evoked Potentials
in Clinical Practice

Evoked potential studies are useful in detecting lesions in multiple sclerosis, as they can provide evidence for lesions in a sensory system when no abnormalities can be detected by neurologic examination. They may be considered as complementary to MR imaging in this sense and provide a measure of the functional status of neural pathways. The characteristic features of an evoked potential abnormality in demyelinating disease is a prolonged latency without loss in amplitude, the latter finding requiring axonal loss. Evoked potentials may be useful in evaluating visual or auditory function in patients who cannot cooperate with more formal testing of vision or hearing such as infants and young children. In conjunction with EEG they can provide useful prognostic information in comatose patients. In intraoperative monitoring they help to ensure integrity of certain neural structures, particularly the spinal cord during major orthopedic or neurosurgical procedures.

NERVE CONDUCTION
STUDIES AND NEEDLE
ELECTROMYOGRAPHY

Electromyography (EMG) refers to the nerve conduction and needle electromyography studies used to evaluate peripheral neuromuscular disorders. These studies derive from electrophysiologic principles and include evaluation of sensory and motor nerve conduction, late responses, neuromuscular transmission, and needle electromyography. Clinicians use these evaluations as an extension of their neurologic examination to confirm clinical findings, localize abnormalities more precisely than possible by neurologic exam,

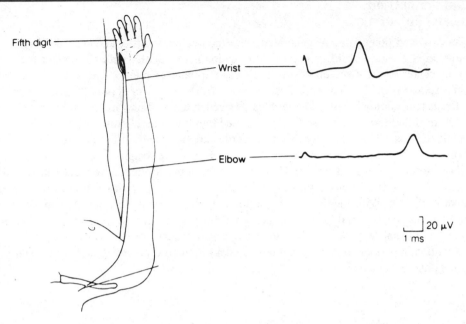

Figure 10-11   Sensory nerve action potentials (SNAPs) recorded following supramaximal percutaneous stimulation of the ulnar nerve at the wrist and elbow, recording from the fifth digit. Calibration: 1 ms and 20 μV. [Reproduced with permission from Albers JW, Leonard JA: Nerve conduction studies and electromyography, in Crockard A, Hayward R, Hoff JT (eds): *Neurosurgery: The Scientific Basis of Clinical Practice,* vol. 2, 2d ed. Oxford, Blackwell Scientific Publication, 1992, p 738.]

and identify the underlying pathophysiology. The primary role of EMG is diagnostic, but the results are occasionally used to monitor disease progression or treatment response.

Nerve Conduction Studies

Nerve conduction techniques are standardized, although minor technical differences exist among laboratories. Normal values usually are reported as three standard deviations from the mean or as the fifth to 95th percentiles, depending on the symmetry of the distribution. Many results are age dependent, and some vary according to patient size (Rivner et al, 1990; Stetson et al, 1992; Bolton and Carter, 1980). Interlaboratory differences reflect use of different fixed distances or different temperatures in determining reference values. Limb temperature is an important source of variability because cooling decreases the rate at which ion channels open, resulting in increased amplitude and decreased conduction velocity. It is standard practice to monitor limb temperatures and warm if necessary to approximately 32 to 36°C.

SENSORY AND MOTOR CONDUCTION STUDIES   Sensory nerve action potentials (SNAPs) and compound muscle action potentials (CMAPs) are recorded with surface electrodes placed on the skin in response to percutaneous electrical stimulation of peripheral nerves. SNAPs are small responses recorded in μV. Typically they are biphasic or triphasic potentials, representing a volume conducted signal as it approaches, passes beneath, and travels beyond the recording electrode (Fig. 10-11). CMAPs are larger than SNAPs and are recorded in millivolts (mV), reflecting the amplification of thousands of muscle fibers innervated by each motor axon. When recorded directly over the muscle end plate, CMAPs are biphasic because the potential originates beneath and travels away from the electrode (Fig. 10-12). The amplitude of sensory or motor responses is important because it reflects in part the number and size of functioning nerve or muscle fibers; loss of axons or muscle fibers results in reduced amplitude.

The speed of action potential conduction can be measured along any accessible nerve. Conduction velocity for the fastest conducting fibers is determined by stimulating the nerve at two sites, measuring the latency from each stimulus to onset of response, and dividing the distance between the two sites by the difference in latency between the two responses. Conduction velocity is expressed in meters per second (m/s). Another measure of conduction speed is the distal latency. This latency reflects the time (ms) that elapses from the stimulus to the response along the end of the nerve. All measures of transmission speed reflect peripheral nerve structure and function, including nerve caliber, myelin integrity, internodal length, axonal resistance, temperature, and age.

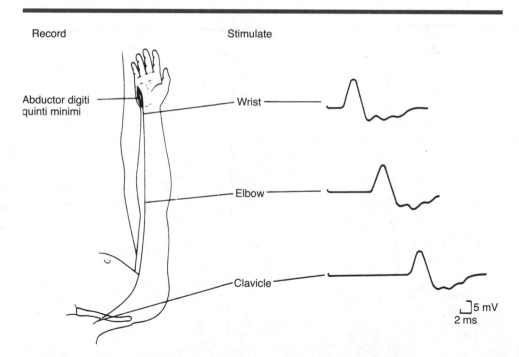

Figure 10-12 Ulnar motor nerve conduction study of the upper extremity. Compound muscle action potentials (CMAPs) recorded following supramaximal percutaneous stimulation of the ulnar nerve at the wrist, elbow, and clavicle, recording from the abductor digiti quinti minimi. Calibration: 2 ms and 5 mV. [Reproduced with permission from Albers JW, Leonard JA: Nerve conduction studies and electromyography, in Crockard A, Hayward R, Hoff JT (eds): *Neurosurgery: The Scientific Basis of Clinical Practice,* vol. 2, 2d ed. Oxford, Blackwell Scientific Publication, 1992, p 738.]

LATE RESPONSES   The F wave is a "late response" recorded from the surface that represents a discharge of one or more motor units. Antidromic stimulation of a motor nerve produces the F wave by generating an action potential traveling toward the spinal cord and away from the muscle. Upon reaching the spinal cord, this action potential activates some of the anterior horn cells, producing an action potential that travels down the same nerve. The latency from stimulation to response is measured, reflecting transmission time along the entire nerve from the stimulation site to the spinal cord and then back down to the muscle. The long conduction distance accentuates minor conduction abnormalities, making F wave latency a sensitive indicator of some peripheral disorders (Fig. 10-13).

The H reflex is a monosynaptic spinal cord reflex analogous to the Achilles muscle stretch reflex, differing only in activation method. The Achilles reflex originates with

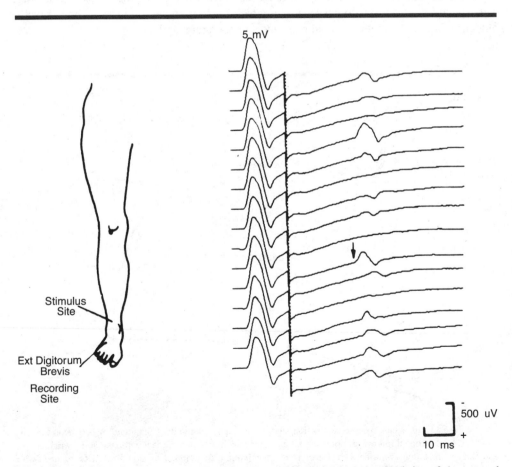

Figure 10-13   Representative F responses following percutaneous antidromic stimulation of the peroneal nerve at the ankle. The resultant F response is shown at the right of the recording. (Reproduced with permission from Albers JW: Clinical neurophysiology of generalized polyneuropathy. *J Clin Neurophysiol* 10:149, 1993.)

activation of length-sensitive intrafusal muscle receptors, whereas the H reflex originates with percutaneous electrical stimulation of afferent tibial nerve fibers. The H reflex
is elicited by stimulating the tibial nerve with a submaximal stimulation and recording
the resultant CMAP from the soleus muscle. Submaximal stimulation preferentially activates large Ia afferents without stimulating the smaller motor axons. The H reflex has
limited clinical application, but it does allow study of conduction along the entire reflex
arc.

Small nerve fibers mediate skin potential responses (SPRs, or sympathetic skin
responses) which provide a measure of autonomic function. They represent the potential
produced by electrically charged sweat as recorded differentially from skin between areas
of high (e.g., palm) and low (e.g., dorsum of hand) sweat gland density. SPRs occur
spontaneously or in response to a variety of stimuli, including percutaneous electrical
stimulation. The stimuli elicit an autonomic response to startle, as opposed to directly
stimulating autonomic nerve fibers.

REPETITIVE MOTOR NERVE STIMULATION   The most common method used
to evaluate neuromuscular transmission is repetitive motor nerve stimulation (Ozdemir
and Young, 1976). This technique identifies failure of neuromuscular transmission as a
CMAP amplitude decrement with repeated stimulation. Normally, there is no variation in
CMAP amplitude or configuration because acetylcholine (ACh) released from the nerve
terminal in response to axonal depolarization produces an end plate potential (EPP) larger
than necessary to generate a muscle fiber action potential (MFAP). The EPP depends on
many factors, including ACh availability, release, and timely inactivation, as well as intact
ACh receptors (AChRs); abnormality of any may impair neuromuscular transmission.
Repetitive motor nerve stimulation at low rates (e.g., 3 Hz) challenges neuromuscular
transmission by taking advantage of the normal decrease in ACh availability prior to re-
plenishment of the immediately available ACh store by mobilization. Because mobilization takes approximately 1 s, a second stimulus delivered before mobilization is complete
releases fewer ACh quanta and evokes a smaller EPP. Whenever the EPP is borderline-
low, further deterioration may elicit a subthreshold response and transmission failure. The
optimal stimulus rate for demonstrating defective neuromuscular transmission of the type
associated with myasthenia gravis is between 2 and 5 Hz. After extended (e.g., 60 s) exercise, the spontaneous release of ACh quanta is temporarily increased and the immediately
available store diminished in 2 to 4 min (postactivation exhaustion) (Magleby, 1979).
During this time ACh availability falls and the EPP amplitude decreases, representing the
optimal time to demonstrate mild defects of neuromuscular transmission (Fig. 10-14).

The interval between repeated stimuli is important in additional ways. If the second
stimulus occurs during the period of postactivation facilitation, neuromuscular transmission is enhanced. After a depolarization, calcium ions persist in the presynaptic terminal
for about 200 ms (Swift, 1981). Because of the persistent calcium, a second impulse
arriving within this time releases a greater percentage of the immediately available store
of ACh than the first impulse, resulting in little or no diminution of the EPP (calcium-
dependent facilitation). Therefore, repetitive stimulation at high rates (10 to 50 Hz) is
useful in facilitating transmission in disorders with defective ACh release such as the
Lambert-Eaton myasthenic syndrome.

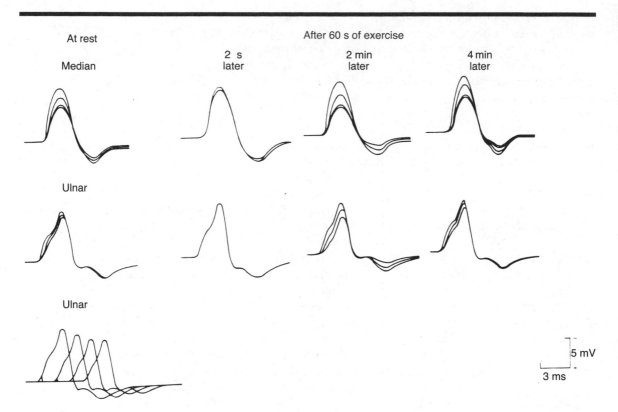

At rest

After 60 s of exercise

Median

2 s later

2 min later

4 min later

Ulnar

Ulnar

5 mV

3 ms

Figure 10-14 Compound muscle action potentials (CMAPs) obtained from a patient with myasthenia gravis during repetitive supramaximal motor nerve stimulation of the median and ulnar nerves at 3 Hz, recording from thenar and hypothenar muscles, respectively. Four superimposed responses are shown at rest and after 60 s of exercise (recording 2 s, 2 min, and 4 min later). The repair of the decrement immediately after exercise reflects postactivation facilitation. The increased decrement 2 min later reflects postactivation exhaustion. (Reproduced with permission from Albers JW, Sanders DB: Repetitive stimulation. American Academy of Neurology Annual Course No. 350. Minneapolis, American Academy of Neurology, 1988.)

Needle EMG

During the needle EMG examination, the electromyographer inserts a sterile needle electrode through the skin into muscle, and electrical signals from muscle at rest and during volitional activation are amplified and monitored on an oscilloscope and a loudspeaker.

INSERTIONAL ACTIVITY Normal muscle is electrically silent away from the end plate region. With electrode movement, normal insertional activity consists of a brief (several hundred milliseconds) electrical discharge. Near the end plate, spontaneous miniature end plate potentials (MEPPs) occur randomly, appearing as small (a few millivolts), irregularly occurring negative potentials. These potentials produce a characteristic "sea shell" sound when heard over the loudspeaker. End plate spikes also are recorded in the end plate region. These potentials may originate from terminal nerve or muscle fibers in response to mechanical stimulation from the recording electrode. They appear as action potentials of 100- to 200-mV amplitude with an initial negative deflection and irregular

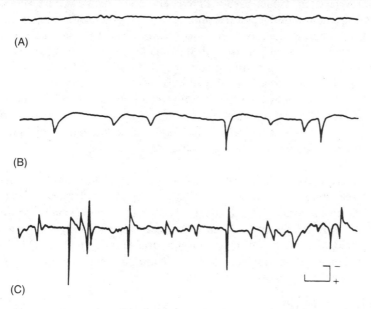

Figure 10-15 EMG needle electrode recordings from muscle at rest. (*A*) Normal muscle with no evidence of abnormal spontaneous activity. (*B*) Abnormal spontaneous activity consisting of positive waves. (*C*) Abnormal spontaneous activity consisting of fibrillation potentials and occasional positive waves. Time marker, 10 ms; voltage marker, 50 μV. (Modified with permission from Bromberg MB, Albers JW: Electromyography in idiopathic myositis. *Mt Sinai J Med* 55: 459, 1988.)

discharge rate. Loss of innervation, regardless of cause, results within weeks in the sequential appearance of increased and prolonged insertional activity, unsustained positive waves and scattered fibrillation potentials, and finally sustained positive waves and spontaneous fibrillation potentials (Fig. 10-15). All of these spontaneous discharges represent involuntary muscle fiber action potentials associated with denervation ACh-hypersensitivity due to proliferation of AChRs on the muscle fiber surface. They are easily recognized, not easily confused with other EMG signals, and not present in normal muscle.

MOTOR UNIT ACTION POTENTIAL The electromyographer inserts an electrode into muscle to record electrical activity from individual motor units. The motor unit action potential (MUAP) is an extracellular summation of the individual MFAPs from a given motor unit. MUAPs are generally triphasic when recorded with a concentric needle electrode, reflecting the distant recording of a monophasic wave in a volume conductor as the potential approaches, passes, and then travels away from the electrode.

Examination of the volitional interference pattern requires evaluation of MUAP size and configuration and the activation pattern. MUAP size and configuration are judged by the amplitude, duration, and number of phases (baseline crossings plus one) or reversals (turns). Because the MUAP is a summation of individual MFAPs, increased muscle fiber density results in increased amplitude, whereas decreased density results in reduced amplitude. The degree of MUAP polyphasia refers to the subjective estimate of the number of phases or reversals and is increased with reinnervation. The MUAP interference pattern refers to the sequential introduction (recruitment) of MUAPs as the subject increases the force of muscular contraction, as well as to MUAP discharge rate and rhythm. Motor units are recruited in a fixed pattern with the smaller motor units recruited before the larger ones. The MUAPs first recruited discharge between 5 and 15 Hz. As the subject increases force, the rate increases until additional MUAPs are activated. Recruitment is decreased from loss of individual motor units (neurogenic pattern) or increased from reduced force generation by individual motor units (myopathic pattern). Estimations of increased recruitment are technically difficult, because the electromyographer must subjectively judge the amount of force generated.

SINGLE FIBER EMG   Single fiber EMG (SFEMG) is a sensitive method for extracellular recording of single MFAPs (Stalberg et al, 1974; Sanders and Stalberg, 1996). The selective recording of individual MFAPs relates to the small recording surface (25 μm) of the SFEMG electrode. SFEMG has been used to study a variety of physiologic and pathologic conditions of neuromuscular transmission and muscle fiber density. The most common application relates to the evaluation of neuromuscular transmission in patients with myasthenia gravis.

JITTER MEASUREMENT   The small recording surface of an SFEMG electrode allows recording from individual MFAPs. When MFAPs are recorded from the same motor unit during minimal volitional activation, small variations occur in the timing of the action potentials. This variation is called jitter, and it reflects the small difference in the time required for an end plate potential to reach threshold. Jitter can be considered a measure of the neuromuscular transmission safety factor. When the safety factor is large (e.g., the end plate potential is well above threshold), jitter values are small, indicating little variability in the timing of MFAP discharge. When the safety factor is small (e.g., the end plate potential is just above the threshold), jitter values are large, reflecting great variability in the timing of MFAP discharge. With substantial neuromuscular transmission impairment, the EPP fails to reach threshold and an MFAP is not generated (blocking). The decremental response recorded in patients with defective neuromuscular transmission during repetitive motor stimulation is related to blocking of individual MFAPs.

    Examples of jitter from three pairs of muscle fibers are shown in Fig. 10-16. The measure used to describe jitter is the mean consecutive interpotential difference (MCD), which is calculated by a variety of formulas, depending on the recording paradigm. Substantial variability occurs in the MCD among normal MFAP pairs, so approximately 20 potential pairs are studied for any muscle and the results expressed as an average MCD, the percentage of pairs having an abnormal MCD, and the percentage of pairs demonstrating intermittent blocking. Normal values vary slightly from laboratory to laboratory, depending on technique, patient age, and the muscle tested.

MUSCLE FIBER DENSITY   SFEMG is occasionally used to determine muscle fiber density. Because the SFEMG electrode records from a very small area relative to a conventional concentric needle electrode, the number of individual MFAPs from a single motor unit can be counted during a single electrode placement, and the average number of

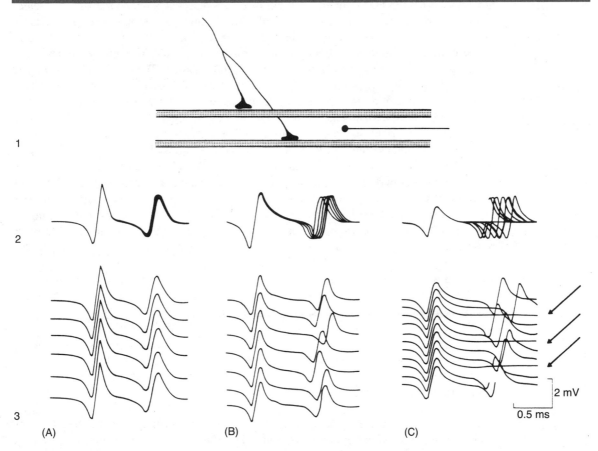

Figure 10-16   SFEMG recording from a patient with myasthenia gravis. The SFEMG electrode and two muscle fibers innervated by the same neuron are shown in row 1. Six consecutive recordings are shown in superimposed (row 2) and raster display (row 3), triggering on the first muscle fiber action potential (MFAP) to demonstrate the variability in the onset of the second MFAP relative to the first. Normal jitter is demonstrated in column A, with increasing jitter in column B, and increased jitter and intermittent blocking (*arrows*) in column C. [Reprinted with permission from the AAEE Glossary of Terms in Clinical Electromyography, compiled by the Nomenclature Committee, American Association of Electrodiagnostic Medicine (formerly the American Association of Electrodiagnostic Medicine): *Muscle Nerve* 10 (Suppl):G51, 1987.]

MFAPs calculated from multiple locations. In association with axonal sprouting and reinnervation, muscle fiber density increases, making SFEMG a sensitive method for identifying previous denervation.

What Can Be Learned from the EMG Examination

This section presents selected clinical problems together with the anticipated electrodiagnostic findings. For each, information is identified that can be obtained from the electrodiagnostic study, as well as the common pitfalls.

MONONEUROPATHY   In the evaluation of a suspected mononeuropathy, the electromyographer must localize the abnormality to a single nerve and perform sufficient evaluation to exclude other localizations. For a mixed nerve, this includes sensory and motor conduction studies, including conduction across points of potential compression. Large sensory fibers are particularly sensitive to compression. The earliest abnormality is slowing across the lesion, followed by evidence of partial conduction block (loss of amplitude with stimulation proximal to the lesion), and loss of sensory or motor amplitude in association with axonal degeneration. The finding of focal slowing or partial conduction block is important in localizing a focal lesion. Evaluation of adjacent and contralateral nerves identifies more widespread abnormalities or mild side-to-side differences. Needle examination of muscles innervated by the involved nerve documents the extent and magnitude of partial denervation. Expected findings include increased insertional activity, positive waves and fibrillation potentials, and MUAP changes associated with axon loss in muscles innervated by the involved nerve. Examination of several muscles innervated by different peripheral nerves and nerve roots, sometimes including the paraspinal muscles, is important to isolate the abnormality.

PLEXOPATHY   Electrodiagnostic findings in plexopathy can usually be distinguished from those of an isolated mononeuropathy or radiculopathy. A key abnormality in plexopathy is an appropriate motor *and* sensory nerve conduction abnormality. When present, a reduced sensory amplitude localizes the lesion to or distal to the dorsal root ganglion, excluding radiculopathy from consideration. The needle examination is important in localizing the lesion to the plexus by demonstrating abnormal findings that are limited to anterior myotome muscles, generally in the distribution of more than one nerve root and peripheral nerve, while sparing paraspinal muscles.

RADICULOPATHY   In radiculopathy, the needle examination demonstrates findings limited to anterior *and* posterior myotome muscles of a single root innervation. Involvement of the paraspinal muscles localizes the problem to the spinal nerve before it separates into its anterior and posterior primary divisions. This localization also accounts for the normal sensory responses despite decreased sensation on clinical examination, because a lesion proximal to the dorsal root ganglion spares the sensory nerve cell bodies and distal axons. In the special case of nerve root avulsion, the SNAP is normal despite the complete absence of sensation. In a chronic radiculopathy, paraspinal abnormalities may be obscured by regeneration of the posterior primary division fibers. Unlike the relatively precise localization possible in some mononeuropathies, localization in radiculopathy is less precise. Localization to a single root does not identify the site of abnormality along that root. Specifically, electrodiagnostic studies alone cannot determine whether the root lesion is extradural (e.g., herniated disc or foraminal stenosis), intradural-extramedullary (e.g., leptomeningeal carcinomatosis), or intramedullary (e.g., anterior horn cell disease). Involvement proximal to the dorsal root ganglion up to and including the anterior horn cell will produce similar findings that cannot be distinguished from radiculopathy (McGonagle et al, 1990).

POLYNEUROPATHY   In patients with polyneuropathy, EMG results allow broad classification into one of several groups depending on the presence of predominant sensory or motor fiber involvement and evidence of primary axonal loss or demyelination (Donofrio and Albers, 1990). In addition, conduction abnormalities distinguish hereditary from acquired demyelination. Evaluation includes motor and sensory nerve conduction studies in the upper and lower extremities to define the type and distribution of abnormality. Selected bilateral studies are needed to evaluate symmetry. Abnormalities are most common in the distal lower extremities. The type and extent of examination required to characterize the polyneuropathy depend on the extent of involvement. In mild disease examination of the most clinically involved sites usually provides the most useful information. In severe disease demonstrating absent distal lower extremity responses gives little help in defining the underlying pathophysiology, and it is often necessary to examine less involved sites. Needle EMG may involve limited evaluation of up to three extremities to define adequately the extent and distribution of axonal degeneration.

Sensorimotor polyneuropathy of the axonal type is common and associated with a variety of toxic, nutritional, metabolic, and genetic etiologies. Treatment of these disorders is often limited. In contrast, sensorimotor polyneuropathy of the demyelinating type is usually treatable or associated with treatable underlying disorders (Donofrio and Albers, 1990; Miller, 1985). Demyelinating neuropathy is characterized by prominent conduction slowing, abnormal temporal dispersion, and partial conduction block. Pure sensory *neuronopathy*, in which the primary insult is to dorsal root ganglion neurons, is uncommon and is usually due to hereditary, inflammatory (e.g., Sjögren syndrome), paraneoplastic, or toxic etiologies. Pure motor polyneuropathy is also uncommon, and consideration of this diagnosis should suggest alternate possibilities such as primary motor neuron disease, polyradiculopathy, or even defective neuromuscular transmission. For some patients clinically thought to have polyneuropathy, asymmetric electrodiagnostic abnormalities suggest the diagnosis of mononeuritis multiplex.

NEUROMUSCULAR JUNCTION Repetitive motor nerve stimulation is the most common method used to demonstrate defective neuromuscular transmission. In myasthenia gravis, the classical finding is decremental response to motor nerve stimulation at low rates (3 Hz) until the third or fourth stimulation, with amplitude stabilization or increase thereafter (the "early dip" phenomenon). The early decrement reflects ACh depletion from the immediately available ACh store and failure of the EPP to exceed threshold in some fibers. The stabilization and partial repair with continued stimulation reflects ACh mobilization. A myasthenic decrement can be completely or partially repaired immediately after brief exercise (postactivation facilitation) and accentuated 2 to 4 min after longer exercise (postactivation exhaustion). A typical response for a patient with moderately severe generalized myasthenia gravis is shown in Fig. 10-14. The best results are obtained from muscles that are easily restrained (e.g., distal muscles). Because facial and proximal muscles are frequently symptomatic, evaluation usually includes study of facial, deltoid, and trapezius muscles.

In the evaluation of suspected myasthenia gravis, electromyographers use SFEMG to demonstrate mild abnormalities because it is more sensitive than repetitive motor nerve stimulation. A representative abnormal SFEMG recording from an extremity muscle of a patient with myasthenia gravis is shown in Fig. 10-16, demonstrating increased jitter and intermittent blocking in column C. Neither the presence of a decremental response nor increased jitter are specific for myasthenia gravis; both simply represent evidence of defective neuromuscular transmission.

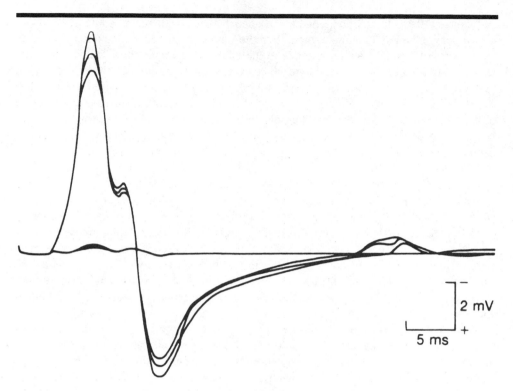

2 mV

5 ms

Figure 10-17   Compound muscle action potentials (CMAPs) evoked by repetitive supramaximal ulnar motor nerve stimulation at 3 Hz, recorded from hypothenar muscle in a patient with Lambert-Eaton myasthenic syndrome. The smaller tracing represents the markedly reduced CMAP amplitude with a small decrement in rested muscle. The superimposed larger tracing recorded immediately after 10 s of maximal voluntary contraction represents marked postexercise facilitation. (Reproduced with permission from Albers JW, Sanders DB: Repetitive stimulation. American Academy of Neurology Annual Course No. 350. Minneapolis, American Academy of Neurology, 1988.)

The Lambert-Eaton myasthenic syndrome (LEMS) is a disorder of neuromuscular transmission sometimes associated with small-cell cancer of the lung or other malignancies. The diagnosis almost always is established in the EMG laboratory. The neuromuscular transmission defect is related to impaired Ca^{2+}-mediated ACh release. CMAP amplitudes are diffusely low, and repetitive motor nerve stimulation at low rates demonstrates a small decrement, similar to that seen with myasthenia gravis. However, postactivation facilitation in response to brief exercise or rapid stimulation (20 to 50 Hz) dramatically increases the CMAP amplitude (greater than 200 percent, Fig. 10-17). The needle examination often shows striking moment-to-moment variability of MUAP amplitude and configuration, reflecting postactivation facilitation.

MYOPATHY   In the evaluation of suspected myopathy, nerve conduction studies have limited application and are used primarily to confirm sparing of sensory nerves and to evaluate neuromuscular transmission. The needle examination is perhaps the most sensitive indicator of myopathy, although certain electrodiagnostic features are common to most myopathies, regardless of etiology. Often only the distribution of abnormality is helpful in establishing a specific diagnosis, although some findings such as myotonic discharges suggest a specific diagnosis. Inflammatory myopathies such as polymyositis demonstrate increased insertional activity, positive waves and fibrillation potentials, complex repetitive discharges, and small-amplitude, short-duration polyphasic MUAPs with increased recruitment. Most symptomatic patients show these findings, particularly in paraspinal muscle. Several metabolic myopathies, such as those associated with corticosteroids, present different abnormalities. In steroid myopathy, MUAP recruitment abnormalities may be profound, yet no abnormalities of insertional activity occur. In this setting the absence of abnormal insertional or spontaneous activity is helpful in differentiating progressive inflammatory myopathy from corticosteroid myopathy.

Indications for EMG Studies

The primary indications for EMG studies are to document a peripheral disorder, localize abnormalities to a degree not possible clinically, and establish the underlying pathophysiology. For many problems, such as suspected carpal tunnel syndrome, nerve conduction studies are used to confirm the clinical suspicion. The studies are therefore considered "permissive" in establishing the diagnosis, meaning that the diagnosis of a median mononeuropathy at the wrist cannot be established with certainty without EMG confirmation. Similarly, evaluation of suspected polyneuropathy almost always includes EMG evaluation because of the sensitivity in diagnosing polyneuropathy and the ability to identify primary demyelination noninvasively. EMG studies are used in patients with sensory loss to localize the lesion proximal or distal to the dorsal root ganglion. Lesions at or distal to the dorsal root ganglia invariably cause SNAP abnormalities; more proximal lesions do not. For other problems, such as suspected radiculopathy, EMG studies are needed to determine the severity of axonal degeneration, and a normal study does not exclude a structural abnormality producing symptomatic radiculopathy. Motor neuron disease and inflammatory myopathy are examples of disorders in which the electrodiagnostic evaluation confirms the clinical findings and establishes evidence of abnormality in clinically normal muscle. In both disorders, the studies also confirm normal sensory nerve function.

There are few absolute contraindications to EMG. Nerve conduction studies are safe in patients with implanted cardiac pacemakers, but studies are not recommended in patients with external cardiac pacemakers or in any patient with an external conductive lead terminating in or near the heart (American Association of Electrodiagnostic Medicine, 1992). Implanted cardiac defibrillators should be deactivated before nerve conduction studies are undertaken. Central venous or arterial catheters predispose patients to ventricular fibrillation from EMG equipment leakage currents. Study of electrically sensitive patients can be performed without risk when the electromyographer gives proper attention to equipment leakage current, location and type of percutaneous catheters, and grounding (American Association of Electrodiagnostic Medicine, 1992). Needle EMG examination of deep muscles such as paraspinal muscles is relatively contraindicated in patients who are anticoagulated or who have substantial thrombocytopenia or other coagulopathies. Platelet counts $< 50,000/mm^3$ and prothrombin or partial thromboplastin times $1\frac{1}{2}$ to 2 times the control value are associated with increased risk of bleeding (American Association of Electrodiagnostic Medicine, 1992). Whenever the study is warranted in view of the potential benefit relative to the risk of intramuscular or other bleeding, superficial and even deep muscles can be examined and hemostasis usually established with prolonged pressure over the examination site. The use of disposable EMG needles or other forms of needle sterilization controls the percutaneous spread of transmissible disease (American Association of Electrodiagnostic Medicine, 1992).

EMG can be useful to estimate the duration of a problem, to establish prognosis, and to monitor treatment. Because EMG abnormalities associated with acute axonal loss typically progress in a predictable manner, frequently it is possible to establish the onset of a peripheral problem with an accuracy of days to weeks. In patients with acute symptoms, EMG is sometimes useful in identifying a preexisting lesion, and this may be valuable in cases with medical-legal implications. In acute nerve injury, identifying even one motor unit under volitional control suggests a more favorable prognosis than finding none. EMG occasionally is used in disorders such as myasthenia gravis and inflammatory neuropathy to monitor disease progression or treatment response.

SUGGESTED READINGS

American Association of Electrodiagnostic Medicine: Guidelines in electrodiagnostic medicine. *Muscle Nerve* 15:229–253, 1992.

Bolton CF, Carter KM: Human sensory nerve compound action potential amplitudes: Variation with sex and finger circumference. *J Neurol Neurosurg Psychiatry* 43:925–928, 1980.

Chiappa KH: *Evoked Potentials in Clinical Medicine*, 3d ed. Philadelphia, Lippincott-Raven, 1997.

Daly DD, Pedley TA (eds): *Current Practice of Clinical Electroencephalography*. New York, Raven, 1990.

Donofrio PD, Albers JW: AAEM minimonograph #34: Polyneuropathy: Classification by nerve conduction studies and electromyography. *Muscle Nerve* 13:889–903, 1990.

Fishman RA: *Cerebrospinal Fluid in Diseases of the Nervous System*, 2d ed. Philadelphia, Saunders, 1992.

Gilman S: Imaging the brain. *N Engl J Med* 333:812–820, 1998; 338:889–896, 1998.

Magleby KL: Facilitation, augmentation, and potentiation of transmitter release, in Tricek S (ed): *Progress in Brain Research: The Cholinergic Synapse*. New York, Elsevier, 1979, pp 175–182.

Masdeu JC, Brass LM, Holman BL, Kushner MJ: Brain single-photon emission computed tomography. *Neurology* 44:1970–1977, 1994.

Mazziotta JC, Gilman S (eds): *Clinical Brain Imaging: Principles and Applications*. Philadelphia, F.A. Davis, 1992.

McGonagle TK, Levine SR, Donofrio PD, et al: Spectrum of patients with EMG features of polyradiculopathy without neuropathy. *Muscle Nerve* 13:63–69, 1990.

Miller RG: Hereditary and acquired polyneuropathies. Electrophysiologic aspects. *Neurol Clin* 3:543–556, 1985.

Ozdemir C, Young RR: The results to be expected from electrical testing in the diagnosis of myasthenia gravis. *Ann NY Acad Sci* 274:203–222, 1976.

Prichard JW, Cummings JL: The insistent call from functional MRI. *Neurology* 48:797–800, 1997.

Quality Standards Subcommittee of the American Academy of Neurology: Practice parameters: Lumbar puncture (summary statement). *Neurology* 43:625–627, 1993.

Rivner MH, Swift TR, Crout BO, et al: Toward more rational nerve conduction interpretations: The effect of height. *Muscle Nerve* 13:232–239, 1990.

Sanders DB, Stalberg EV: AAEM Minimonograph #25: Single-fiber electromyography. *Muscle Nerve* 19:1069–1083, 1996.

Stalberg E, Ekstedt J, Broman A: Neuromuscular transmission in myasthenia gravis studied with single fibre electromyography. *J Neurol Neurosurg Psychiatry* 37:540–547, 1974.

Stetson DS, Albers JW, Silverstein BA, et al: Effects of age, sex, and anthropometric factors on nerve conduction measures. *Muscle Nerve* 15:1095–1104, 1992.

Swift TR: Disorders of neuromuscular transmission other than myasthenia gravis. *Muscle Nerve* 4:334–353, 1981.

Therapeutics and Technology Assessment Subcommittee, American Academy of Neurology: Assessment of brain SPECT. *Neurology* 46:278–285, 1996.